1991
YEAR BOOK OF
VASCULAR SURGERY®

The 1991 Year Book® Series

Year Book of Anesthesia®: Drs. Miller, Kirby, Ostheimer, Roizen, and Stoelting

Year Book of Cardiology®: Drs. Schlant, Collins, Engle, Frye, Kaplan, and O'Rourke

Year Book of Critical Care Medicine®: Drs. Rogers and Parrillo

Year Book of Dentistry®: Drs. Meskin, Currier, Kennedy, Leinfelder, Matukas, and Rovin

Year Book of Dermatology®: Drs. Sober and Fitzpatrick

Year Book of Diagnostic Radiology®: Drs. Reed, Hendee, Keats, Kirkpatrick, Miller, Osborn, and Thompson

Year Book of Digestive Diseases®: Drs. Greenberger and Moody

Year Book of Drug Therapy®: Drs. Lasagna and Weintraub

Year Book of Emergency Medicine®: Drs. Wagner, Burdick, Davidson, Roberts, and Spivey

Year Book of Endocrinology®: Drs. Bagdade, Braverman, Halter, Horton, Kannan, Molitch, Morley, Odell, Rogol, Ryan, and Sherwin

Year Book of Family Practice®: Drs. Berg, Bowman, Dietrich, Green, and Scherger

Year Book of Geriatrics and Gerontology®: Drs. Beck, Abrass, Burton, Cummings, Makinodan, and Small

Year Book of Hand Surgery®: Drs. Dobyns, Chase, and Amadio

Year Book of Health Care Management: Drs. Heyssel, King, and Steinberg, Ms. Avakian, and Messrs. Berman, Brock, Kues, and Rosenberg

Year Book of Hematology®: Drs. Spivak, Bell, Ness, Quesenberry, and Wiernik

Year Book of Infectious Diseases®: Drs. Wolff, Barza, Keusch, Klempner, and Snydman

Year Book of Infertility: Drs. Mishell, Paulsen, and Lobo

Year Book of Medicine®: Drs. Rogers, Des Prez, Cline, Braunwald, Greenberger, Utiger, Epstein, and Malawista

Year Book of Neonatal and Perinatal Medicine: Drs. Klaus and Fanaroff

Year Book of Neurology and Neurosurgery®: Drs. Currier and Crowell

Year Book of Nuclear Medicine®: Drs. Hoffer, Gore, Gottschalk, Sostman, Zaret, and Zubal

Year Book of Obstetrics and Gynecology®: Drs. Mishell, Kirschbaum, and Morrow

Year Book of Occupational and Environmental Medicine: Drs. Emmett, Brooks, Harris, and Schenker

Year Book of Oncology: Drs. Young, Longo, Ozols, Simone, Steele, and Weichselbaum

Year Book of Ophthalmology®: Drs. Laibson, Adams, Augsburger, Benson, Cohen, Eagle, Flanagan, Nelson, Reinecke, Sergott, and Wilson

Year Book of Orthopedics®: Drs. Sledge, Poss, Cofield, Frymoyer, Griffin, Hansen, Johnson, Springfield, and Weiland

Year Book of Otolaryngology–Head and Neck Surgery®: Drs. Bailey and Paparella

Year Book of Pathology and Clinical Pathology®: Drs. Brinkhous, Dalldorf, Grisham, Langdell, and McLendon

Year Book of Pediatrics®: Drs. Oski and Stockman

Year Book of Plastic, Reconstructive, and Aesthetic Surgery: Drs. Miller, Cohen, McKinney, Robson, Ruberg, and Whitaker

Year Book of Podiatric Medicine and Surgery®: Dr. Kominsky

Year Book of Psychiatry and Applied Mental Health®: Drs. Talbott, Frances, Freedman, Meltzer, Perry, Schowalter, and Yudofsky

Year Book of Pulmonary Disease®: Drs. Green, Loughlin, Michael, Mulshine, Peters, Terry, Tockman, and Wise

Year Book of Speech, Language, and Hearing: Drs. Bernthal, Hall, and Tomblin

Year Book of Sports Medicine®: Drs. Shephard, Eichner, Sutton, and Torg, Col. Anderson, and Mr. George

Year Book of Surgery®: Drs. Schwartz, Jonasson, Robson, Shires, Spencer, and Thompson

Year Book of Urology®: Drs. Gillenwater and Howards

Year Book of Vascular Surgery®: Drs. Bergan and Yao

Roundsmanship '91: A Year Book® Guide to Clinical Medicine: Drs. Dan, Feigin, Quilligan, Schrock, Stein, and Talbott

1991
The Year Book of VASCULAR SURGERY®

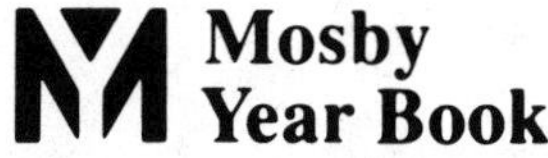

St. Louis Baltimore Boston Chicago London Philadelphia Sydney Toronto

Editor-in-Chief, Year Book Publishing: Nancy Gorham
Sponsoring Editor: Carla L. White
Manager, Medical Information Services: Edith M. Podrazik
Senior Medical Information Specialist: Terri Strorigl
Assistant Director, Manuscript Services: Frances M. Perveiler
Associate Managing Editor, Year Book Editing Services: Elizabeth Fitch
Production Coordinator: Max F. Perez
Proofroom Manager: Barbara M. Kelly

A Year Book Medical Publishers imprint of Mosby-Year Book, Inc.

Mosby-Year Book, Inc.
11830 Westline Industrial Drive
St. Louis, MO 63146

Editorial Office:
Mosby-Year Book, Inc.
200 North LaSalle St.
Chicago, IL 60601

International Standard Serial Number: 0749-4041
International Standard Book Number: 0-8151-0680-7

Editors

John J. Bergan, M.D., F.A.C.S., Hon. F.R.C.S. (Eng)

Clinical Professor of Surgery, University of California, San Diego; Clinical Professor of Surgery, Uniformed Services, University of Health Sciences, Washington, D.C.; Professor of Surgery, Emeritus, Northwestern University Medical School, Chicago

James S. T. Yao, M.D., Ph.D.

Magerstadt Professor of Surgery; Chief, Division of Vascular Surgery, Northwestern University Medical School

Contributing Editors

Ralph G. DePalma, M.D.
Professor and Chairman, Department of Surgery, George Washington University Medical Center, Washington, D.C.

Julie Freischlag, M.D.
Assistant Professor of Surgery, University of California, Los Angeles

Kaj Johansen, M.D.
Harbor View Medical Center, Seattle, Washington

Luis A. Queral, M.D.
Director, Maryland Vascular Institute, Baltimore, Maryland

David B. Roos, M.D.
Denver, Colorado

Harris B. Schumacher, M.D.
Indianapolis, Indiana

Ronald J. Stoney, M.D.
Professor of Surgery, University of California, San Francisco

Thoralf M. Sundt, Jr., M.D.
Chairman, Department of Neurologic Surgery, Mayo Clinic, Rochester, Minnesota

Lloyd M. Taylor, M.D.
Associate Professor of Surgery, Division of Vascular Surgery, Oregon Health Sciences University, Portland, Oregon

Table of Contents

The material covered in this volume represents literature reviewed through July 1990.

Journals Represented

Mosby–Year Book subscribes to and surveys nearly 850 U.S. and foreign medical and allied health journals. From these journals, the Editors select the articles to be abstracted. Journals represented in this YEAR BOOK are listed below.

Acta Chirurgica Scandinavica
Acta Neurochirurgica
Acta Obstetricia et Gynecologica Scandinavica
American Heart Journal
American Journal of Cardiology
American Journal of Epidemiology
American Journal of Medicine
American Journal of Obstetrics and Gynecology
American Journal of Pathology
American Journal of Public Health
American Journal of Roentgenology
American Journal of Surgery
American Review of Respiratory Disease
American Surgeon
Anesthesiology
Angiology
Annals of Emergency Medicine
Annals of Internal Medicine
Annals of Surgery
Annals of Thoracic Surgery
Annals of Vascular Surgery
Annals of the Royal College of Surgeons of England
Archives of Internal Medicine
Archives of Neurology
Archives of Pathology and Laboratory Medicine
Archives of Surgery
Arteriosclerosis
Atherosclerosis
Blood
British Journal of Radiology
British Journal of Surgery
British Medical Journal
Canadian Journal of Surgery
Canadian Medical Association Journal
Cardiovascular and Interventional Radiology
Catheterization and Cardiovascular Diagnosis
Chirurg
Circulation
Clinical Nuclear Medicine
Clinical Physiology
Clinical Radiology
Clinical Science
Dermatologica
Deutsche Medizinische Wochenschrift
Endoscopy
European Heart Journal
European Journal of Applied Physiology and Occupational Physiology
European Journal of Vascular Surgery

Experimental and Molecular Pathology
Human Pathology
Hypertension
International Journal of Epidemiology
International Journal of Radiation, Oncology, Biology, and Physics
Journal de Chirurgie
Journal de Radiologie
Journal of Biomechanics
Journal of Bone and Joint Surgery (British Volume)
Journal of Cardiac Surgery
Journal of Cardiovascular Surgery
Journal of Clinical Epidemiology
Journal of Clinical Microbiology
Journal of Computer Assisted Tomography
Journal of Dermatologic Surgery and Oncology
Journal of Internal Medicine
Journal of Interventional Radiology
Journal of Neurology, Neurosurgery and Psychiatry
Journal of Neurosurgery
Journal of Nuclear Medicine
Journal of Pathology
Journal of Reconstructive Microsurgery
Journal of Surgical Research
Journal of Thoracic and Cardiovascular Surgery
Journal of Trauma
Journal of Urology
Journal of Vascular Surgery
Journal of the American Academy of Dermatology
Journal of the American College of Cardiology
Journal of the American Medical Association
Journal of the Canadian Association of Radiologists
Journal of the Royal College of Surgeons of Edinburgh
Journal of Ultrasound in Medicine
Journal of Vascular Technology
Laboratory Investigation
Lancet
Laryngoscope
Neurosurgery
New England Journal of Medicine
Pace
Pathologe
Pediatric Radiology
Pediatrics
Plastic and Reconstructive Surgery
Presse Medicale
Psychophysiology
Radiology
Reviews of Infectious Diseases
ROFO
Schweizerische Medizinische Wochenschrift
Science
Semaine des Hopitaux

Southern Medical Journal
Stroke
Surgery
Surgery, Gynecology and Obstetrics
Surgical Research Communications
Texas Heart Institute Journal
Thrombosis and Haemostasis
VASA: Zeitschrift fur Grefasskrankheiten
Wiener Klinische Wochenschrift
World Journal of Surgery

Standard Abbreviations

The following terms are abbreviated in this edition: acquired immunodeficiency syndrome (AIDS), central nervous system (CNS), cerebrospinal fluid (CSF), computed tomography (CT), electrocardiography (ECG), and human immunodeficiency virus (HIV).

Introduction

Just as a mirror reflects the contents of a room, this edition of the YEAR BOOK OF VASCULAR SURGERY reflects the status of this subspecialty's particular interests at the beginning of the last decade of the 20th century.

When one looks in a mirror, attention is drawn to the largest objects. Similarly, in this volume, the most apparent aspects of vascular surgery capture attention early. The largest chapter is concerned with cerebrovascular problems. It explores diagnosis by advanced techniques, including color Doppler, transcranial Doppler, and magnetic resonance imaging. And, it hints at the miracles of magnetic resonance arteriography and perhaps eventual replacement of contrast arteriography by this truly noninvasive technique.

Problems of the operations to correct cerebrovascular insufficiency are explored. Prevention of these by electroencephalography and treatment when neurologic deficit has occurred are discussed here. The short- and long-term outcomes of carotid surgery are documented thoroughly. Also, the short- and long-term effects of spontaneous carotid artery dissection are described.

Other major items of interest are reflected in this volume. Among these are aortic surgical problems, including the various forms of aortic aneurysms and variations of aortoiliac occlusive disease. Standard methods of treatment by grafting as well as futuristic ideas, including two-balloon dilatation and stent placement, find room for discussion here. Attempts at solution of specific problems are also discussed. These include prevention of paraplegia in thoracoabdominal aortic surgery and attempts to minimize the trauma of necessary aortic surgery by alternative approaches to the aorta. The particular problem of contamination of an existing aortic aneurysm by opportunistic bacteria also receives appropriate attention.

The mirror of this YEAR BOOK reflects the practice of vascular surgery in the far distal arterial segments of the extremities as well. Here one sees decreased interest in the laser, the disappointments of balloon angioplasty in the far distal circulation, and a beginning definition of the outer limits of revascularization that is carried to the ankle and foot. As the boundaries of far distal arterial reconstruction are being laid out, one cannot help but be amazed at the success and durability of revascularization to small plantar arteries and the possibilities of tissue coverage by free flaps and grafts. Imaginative reconstructions are succeeding in decreasing the need for amputation just as vascular surgery is realizing that reconstruction of the distal circulation succeeds in diabetics as well as, or better than, in nondiabetics.

Although in some ways the messages appearing in this YEAR BOOK OF VASCULAR SURGERY are much like those of a minister preaching to the choir, it is the hope of the editors that the various messages included here will be conveyed to our friends in family practice and in internal medicine.

In reflecting on the mirror that shows contents of a room, after passing over the large items, details and curiosities of ornamentation finally capture attention. Likewise, within this volume certain interesting entities such as the throbbing buttocks syndrome are seen. Also, curiosities such as aneurysms of the digestive system, microemboli to digits, and an interesting pattern of rupture of small arteriolar aneurysms as they occur in pregnancy, after renal transplantation, and in polyarteritis nodosa. As one's attention is drawn to these latter phenomena, one cannot help but think that there is a message there—one that might lead to the fundamental causes of aneurysms, their enlargement, and rupture. If only this mystery could be unraveled, prevention of the devastating consequences of arterial rupture and internal hemorrhage could be avoided.

The disappointments of endovascular surgery diminish the space occupied by those techniques, but a resurgence of interest in problems of the venous system rises to fill it. Manifold differing problems of the venous system are thoroughly reflected in this YEAR BOOK as it mirrors vascular practice.

Thromboembolism continues to occupy much attention. Within that special entity echoes of practice in other countries is heard. These teach the virtues of venous thrombectomy for acute thrombosis, creation of arteriovenous fistulas to improve results of surgery for that problem, and the closure of such arteriovenous connections by minimally invasive radiologic techniques rather than surgery. Further, investigations into problems of the swollen leg are reported here, as are the results of surgery for severe venous stasis disease and treatment of the cosmetic problems of venous stasis by sclerotherapy. Surgery for the varicosities of primary venous stasis is discussed. One also sees in this volume an increasing interest in reconstruction of the vena cava. This, in turn, is brought about by the increasing incidence of the superior vena cava syndrome produced by malignant and benign disease as well as by the iatrogenic introduction of electrodes and catheters.

Although vascular surgery is thought to be a small subspecialty within surgery, in fact, as reflected in this volume of the YEAR BOOK, there are a startling number of differing problems of the arterial and venous systems that command attention. Their diagnosis by increasingly accurate imaging techniques, their study by innovative methods of measurement, and their treatment by a wide variety of surgical procedures are reflected here. These suggest correctly that the subspecialty of vascular surgery is intellectually challenging. Experts who practice this art must remain well informed about an increasingly large number of differing conditions.

It is the hope of the editors of this YEAR BOOK that an exploration of the details displayed on the pages of this volume will be of interest and utility to our colleagues in this very special field.

John J. Bergan, M.D., Hon. F.R.C.S.
James S. T. Yao, M.D., PhD.

1 Basic Considerations

Peripheral Arterial Disease in Large Vessels Is Epidemiologically Distinct From Small Vessel Disease: An Analysis of Risk Factors

Criqui MH, Browner D, Fronek A, Klauber MR, Coughlin SS, Barrett-Connor E, Gabriel S (Univ of California, San Diego, La Jolla)

Am J Epidemiol 129:1110–1119, 1989 1–1

Peripheral arterial disease affects many elderly individuals. Noninvasive techniques were used to evaluate peripheral arterial disease and to distinguish large from small vessel arterial disease in 565 patients aged 38–82 years. A series of noninvasive tests, including flow velocity by Doppler ultrasound, were performed.

Of 69 patients with large vessel peripheral arterial disease, 19 had severe disease. Ninety patients had isolated small vessel peripheral arterial disease. Large vessel peripheral arterial disease in men was significantly associated with age, pack-years of cigarettes smoked, systolic blood pressure, fasting plasma glucose, and marginally with obesity. Significant associations in women were age and systolic blood pressure, although an association was suggested for pack-years of cigarettes, obesity, and low-density lipoprotein. Isolated small vessel peripheral arterial disease was not significantly related to any of the main cardiovascular disease risk factors, including carbohydrate metabolism, fasting plasma glucose, and glycosylated hemoglobin.

When valid and reliable noninvasive techniques are used independently to assess isolated small vessel peripheral arterial disease and large vessel peripheral arterial disease, the former appears unrelated to traditional cardiovascular disease risk factors. Large vessel peripheral arterial disease and isolated small vessel peripheral arterial disease appear to be epidemiologically and pathophysiologically distinct entities.

▶ Noninvasive testing has made an epidemiologic study such as this one possible. However, vascular surgical input was lacking. The authors of this study failed to differentiate between large vessel aortoiliac occlusive disease and large vessel femoropopliteal occlusive disease. Furthermore, small vessel peripheral arterial disease was defined as occlusive disease in vessels less than 2 mm in diameter and was detected by isolated toe pressure abnormalities or abnormalities of reactive hyperemia. One would hope that future analysis of data from this group or others would include input from the peripheral vascular community. Vascular surgeons are aware of the fact that isolated small vessel peripheral arterial disease is vastly different from large vessel occlusive disease. The conclusion of this study, that small vessel occlusive disease is not associated with abnormalities of glycosylated hemoglobin, is in fact consistent with those published by LoGerfo and Coffman just a few years ago (1).

Reference

1. LoGerfo FW, Coffman JD: *N Engl J Med* 311:1615, 1984.

Fish Intake and Arterial Wall Characteristics in Healthy People and Diabetic Patients

Wahlqvist JL, Lo CS, Myers KA (Monash Univ; Prince Henry's Hosp, Melbourne)

Lancet 2:944–946, 1989 1–2

Epidemiologic studies have indicated that diets rich in fish or marine oil may reduce the incidence of occlusive vascular disease. The relationship between fish consumption and arterial wall characteristics was investigated in 31 healthy persons and 22 patients with non-insulin-dependent diabetes mellitus (NIDDM).

Arterial compliance, as measured by Doppler ultrasonography, was significantly lower in nonfish eaters than among fish eaters in the healthy group, the NIDDM group, and the 2 groups combined. An increase in mean proximal resistance at the common femoral artery and posterior tibial artery in nonfish eaters was significant only in the combined group and in the healthy group, respectively.

Fish consumption may be important for better arterial wall characteristics. Several studies have suggested that diets rich in fish oil or ω-3 fatty acids significantly reduce plasma concentrations of cholesterol and triglyceride, improve fat tolerance, prolong bleeding time, reduce platelet count, and decrease platelet adhesiveness. Dietary n-3 polyunsaturated fatty acids that are abundant in marine organisms may retard the development of arteriosclerotic cardiovascular disease.

▶ It is interesting in this study that the method used to determine arterial wall compliance and proximal resistance assesses both the aortoiliac segment and the segment of artery proximal to the posterior tibial. This study suggests that as little as 2 fish dishes per week improves aortoiliac arterial compliance and supports the findings of the lower incidence of ischemic heart disease in long-term fish diet consumers.

Smoking and Atherosclerosis

Kunze M, Schwarz B (Universität Wien, Vienna)

Wien Klin Wochenschr 101:683–687, 1989 1–3

Smoking, hyperlipidemia, and hypertension are the 3 major cardiovascular risk factors. More than 50% of all deaths are caused by cardiovascular disease. Approximately 33% of all atherosclerotic diseases and 30% of all cardiovascular diseases are caused by smoking. Smoking also significantly contributes to respiratory diseases. Furthermore, smoking is a major cause of malignant diseases.

In Austria the number of persons who smoke has steadily increased from 27.7% of the total population in 1972 to 30% in 1986. As the number of ex-smokers has slightly increased from 11.5% in 1972 to 13% in 1986, the increase in the number of smokers can be attributed to new smokers. Among women, the number of smokers has drastically increased, from 13% in 1972 to 21% in 1986. The highest increase is seen in girls younger than age 15 years, who also smoke more frequently than those in other age groups.

Because of the known association between the use of oral contraceptives and stroke, the sharp increase in the number of women who smoke represents a substantial increase in the number of women at risk. In contrast, the number of men who smoke decreased from 45% in 1972 to 40% in 1986. The number of boys younger than age 15 years who start smoking is also declining. An Austrian survey of smoking habits among children aged 11–15 years showed that among 15-year-old children, 17% of the boys and 19% of the girls smoked regularly. Among 13-year-old children, 7% of the boys and 5% of the girls smoked regularly.

Since 1974 numerous programs to decrease tobacco consumption have been initiated. Most are based on established international guidelines to reduce smoking. Increasing the price of tobacco products is one of the more effective measures to decrease tobacco consumption in Austria. The best preventive measure for keeping children from starting the smoking habit appears to be promoting the concept that smoking is socially unacceptable. Austrian physicians need to realize more that the treatment of nicotine addiction should be taken as seriously as the treatment of addiction to other psychotropic substances.

▶ The epidemiologic observations described here from Austria are similar to those observed in our own hospitals in the United States where the nursing staff, especially the operating room nurses, continue to smoke while the physician staff increasingly abstains. The worldwide problem of nicotine addiction is slowly coming under control.

The Influence of Age, Sex, Smoking, and Diabetes on Lower Limb Transcutaneous Oxygen Tension in Patients With Arterial Occlusive Disease

Rooke TW, Osmundson PJ (Mayo Clinic and Found)

Arch Intern Med 150:129–132, 1990 1–4

Transcutaneous oxygen tension ($TcPo_2$) measurement is an increasingly popular method for assessment of cutaneous blood flow. Data on 129 patients with unilateral or bilateral lower limb arterial occlusive disease were studied retrospectively to assess the effects of age, sex, smoking, and diabetes on lower limb $TcPo_2$. The severity of lower limb arterial occlusive disease was estimated using the clinical signs and symptoms of disease or the ankle/brachial blood pressure indices.

Age, sex, and smoking had no significant effects on $TcPo_2$ and disease severity. In contrast, both $TcPo_2$ and disease severity were adversely af-

Effect of Diabetes and Ankle/Brachial Blood Pressure Index on Transcutaneous Oxygen Tension ($TcPo_2$)

				Supine		Elevated	
Ankle/ Brachial Index	N*	Diabetes	Average Ankle/Brachial Index	$TcPo_2$ (Foot) mm Hg	Regional Perfusion Index	$TcPo_2$ (Foot) mm Hg	Regional Perfusion Index
All	76	+	0.58±0.29	34.6±22.2	0.55±0.37	25.0±21.3	0.38±0.32
patients	166	−	0.59±0.28	46.9±21.5†	0.75±0.35†	35.7±22.5†	0.55±0.34†
>0.8	19	+	0.96±0.18	43.8±18.2	0.73±0.33	33.7±17.1	0.53±0.28
	37	−	1.03±0.14	55.9±12.8‡	0.88±0.20§	49.1±14.5†	0.74±0.23†
0.45-0.8	29	+	0.60±0.09	39.9±20.6	0.65±0.35	31.1±22.4	0.48±0.33
	72	−	0.57±0.09	52.3±19.7‡	0.83±0.32‡	39.5±21.5	0.60±0.32
<0.45	28	+	0.30±0.11	23.0±21.7	0.34±0.32	12.8±17.3	0.18±0.24
	56	−	0.33±0.09	33.8±22.3§	0.55±0.37‡	22.0±21.0§	0.34±0.32§

*Fifteen limbs (8 diabetic, 7 nondiabetic) included in the table are not included here because of an ankle/brachial index of more than 1.5.
†Differs from diabetic, $P < .005$.
‡Differs from diabetic, $P < .01$.
§Differs from diabetic, $P < .05$.
(Courtesy of Rooke TW, Osmundson PJ: *Arch Intern Med* 150:129–132, 1990.)

fected by diabetes. When limbs with similar signs and symptoms or similar ankle blood pressure indices were compared, TcP_{O_2} remained significantly lower in patients with diabetes than in nondiabetic persons (table).

Regardless of the severity of arterial occlusive disease, patients with diabetes have significantly lower TcP_{O_2} in the feet than nondiabetics. Further studies are needed to define the nature and clinical significance of these findings. Measurement of TcP_{O_2} is a valuable noninvasive test to assess the functional status of cutaneous blood flow.

▶ The question is, Is this useful information or merely interesting?

Cigarette Smoking-Associated Changes in Blood Lipid and Lipoprotein Levels in the 8- to 19-Year-Old Age Group: A Meta-Analysis

Craig WY, Palomaki GE, Johnson AM, Haddow JE (Found for Blood Research, Scarborough, Maine)

Pediatrics 85:155–158, 1990 1–5

Most smoking-associated changes in serum lipid and lipoprotein levels in children are in the direction of increased coronary disease risk, as in adults. Lipid changes were quantified in smokers and nonsmokers of both sexes aged 8–19 years. Serum levels of triglycerides, very-low-density lipoprotein (VLDL) cholesterol, and low-density lipoprotein cholesterol were significantly increased in smokers, whereas total cholesterol and high-density lipoprotein cholesterol were significantly reduced compared with levels in nonsmokers. Except for VLDL cholesterol, the changes were more marked than in adults. Serum total cholesterol is increased in adult smokers.

Because coronary disease begins to develop in childhood in Western populations, it is important to identify potential risk factors at a time when prophylactic measures might be most effective. The finding that smoking causes lipid and lipoprotein changes in children that resemble those seen in adults emphasizes the need for interventions to end cigarette consumption.

▶ Although the data in this study suggest that young smokers are at increased risk for coronary artery disease, in fact, the high triglyceride levels suggest that they may be at even greater risk for peripheral arterial occlusive disease.

Are Passive Smokers at Greater Risk of Thrombosis?

Sinzinger H, Virgolini I (Österreichischen Akademie der Wissenschaften Wien, Vienna)

Wien Klin Wochenschr 101:694–698, 1989 1–6

The association between cigarette smoking and vascular injury has been well documented, but a similar relationship between passive smoking and vascular injury has not been confirmed. Nicotine is a naturally-occurring alkaloid having a structure similar to that of aspirin and indomethacin, which are known prostaglandin synthesis inhibitors. Prostaglandin I_2 (PgI_2) exerts an antiaggregatory effect on platelets. In laboratory animals, the nicotine and carbon monoxide in cigarette smoke inhibits PgI_2 synthesis and increases secretion of thromboxane A_2 which is a known platelet aggregation factor (Fig 1–1). These findings were later confirmed in adult smokers. However, no data are available on the relationship between passively inhaled cigarette smoke and PgI_2 synthesis inhibition or thromboxane A_2 secretion.

To assess the acute and chronic effects of passive smoking on the vessel wall, platelet function, and the PgI_2 system, 8 smokers aged 22–30 years smoked a total of 30 cigarettes in a large enclosed room kept at 22 C and

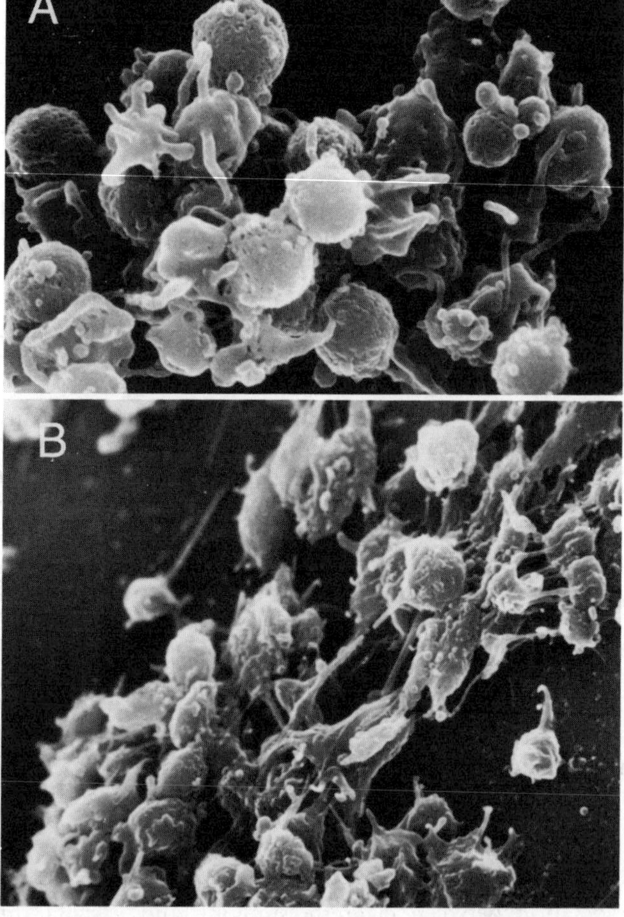

Fig 1–1.—Electronmicroscopic image of human platelets. **A**, "resting" (before), and (**B**) activated platelets from a nonsmoker (after passive smoking) under identical work loads (original magnification, ×6800). (Courtesy of Sinzinger H, Virgolini I: *Wien Klin Wochenschr* 101:694–698, 1989.)

60% relative humidity. Eight nonsmoking volunteers aged 24–30 years stayed for 60 minutes in the smoke-filled room. The smoking and smoke exposure experiments were repeated daily for a total of 5 days. Blood samples were collected at baseline, immediately after, 20 and 60 minutes after, and 6 hours after passive exposure to cigarette smoke.

Passive exposure to cigarette smoke decreased PgI_2 activity and stimulated platelet activity as if the nonsmokers had been smoking, but to a lesser degree. However, within 6 hours after exposure all measured parameters had returned to normal. After 5 days of daily exposure to cigarette smoke, baseline values of platelet function parameters approached those measured in smokers. Baseline values of platelet function in chronic smokers did not change throughout the study. Nonsmokers with atherogenic risk factors who are chronically exposed to passive cigarette smoke may be at increased risk of having atherosclerosis, thrombosis, or other disorders associated with abnormal platelet function.

▶ It appears that for individuals condemned to passive smoking, antiplatelet therapy might be quite appropriate.

Prevalence of Hyperhomocyst(e)inemia in Patients With Peripheral Arterial Occlusive Disease

Malinow MR, Kang SS, Taylor LM, Wong PWK, Coull B, Inahara T, Mukerjee D, Sexton G, Upson B (Oregon Primate Research Ctr, Beaverton; Oregon Health Sciences Univ, Portland; St Vincent Hosp and Med Ctr, Portland, Ore; Rush-Presbyterian-St Luke's Med Ctr, Chicago)

Circulation 79:1180–1188, 1989 1–7

Several studies have suggested that abnormalities of homocyst(e)ine [H(e)] metabolism may be implicated in the pathogenesis of atherosclerosis and thrombosis. A micromethod adapted for automated determinations was used to measure basal plasma levels of H(e), which included the sum of free and bound forms of homocysteine, its disulfide oxidation product, homocystine, and the homocysteine-cysteine-mixed disulfide. Two groups were studied: 103 apparently healthy individuals (controls) and 47 patients with peripheral arterial occlusive disease (PAOD). Because the patients were older than the controls, the latter were subdivided into younger (age 60 years or younger) and older (older than age 60 years) subgroups.

Among younger controls, the mean levels of H(e) were 11.18 nmol/mL and 8.58 nmol/mL in men and women, respectively; in the older group, mean levels of H(e) were 10.74 nmol/mL and 9.04 nmol/mL, respectively. Mean levels of H(e) correlated significantly with age in the younger control women, but not in the other 3 subgroups. Mean levels of H(e) in patients with PAOD of 15.44 nmol/mL in men and 17.04 nmol/mL in women were considerably higher than those in controls. In patients with PAOD, age, cholesterolemia, and the prevalence of smoking and diabetes were similar among those with normal or elevated levels of

H(e), but hypertension was more frequent in those with high levels of H(e).

Hyperhomocyst(e)inemia is common in patients with PAOD and is an independent risk factor for arterial occlusive disease. This condition can damage vascular endothelium, promote thrombosis, oxidize low-density lipoproteins, and thus influence atherogenesis.

▶ This study is of particular interest because it is well known that homocysteinuric patients exhibit premature arteriosclerotic changes as early as 8 weeks of age. In patients with peripheral arterial occlusive disease, multiple mechanisms may be present that lead to damaged vascular endothelium, which promotes thrombosis, oxidizes low-density lipoprotein, and increases atherogenesis.

Homocysteine, an Atherogenic Stimulus, Reduces Protein C Activation by Arterial and Venous Endothelial Cells

Rodgers GM, Conn MT (Univ of Utah)

Blood 75:895–901, 1990 1–8

Endothelial cells express several antithrombotic properties that maintain vessel wall thromboresistance. One of these properties, thrombomodulin (TM), is an integral endothelial cell membrane protein involved in the protein C pathway of coagulation. Abnormalities in TM activity may predispose to a thrombotic tendency. A study was conducted to determine whether homocysteine-treated endothelial cells exhibit reduced TM activity and, if so, by what mechanism(s).

Increased blood levels of homocysteine are associated with atherosclerosis and thrombotic disease. Results of previous studies have shown that treatment of cultured endothelial cells with homocysteine increased endogenous factor V activity by activation of the cofactor. In these experiments, both arterial and venous endothelial cells activated protein C; homocysteine, .6 mmol/L, reduced endothelial cell protein C activation by 12%. The maximal inhibition (90%) of protein C activation occurred with homocysteine, 7.5–10 mmol/L, after 6–9 hours of incubation.

Cultured endothelial cells did not accelerate the metabolism of homocysteine. In low concentrations the metabolite acted as a competitive inhibitor to thrombin, rather than inducing an inhibitor to activated protein C. These findings suggest that the effects of homocysteine on the vascular endothelial cell protein mechanism may contribute to the thrombotic tendency observed in patients with increased blood levels of this metabolite.

▶ Atherosclerosis is almost uniformly present in aged individuals in Western countries. Thus, current research must determine why some persons with extensive atherosclerosis have severe symptoms and rapid disease progression, whereas others with similar lesions remain asymptomatic. Elevated plasma homocysteine is an established risk factor for symptomatic atherosclerosis and for rapidly progressive atherosclerosis. In this paper, Rodgers and Conn demonstrate a possible mechanism explaining this association: inhibition of protein C activation in endothelial cell cultures exposed to homocysteine. This significant decrease in natural antithrombotic potential may partly explain why symptoms occur related to atherosclerotic plaques in some, but by no means in all, individuals. Homocysteine is interesting because elevated levels can be reduced by administration of nontoxic substances such as folic acid, pyridoxine, and vitamin B_{12}. This paper adds weight to the evidence that homocysteine itself is toxic, rather than a simple marker, and that therapy to reduce plasma levels of this substance is rational and may be anticipated to be beneficial.—Lloyd M. Taylor, M.D., Associate Professor of Surgery, Division of Vascular Surgery, Department of Surgery, Oregon Health Sciences University, Portland, Oregon

---

Impaired Homocysteine Metabolism in Early-Onset Cerebral and Peripheral Occlusive Arterial Disease: Effects of Pyridoxine and Folic Acid Treatment

Brattström L, Israelsson B, Norrving B, Bergqvist D, Thörne J, Hultberg B, Hamfelt A (Univ of Lund; Malmö Gen Hosp; Sundsvall Hosp, Lund, Sweden)

Atherosclerosis 81:51–60, 1990 1–9

Marked homocysteinemia caused by either cystathionine β-synthase deficiency or genetic defects of vitamin B_{12} or folate metabolism is associated with vascular disease of very early onset. Homocysteine metabolism was examined in 72 patients seen before age 55 years with occlusive disease of cerebral, carotid, or aortoiliac vessels. Thirty-one patients were hypertensive. None had liver or kidney disease or diabetes. Twenty parents of patients with homocysteinuria also were studied.

Twenty patients (28%) had basal homocysteinemia and another 26 (36%) had abnormal increases in plasma homocysteine after methionine loading orally. Their levels were within the range for 20 obligate heterozygotes for homocysteinuria resulting from cystathionine β-synthase deficiency. The basal plasma homocysteine level correlated negatively with the vitamin B_{12} and folate concentrations.

Twenty patients received pyridoxine in a dose of 240 mg daily and folic acid in a dose of 10 mg daily. Fasting homocysteine levels fell by a mean of 53% after 4 weeks, and the methionine response fell by a mean of 39%. Changes in basal homocysteine were most marked in patients with subnormal folate levels.

A substantial number of patients with early-onset vascular disease have impaired homocysteine metabolism. The impairment is readily reversed by vitamin treatment, so that it might be productive to screen such patients for impaired homocysteine metabolism.

► If, in fact, a large number of patients with early-onset or precocious arterial occlusive disease have impaired homocysteine metabolism, screening by the simple methods described might be valuable. Treatment with vitamin therapy could be done quite simply.

Localization of PDGF-B Protein in Macrophages in All Phases of Atherogenesis

Ross R, Masuda J, Raines EW, Gown AM, Katsuda S, Sasahara M, Malden LT, Masuko H, Sato H (Univ of Washington; Research Inst, Osaka; Mochida Pharmaceutical Co, Tokyo)

Science 248:1009–1012, 1990 1–10

Migration of medial smooth muscle cells into the intima is one of the basic processes underlying atherosclerosis. Platelet-derived growth factor (PDGF) may be involved in both the migration and proliferation of intimal smooth muscle cells. Platelet-derived growth factor B chain protein was identified in macrophages at all stages of lesion development in both primate and human vessels. Advanced lesions of induced atherosclerosis in primates contained increased amounts of PDGF-B, the receptor for colony-stimulating factor type 1, the β subunit of PDGF receptor, interleukin-1, and transforming growth factor β1. Macrophages in atherosclerotic lesions obtained from patients at surgery also contained PDGF-B. Smooth muscle cells were negative for PDGF-B.

These findings suggest that the entry of monocytes into the artery and their differentiation into macrophages may stimulate PDGF-B gene expression and protein synthesis. Interactions among monocytes, T cells, and endothelium may lead to the formation and release of growth-regulating and other bioactive molecules and thereby to further migration of smooth muscle cells into the arterial intima.

▶ The "response to injury" hypothesis of atherosclerosis has required modification because endothelial changes and platelet interactions observed at branches and bifurcations of arteries are not uniformly present. On the other hand, the observations in this report demonstrate the presence of PDGF-B chain in macrophages during all stages of human and nonhuman primate atherogenesis. This is consistent with the chronic inflammatory and focal nature of the lesions of atherosclerosis.

Detection of Activated T Lymphocytes in the Human Atherosclerotic Plaque

Hansson GK, Holm J, Jonasson L (Gothenburg Univ, Sweden)

Am J Pathol 135:169–175, 1989 1–11

The finding of significant quantities of T cells in human atherosclerotic plaque, in which smooth muscle cells express major histocompatibility complex class II (Ia) antigens, suggests the possibility of a local immune response. To determine whether specific T cells are activated locally immunofluorescent techniques were used on cryostat sections from carotid endarterectomy specimens and on isolated plaque cells.

Of cells in atherosclerotic plaques that stained positive for T-cell-specific surface protein CD3, a mean of 6.4% expressed interleukin-2 receptor. Analysis of isolated plaque cells demonstrated that 10% of E receptor-positive cells expressed interleukin-2 receptor. Approximately one third of the T cells isolated from plaque expressed HLA-DR and very late activation antigen 1. These activation markers were also observed with similar frequency in plaque sections.

The pathogenesis of atherosclerosis may involve an immune response. The activation pattern of many T cells in atherosclerotic plaques is a type similar to that seen in connective tissue diseases. Significant paracrine secretion of lymphokines may occur in the plaque. Activation of T cells by class II major histocompatibility complex antigens, therefore, may have importance not only in the pathogenesis of atherosclerosis but also in the function of other types of plaque cells.

▶ The observations in this study are consistent with other observations in which cyclosporine A, which is an inhibitor of T cell activation, significantly reduced the arterial intimal proliferation occurring after mechanical injury.

Atherosclerotic Lesions in Humans: In Situ Immunophenotypic Analysis Suggesting an Immune Mediated Response

Wal AC van der, Das PK, Berg DB van de, Loos CM van der, Becker AE (Univ of Amsterdam; Academic Med Ctr, Amsterdam)

Lab Invest 61:166–170, 1989 1–12

Although recent immunocytochemical investigations have shown unequivocally the presence of lymphocytes in atherosclerotic lesions, not much has been done to assess the role of an immune-mediated process in atherogenesis. The in situ immunophenotypical characterization of cellular infiltrates in different types of human atherosclerotic lesions, including diffuse intimal thickening, was analyzed using monoclonal antibodies in specimens obtained at autopsy. Particular emphasis was given to monocytes/macrophages and lymphocytes and their possible interactions using immuno-double staining techniques.

T lymphocytes and macrophages were detected in diffuse intimal thickening, fatty streaks, and atheromatous plaques. Some infiltrates contained predominantly T suppressor/cytotoxic cells, whereas others showed mixtures of T suppressor/cytotoxic cells and T helper/inducer cells in ratios varying from 1:1 to 4:1. A substantial number of T cells and macrophages were considered to be immunoactivated because of their expression of HLA-DR; some cells also expressed strong I12 receptor activity. The activation was particularly noticeable at sites of close cell-to-cell contact between monocytes/macrophages and lymphocytes.

A specific in situ immune-mediated hypersensitivity reaction appears to be associated with the development of atherosclerosis.

▶ The observations of this study suggest that diffuse intimal thickening sets the scene for an immune-mediated hypersensitivity response that contributes to the full-blown atherosclerotic lesion.

Rapidly Progressive Atherosclerosis in Aortocoronary Saphenous Vein Grafts: Possible Immune-Mediated Disease
Ratliff NB, Myles JL (Cleveland Clinic Found)
Arch Pathol Lab Med 113:772–776, 1989 1–13

Atherosclerosis becomes a prominent problem with saphenous vein coronary bypass grafts after 5 years. A total of 115 aortocoronary saphenous vein grafts from 100 consecutive reoperations were examined, and coronary arteries with severe atherosclerosis were examined during 20 autopsies.

Diffuse intimal fibroplasia was a nearly universal finding in the vein grafts. Lipid-laden foam cells or necrotic lipid debris were observed in 46% of grafts, which were thus classified atherosclerotic. Atherosclerosis was concentric in more than three fourths of the patients. The atherosclerotic grafts were fragile. Whereas recent thrombi were about equally frequent in grafts with and without atherosclerosis, remote thrombi were more frequent in grafts without atherosclerosis.

Both intimal fibroplasia and atherosclerosis in aortocoronary saphenous vein grafts closely resemble immune-mediated atherosclerosis. Vein graft changes may be immune-mediated lesions, possibly triggered by graft injury during operation.

▶ If rapidly progressive atherosclerosis in saphenous vein grafts is immune mediated, what will be the therapeutic consequences of these observations?

Detection and Quantification of Lipoprotein(a) in the Arterial Wall of 107 Coronary Bypass Patients
Rath M, Niendorf A, Reblin T, Dietel M, Krebber H-J, Beisiegel U (Universitäts-Krankenhaus Eppendorf, Hamburg, Germany)
Arteriosclerosis 9:579–592, 1989 1–14

Epidemiologic studies suggest a positive correlation between high serum lipoprotein[a] (Lp[a]) levels and coronary heart disease. To define the role of Lp[a] in atherogenesis, lipid and lipoprotein parameters were analyzed in routine biopsy specimens taken from the ascending aorta in 107 patients undergoing aortocoronary bypass surgery and correlated with serum levels.

Bypass patients had significantly higher serum Lp[a] levels compared with an age-matched control group. There was a significant positive correlation between serum Lp[a] and arterial wall apolipoprotein (apo [a]). The apo[a]-linked apo B in the arterial wall correlated with serum Lp[a] levels, indicating that high serum Lp[a] levels could contribute significantly to the deposition of apo B in the arterial wall. In contrast, no significant correlation was found between serum and arterial wall apo B. Apo[a] was detected in the arterial wall as an intact protein, whereas apo B was partially linked to apo[a] in the aortic wall. Furthermore, the apo[a] isoform pattern in the arterial wall was comparable to the serum pattern. Both apo[a] and apo B co-localized in the arterial wall, predominantly in the intima and extracellularly. Increased cholesterol, apo[a], and apo B levels were noted in arterial walls with >50% visible plaques compared with those with <50% plaque area. Density gradient ultracentrifugation showed that Lp[a]-like particles could be isolated from plaque tissue. It would appear that Lp[a] accumulates in the arterial wall as apo[a] and apo B and partly in the form of lipoprotein-like particles, contributing to plaque formation and coronary heart disease.

▶ This appears to be the first study showing the positive correlation of Lp[a] serum levels with apo(a) and apo(B) accumulation in the arterial wall.

Quantitation and Localization of Apolipoproteins [a] and B in Coronary Artery Bypass Vein Grafts Resected at Re-Operation

Cushing GL, Gaubatz JW, Nava ML, Burdick BJ, Bocan TMA, Guton JR, Weilbaecher D, DeBakey ME, Lawrie GM, Morrisett JD (Baylor College of Medicine; Methodist Hosp, Houston)

Arteriosclerosis 9:593–603, 1989 1–15

The plasma concentration of lipoprotein[a] (Lp[a]) correlates highly with cardiovascular disease. To assess the role of Lp[a] in vein graft atherosclerosis, tissue levels of apo[a] and apo B, the 2 major apoproteins of Lp[a], were measured in saphenous vein bypass grafts in patients undergoing coronary re-bypass surgery and correlated with graft duration, pathologic findings, and plasma levels of apoLp[a].

In 17 patients (mean age, 63 years) with grafts of a mean 112 months' duration before resection, the mean total plasma cholesterol level was 221 mg/dL, the mean high-density-lipoprotein cholesterol level was 31 mg/dL, and the mean plasma triglyceride level was 228 mg/dL. Whereas the tissue level of mean apoLp[a] was below measurable limits (<2 ng/mg) and the apo B level was very low (3.3 ng/mg) in normal saphenous veins, mean tissue levels in resected grafts were 32 ng/mg and 70 ng/mg, respectively. In a subgroup of 28 patients in whom 59 grafts were resected and 77 tissue segments were analyzed, the tissue apoLp[a]:apo B ratio was .313. This was 56% higher than the plasma apoLp[a]:apo B ratio (.132) in the same patients.

There was a positive correlation between plasma and tissue levels of apoLp[a] and apo B. Immunochemical localization of the apoproteins showed that both apo[a] and apo B co-localized in areas of atherosclerosis and were absent in normal fresh saphenous veins. Tissue apo B, but not apoLp[a], correlated positively with measurements of atherosclerosis, including percent of the luminal area occupied by lipid-rich core regions and characteristic fibrous proliferation plus lipid, whereas presence of foam cells correlated positively with apoLp[a].

There appears to be a net accumulation of apoLp[a] and apo B in saphenous vein bypass grafts from the time of their grafting into the arterial bed. Thus these lipoproteins play an important role in vein graft atherosclerosis.

▶ In addition to the findings of this study is the link between lipid levels and graft failure. Hypertriglyceridemia has been documented repeatedly in association with early vein graft occlusion.

Premature Arterial Disease Associated With Familial Antithrombin III Deficiency

Johnson EJ, Prentice CRM, Parapia LA (Bradford Royal Infirmary; Leeds Gen Infirmary, West Yorkshire, England)

Thromb Haemost 63:13–15, 1990 1–16

Antithrombin III (ATIII) is an inhibitor of coagulation. Patients with inherited ATIII deficiency are predisposed to venous embolism but have not been reported to be predisposed to arterial occlusive disease. Findings were evaluated in members of a family with ATIII deficiency who had severe arterial thrombosis.

Woman, 27, was admitted to the emergency department with bilateral rest pain resulting from ischemia caused by peripheral artery insufficiency. Popliteal and pedal pulses were absent bilaterally. Aortograpy revealed blockage of both distal superficial femoral arteries. The day after aortography a stroke occurred that resulted in hemiparesis. The ATIII level was 12 mg/dL. Warfarin therapy was initiated. Ischemia improved, and some of the paralysis abated over the course of the next year.

Antithrombin III deficiency is a potentially preventable cause of thromboembolic disease. It should be considered in all patients with arterial, as well as venous, thromboembolic disease, especially if it occurs at an early age. Such patients should be counseled against smoking to further reduce the risk factors for thromboembolic disease.

▶ Among coagulation abnormalities only hyperfibrinogenemia and factor VII levels had been implicated in atherosclerotic occlusive disease. This study seems to add antithrombin III as another risk factor.

Immunoelectron-Microscopic Localization of S-Protein/Vitronectin in Human Atherosclerotic Wall

Niculescu F, Rus HG, Poruţiu D, Ghiurca V, Vlaicu R (School of Medicine, Romania)
Atherosclerosis 78:197–203, 1989 1–17

S-protein/vitronectin is a multifunctional 75-kDa protein found in serum and plasma at levels of 200–300 μg/mL. The protein interacts with both complement activation and coagulation pathways. It inhibits complement system activation by preventing insertion of C5b-9 into the cell membrane. It may regulate coagulation by preventing inactivation of thrombin and reducing factor Xa inhibition by antithrombin III.

Immunoelectron-dense deposits of S-protein/vitronectin were localized in atherosclerotic femoral and iliac arteries taken at surgery, using an affinity-purified rabbit IgG specific for the human protein. Deposits occurred in both intimal thickenings and fibrous plaques. S-protein/vitronectin was not seen in intact cells or in cholesterol clefts. Cell debris was negative for S-protein/vitronectin but positive for C5b-9.

S-protein/vitronectin may have a role in defense of the arterial wall by limiting the extent of complement activation. Such activation is an important part of inflammatory events in atherogenesis.

▶ This abstract suggests that the S protein vitronectin acts in defense against the inflammation, which is an important component of the atherogenesis phenomenon, by restricting the extent of complement activation.

Heparin Kinetics in Vascular Surgery

Williams NN, Broe PJ, Burke P, Meagher EA, O'Donoghue C, Otridge B, Bouchier-Hayes D (Beaumont Hosp, Dublin)
Eur J Vasc Surg 3:493–496, 1989 1–18

The kinetics of heparin therapy during vascular surgery was studied in 9 patients undergoing major vascular surgery, including 1 carotid, 1 common iliac, and 7 aortic operations. After baseline blood samples were obtained for determinations of plasma heparin levels and activated partial thromboplastin time (APTT), each patient received a bolus dose of heparin, 100 units per kg. A second dose of heparin was administered intraoperatively 5 minutes before cross-clamping. Plasma heparin levels and APTT levels were measured at 10-minute intervals for 1 hour and at 20-minute intervals for the second hour after each dose of heparin.

Heparin doses ranged from 4,500 to 8,600 units (mean, 6,500 units). Maximal heparin levels of .83 × .04 units per mL were achieved within 10 minutes of heparin administration and were almost identical in the pre- and intraoperative periods. The decay curves for heparin in both periods displayed first-order kinetics with a half-life of 110 minutes. Mean APTT levels at 10 minutes attained maximal values of 6.6 and 8.8 times the controls, respectively. At the end of the 2 hours the mean APTT remained more than twice the control at both pre- and intraoperative periods.

Heparin kinetics is not adversely affected by surgical trauma. Because the use of standard dose schedules of heparin may lead to excessive peak levels, preoperative heparin testing is recommended to increase the safety of heparin administration during vascular surgery. This protocol involves measurement of APTT 10 minutes after the administration of heparin, 50 units per kg; the same dose of heparin is used during surgery if the APTT is more than twice the control and increased when APTT is less than twice the control.

▶ The very practical observations in this abstract suggest that peak values of heparin are achieved at 10 minutes, that the decay curves suggest a half-life of 110 minutes, and that these values are not adversely affected by the surgical event.

Heparin-Induced Thrombocytopenia

Becker PS, Miller VT (Johns Hopkins Univ; Northwestern Univ)

Stroke 20:1449–1459, 1989 1–19

More than half of the nearly 600 reported patients with heparin-induced thrombocytopenia (HITP) have had thromboembolism, including both venous and arterial embolism. Type I HITP is characterized by a significant fall in the platelet count, but levels usually remain above $50{,}000/mm^3$. The fall is evident within 1–5 days after the start of treatment, and counts often return to normal despite ongoing heparin therapy. Type II HITP is more severe, has a later onset, and thromboembolic complications are more frequent.

The relationship between heparin dose and the incidence or severity of HITP remains uncertain. Platelet production is normal or increased, so that increased platelet loss must be responsible for the thrombocytopenia. A direct platelet-aggregating effect may cause type I HITP. Type II cases may be immune mediated, but the precise relationship between platelets, antiplatelet antibodies, and heparin require further study. It is not clear why certain patients with HITP have thromboembolic complications. Stroke apparently resulting from heparin therapy has been reported 29 times.

Platelet counts should be monitored in heparin-treated patients, but the optimal frequency of monitoring remains to be established. Heparin should be stopped immediately if HITP and thrombosis develop. Promising results have been obtained in animal studies of synthetic low-molecular-weight heparin. Platelet transfusions have generally not given impressive results in patients with severe HITP. More rapid recovery has been described in patients given aspirin or dextran.

▶ Because of the importance of heparin-induced thrombocytopenia, this abstract is presented more as a reference or progress review than as definitive information.

Effect of Heparin on Adaptation of Vein Grafts to Arterial Circulation
Kohler TR, Kirkman T, Clowes AW (Univ of Washington)
Arteriosclerosis 9:523–528, 1989 1–20

The thickening of vein grafts inserted into the arterial circulation is a consequence of smooth muscle cell (SMC) hyperplasia and of synthesis and deposition of extracellular matrix. This process is thought to be similar to that which causes arterial wall thickening. Heparin inhibits intimal thickening in injured arteries. To determine whether heparin might inhibit vein-graft hyperplasia as well, 25 New Zealand rabbits were subjected to common carotid artery injuries by passing a balloon embolectomy catheter. A second group of 43 rabbits received interposition vein grafts in the right common carotid artery. All animals received either continuous intravenously administered heparin or saline solution. A third group of 10 rabbits underwent vein grafting and placement of infusion pumps containing either heparin or saline.

Heparin treatment in balloon-injured rabbit carotid arteries resulted in a significant reduction in intimal cross-sectional area at 1 week and 2 weeks. In contrast, the carotid arteries of the saline-treated controls showed significant intimal thickening at 1 week and 2 weeks. Heparin treatment in rabbits with vein grafts resulted in only a slight reduction in intimal cross-sectional area at 2 weeks but no reduction in wall thickness at any other time and no reduction in SMC proliferation at 1, 2, or 4 weeks. Either SMC in veins are less susceptible to heparin than are SMC in arteries, or the mechanism of wall thickening in vein grafts differs substantially from the mechanism responsible for wall thickening in arteries.

▶ The heparin effect on vein grafts observed in this study is quite disappointing.

Localized Release of Perivascular Heparin Inhibits Intimal Proliferation After Endothelial Injury Without Systemic Anticoagulation
Okada T, Bark DH, Mayberg MR (Univ of Washington)
Neurosurgery 25:892–898, 1989 1–21

Endothelial injury triggers hyperplasia of vascular smooth-muscle cells (SMC) by initiating platelet adherence and aggregation and releasing SMC mitogen platelet-derived growth factor (PDGF). Exposure of the media to serum components normally excluded may also initiate SMC proliferation and migration after endothelial injury. Although heparin may diminish myointimal proliferation either by preventing platelet aggregation or by direct inhibition of PDGF release, systemic heparin administration is associated with a considerable risk of hemorrhage, and its use in a clinical setting is therefore limited.

Polyvinyl alcohol (PVA) is a water-soluble, nontoxic polymer used in continuous-release drug delivery systems. In previous experiments, heparin mixed in PVA was applied locally to the adventitia of injured vessels

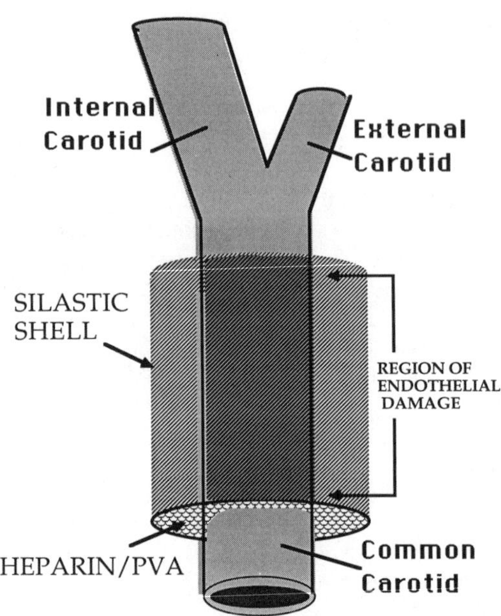

Fig 1–2.—Schematic representation of continuous heparin delivery system. Heparin is mixed with PVA and applied to the adventitial surface of the de-endothelialized rat common carotid artery. A Silastic cuff retards permeation of the heparin into nearby tissue. (Courtesy of Okada T, Bark DH, Mayberg MR: *Neurosurgery* 25:892–898, 1989.)

where it exerted a localized acute antithrombotic effect without systemic anticoagulation. Heparin in PVA was tested in a chronic model of rat carotid endothelial injury.

Using a balloon catheter technique, consistent SMC proliferation was produced in the common carotid artery (CCA) of 30 rats. In 15 rats, heparin/PVA gel was applied to the adventitial surface of the de-endothelialized CCA and surrounded by a Silastic shell to prevent release into adjacent tissue (Fig 1–2). In the other 15 rats PVA gel without heparin was similarly applied. Animals in both groups were killed at 5, 10, and 20 days after endothelial injury and the carotid vessels were examined by light microscopy, scanning electron microscopy, and immunohistochemical studies.

Control vessels showed prominent proliferation and migration of medial SMC into the intima over the study period. Immunohistochemical analysis identified the presence of actin in the proliferating intimal cells, suggesting their derivation from SMC. Application of continuous-release heparin to the adventitial surfaces of de-endothelialized CCA markedly inhibited myointimal proliferation and prevented luminal narrowing at all time periods without changing any of the systemic coagulation parameters.

Selective application of heparin in a PVA polymer application to damaged adventitial surfaces after endothelial injury inhibits SMC proliferation. The technique may have application in research as well as in a clinical setting.

▶ Innovative delivery systems may play a part in the ultimate conquering of the process of precocious myointimal hyperplasia.

Inhibition of Myointimal Proliferation of the Rat Carotid Artery by the Peptides, Angiopeptin, and BIM 23034

Lundergan C, Foegh ML, Vargas R, Eufemio M, Bormes GW, Kot PA, Ramwell PW (Georgetown Univ)

Atherosclerosis 80:49–55, 1989 1–22

Coronary artery restenosis, which is common after coronary bypass and angioplasty, is caused by myointimal proliferation. The effects of 5 synthetic somatostatin analogues on this process were tested in vivo on smooth muscle cells in rat coronary arteries subjected to endothelial injury by air drying.

When rats were pretreated 2 days before and for 5 days after endothelial injury, morphometric analysis showed significant inhibition of myointimal thickening by angiopeptin, 20 μg/kg/day and 50 μg/kg/day, and BIM 23034, a closely related octapeptide, given subcutaneously. Angiopeptin also had such an inhibitory effect when administered only 30 minutes before injury and for 5 days afterward. Angiopeptin, 100 μg/kg/day given subcutaneously 2 days before and for 5 days after endothelial injury, inhibited uptake of thymidine as well.

Angiopeptin and its congener BIM 23034 inhibit myointimal proliferation. Because all of the tested peptides inhibit secretion of growth hormone, the antiproliferative effect of angiopeptin is more likely to be the result of direct action on the blood vessel. Angiopeptin may be useful in prevention of restenosis after coronary artery bypass grafting or angioplasty.

▶ Perhaps peptides rather than heparin may be the ultimate answer in shutting down the myointimal response.

Inhibitors of Angiotensin-Converting Enzyme Prevent Myointimal Proliferation After Vascular Injury

Powell JS, Clozel J-P, Müller RKM, Kuhn H, Hefti F, Hosang M, Baumgartner HR (Hoffmann-La Roche Ltd, Basel, Switzerland)

Science 245:186–188, 1989 1–23

Proliferation of smooth muscle cells in the intima of muscular arteries and formation of extracellular matrix are major processes that lead to vascular stenosis in arteriosclerosis, after vascular surgery, and after coronary angioplasty. Because angiotensin-converting enzyme is present in vessel walls and medial smooth muscle cells have specific angiotensin receptors, a local angiotensin system may have a role in regulating the vascular response to arterial injury.

The angiotensin-converting enzyme inhibitor cilazapril was given to rats that had a carotid artery denuded of endothelium and injured by balloon catheterization. Control animals had marked intimal thickening and luminal narrowing after 2 weeks as a result of proliferation of smooth muscle cells, migration of smooth muscle cells from the media to the intima, and synthesis of extracellular matrix. Treated animals had 80% less formation of neointima and no luminal compromise. Similar results were obtained when captopril was given with food from 6 days before to 2 weeks after balloon injury. Verapamil also suppressed myointimal proliferation.

A local angiotensin system may contribute to the myointimal proliferative response of the vascular wall to injury. Inhibition of angiotensin-converting enzyme may have therapeutic value in preventing the proliferative lesions that follow coronary angioplasty and vascular surgery. Possibly, converting enzyme inhibition can act synergistically with heparin to prevent proliferative responses.

▶ Clearly, a great deal of energy is being expended in finding the antidote to myointimal hyperplasia.

Intimal Fibromuscular Hyperplasia at the Venous Anastomosis of PTFE Grafts in Hemodialysis Patients: Clinical, Immunocytochemical, Light and Electron Microscopic Assessment

Swedberg SH, Brown BG, Sigley R, Wight TN, Gordon D, Nicholls SC (Univ of Washington, Swedish Hosp, Seattle)

Circulation 80:1726–1736, 1989 1–24

The most common cause of failure of Brescia-Cimino arteriovenous fistulas or polytetrafluoroethylene (PTFE) grafts used for chronic hemodialysis is progressive venous stenosis, occurring just downstream of the anastomosis. A total of 116 patients receiving chronic hemodialysis were followed during sequential 5-year periods to define the clinical, immunocytochemical, and light and electron microscopic characteristics of this accelerated venous stenosis.

Venous stenosis, as the cause of failure of the arteriovenous anastomosis, occurred significantly more frequently (45% vs. 16%) and somewhat earlier (16 vs. 22 months) in PTFE grafts than in Brescia-Cimino fistulas. Proximal vein segments were removed from 5 failed PTFE grafts and 2 functioning PTFE grafts. Light microscopic studies showed marked intimal hyperplasia in all failed PTFE grafts, in contrast to the minimal intimal thickening noted on functioning grafts. Immunocytochemical staining showed that the intimal hyperplasia consisted almost exclusively of smooth muscle cells. Extracellular and intracellular lipid, foam cells, and intimal macrophages were absent.

Ultrastructural examination revealed a large proportion of extracellular matrix separating the smooth muscle cells in the neointima. Collagen fibrils and elastin bundles were most abundant deeper in the intima, whereas the matrix was strikingly rich in proteoglycan near the lumen. Consistent signs of luminal and intimal fibrin or hemosiderin accumulation were absent.

The uniform intimal gradients in smooth muscle actin content and extracellular matrix composition suggest that the hyperplastic response is steadily progressive, rather than episodic. That response is stimulated by conditions present near the PTFE-to-vein anastomosis and is apparently not mediated by thrombogenic processes or lipid accumulation. On the basis of the clinical and histologic observations and analysis of the hemodynamic stresses, it is hypothesized that the platelet activation associated with turbulent shear stresses or repeated thrombus formation after needle puncture in the PTFE graft releases platelet-derived growth factor that promotes downstream smooth muscle proliferation. This myointimal proliferative response provides a readily accessible model of fibromuscular dysplasia in humans and may provide clues to the pathogenesis of arteriosclerosis.

▶ The biointimal hyperplastic response is indeed steadily progressive, not episodic, stimulated by activity at the graft-native vessel junction, but what really needs to be known is what will shut the process down once it has been initiated?

Regrowth of Arterial Endothelium: Denudation With Minimal Trauma Leads to Complete Endothelial Cell Regrowth

Lindner V, Reidy MA, Fingerle J (Univ of Washington; Universität Tübingen, Germany)

Lab Invest 61:556–563, 1989 1–25

Complete reendothelialization occurs after small denuding injuries, whereas endothelial cells are incapable of sustaining regrowth after widespread denudation. To elucidate further, endothelial regeneration in the rat carotid artery was investigated using 2 different techniques of denudation. In 1 group of animals the endothelium was removed by balloon catheter denudation and in the other group the endothelium was removed using a loop of nylon filament. In addition, endothelial cell proliferation was correlated with the presence or absence of factors known to influence endothelial cell growth, [e.g., basic fibroblast growth factor (bFGF), β-type transforming growth factor (TGF-β), and fibronectin].

With the filament loop that removed the endothelium without damaging the media, complete endothelial regrowth was achieved by about 10 weeks. In contrast, with balloon catheter denudation, medial cell death occurred and endothelial regrowth was much slower and stopped by about 6 weeks. A large area devoid of epithelium was left. After denudation, large platelet thrombi were seen on the subendothelial surface of vessels denuded with the filament loop, whereas only a monolayer of platelets was evident on the luminal surface of arteries after balloon catheter denudation.

Within the first few weeks after denudation with either technique, the regenerating endothelial cells stained strongly for bFGF, a known endothelial cell mitogen. Whereas the regenerating endothelial cells after filament denudation stained strongly for bFGF at both early and late times, the balloon catheter-denuded vessels did not stain with this antibody at later times when replication of endothelium had stopped. Both groups showed TGF-β in the developing intima and especially on the apical surface of the luminal smooth muscle cells. The surface of these luminal smooth muscle cells also stained with antibody to fibronectin.

Endothelial cell regrowth over the exposed subendothelium of rat carotid arteries depends significantly on the severity of trauma induced by denudation and presence of bFGF. Total regrowth of endothelium can occur over large denuded areas despite the presence of TGF-β and fibronectin on these surfaces.

▶ Sustained endothelial regrowth would be desirable to effect graft coverage, and it may be that endothelial regrowth requires a mitogenic stimulus.

2 New Developments

Transluminal Atherectomy for Occlusive Peripheral Vascular Disease
Graor RA, Whitlow PL (Cleveland Clinic Found)
J Am Coll Cardiol 15:1551–1558, 1990 2–1

The results of percutaneous atherectomy, alone or combined with urokinase for thrombolysis, were assessed in 112 patients who had stenosis or occlusion of the superficial femoral artery. Atherectomies were

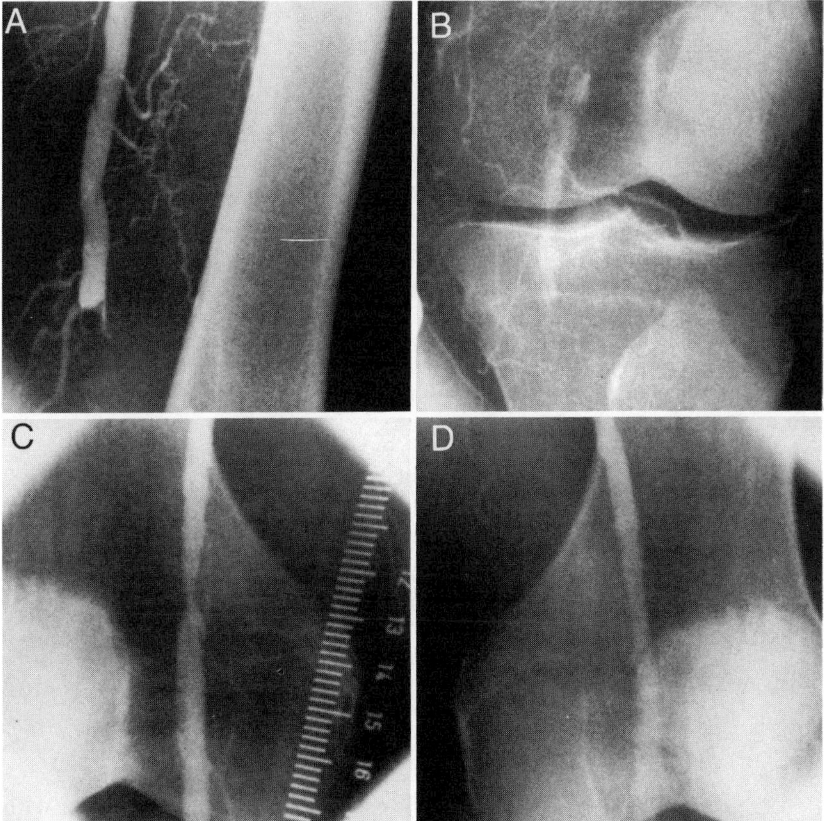

Fig 2–1.—**A**, occlusion of superficial femoral artery at adductor canal documented by angiography. **B**, delayed films demonstrated isolated popliteal artery segment. There was no evidence of a contiguous artery patent from the adductor canal to tibial arteries before infusion of urokinase. After infusion, patency of superficial femoral and popliteral arteries was easily identified, disclosing a short stenotic lesion in the midpopliteal artery (**C**), which was easily treated with a 9F atherectomy device (**D**). This demonstrates conversion of a complex, mainly thrombotic lesion to a simple atherosclerotic lesion. (Courtesy of Graor RA, Whitlow PL: *J Am Coll Cardiol* 15:1551–1558, 1990.)

done in the superficial femoral and popliteal arteries. Sixteen patients received urokinase as an adjunct. The procedure was considered successful if less than 20% stenosis remained after atherectomy. Eighty-four patients had complex lesions exceeding 5 cm in length.

The 30-day patency rate was 93% in patients with complex lesions and 100% in those with simple lesions. After a mean follow-up of 1 year the respective rates were 86% and 93%. Major complications occurred in 7% of patients and included a fatal myocardial infarction. Most complications were associated with hematoma at the entry site of the catheter. Urokinase occasionally converted a complex thrombotic lesion to a simple atherosclerotic lesion (Fig 2–1).

Femoropopliteal atherectomy is an effective procedure that is associated with low rates of morbidity and mortality. It may be a good alternative to conservative management for mildly symptomatic patients. For those with complex symptomatic lesions, atherectomy is more promising than percutaneous transluminal angioplasty and is a reasonable alternative to surgery.

▶ Although vascular surgeons have learned that early results of any procedure are rarely related to long-term acceptance of new techniques, in fact, this study suggests that atherectomy produces better clinical results at 1 year than balloon angioplasty or laser-assisted balloon angioplasty.

Vascular surgeons should not ignore the fact that this article on femorodistal arterial revascularization is published in the *Journal of the American College of Cardiology!*

Percutaneous Peripheral Atherectomy: Angiographic and Clinical Follow-Up of 60 Patients

von Pölnitz A, Nerlich A, Berger H, Höfling B (Ludwig-Maximilians-Univ München, Munich, Germany)

J Am Coll Cardiol 15:682–688, 1990 2–2

Acute reocclusion and the relatively high long-term restenosis rate after an initial successful intervention may limit the percutaneous treatment of vascular disease with balloon angioplasty. New technologies using mechanical or other energy forms that attempt to remove obstructive plaque material are being developed. The long-term clinical and angiographic results were evaluated in patients with symptomatic peripheral vascular disease treated with the Simpson peripheral atherectomy catheter.

The Simpson atherectomy catheter was used to treat 60 patients with 94 lesions comprising 63 stenoses and 31 occlusions of the superficial femoral, popliteal, iliac, and anterior tibial arteries. The immediate angiographic success rate was 90% for occlusions and stenoses, and clinical success was achieved in 82% of the patients. Stenoses were reduced from 83% to 17% acutely and to 31% at 6 months; the

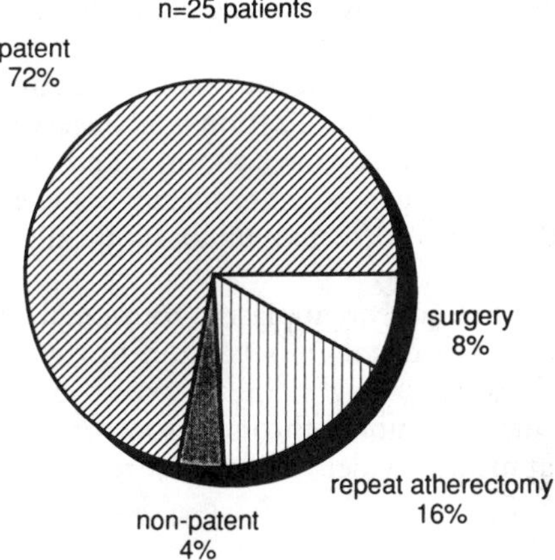

Fig 2–2.—One-year follow-up data in 25 patients after successful atherectomy: clinical patency was achieved in 18, 4 underwent repeated atherectomy, 2 underwent a surgical procedure, and 1 patient with clinical restenosis remained in stable condition without further intervention. (Courtesy of von Pölnitz A, Nerlich A, Berger H, et al: *J Am Coll Cardiol* 15:682–688, 1990.)

occlusions were reduced from 100% to 9% in the short term and to 60% at 6 months. Angiographic restenosis occurred in 24% of the lesions: 23% in concentric and 11% in eccentric lesions and 47% in total occlusions. At 1 year 72% of the patients had clinically patent arteries with maintained Doppler index and walking distance (Fig 2–2). Of 4 patients who had a repeated atherectomy, 3 had a second restenosis.

The use of the Simpson peripheral atherectomy catheter is safe and effective in the treatment of peripheral vascular disease. The procedure seem particularly to benefit patients with eccentric stenoses. It is not limited by the presence of calcification.

▶ Repeated observations have shown atherectomy to be safe and effective in eccentric stenoses, but the fundamental question is whether or not it is durable.

Distal Embolization During Mechanical Thrombolysis: Rotational Thrombectomy Vs Balloon Angioplasty
Titus BG, Auth DC, Ritchie JL (Univ of Washington; VA Med Ctr, Seattle)
Cathet Cardiovasc Diagn 19:279–285, 1990 2–3

The rotational thrombectomy catheter removes fibrin selectively from fresh thrombi and, for this reason, distal embolization may be less frequent than when conventional balloon angioplasty is performed. Distal embolization was estimated in a canine model of thrombotic occlusion. Eleven occluded arterial segments were managed by rotational thrombectomy and 10 others were treated by conventional balloon angioplasty.

The 2 methods were equally effective in recanalizing occluded vessels and reducing stenosis. Distal embolization was observed in all arteries recanalized by rotational thrombectomy and in all but 1 of those treated by balloon angioplasty; the mean weights of emboli were similar in the 2 groups. Residual thrombus, detected angiographically, was less frequent after rotational thrombectomy.

Like conventional balloon angioplasty, rotational thrombectomy frequently is associated with distal embolization of thrombotic debris. The latter procedure, however, may help to avoid embolization of large thrombotic fragments. Rotational thrombectomy also is less often associated with angiographically evident residual thrombus at the site of arterial injury.

▶ Thrombolytic therapy may be improved by the use of rotational atherothrombectomy as described here. Certainly, improved results would be most welcome.

Removal of Intimal Hyperplasia in Vascular Endoprostheses by Atherectomy and Balloon Dilatation

Vorwerk D, Guenther RW (Technical Univ of Aachen, Germany)

AJR 154:617–619, 1990 2–4

A vascular endoprosthesis used as an adjunct to transluminal dilatation may be obstructed by hyperplastic intima. Balloon dilatation has not been as effective as in treating unstented vessels because the stent is not able to expand like a native artery. The Simpson atherectomy catheter was used to treat restenosis within an endovascular stent in 7 patients with reobstruction of a Wallstent implant. A 7F device was used in each case. Patients were followed for 3–12 months.

Hyperplastic intima was easily removed from stents in implant shunts or arteries (Fig 2–3), but residual stenoses at the proximal and distal ends of the stent required subsequent balloon dilatation. In 1 instance the 7F atherectomy device failed to remove all stenosing material from inside the stent. No perforation or embolization followed atherectomy. Heparin treatment accompanied the procedure, and patients with stents also received aspirin. One of 2 patients with restenosis on follow-up underwent repeat atherectomy.

Percutaneous removal of hyperplastic intima from endovascular stents, using the Simpson catheter, is a technically effective means of recanalizing self-expanding stents in peripheral vessels. When stenosis is present at the ends of a stent, adjunctive balloon dilatation may be necessary.

▶ It seems a little incongruous to use an atherectomy device to correct the errors of a stent.

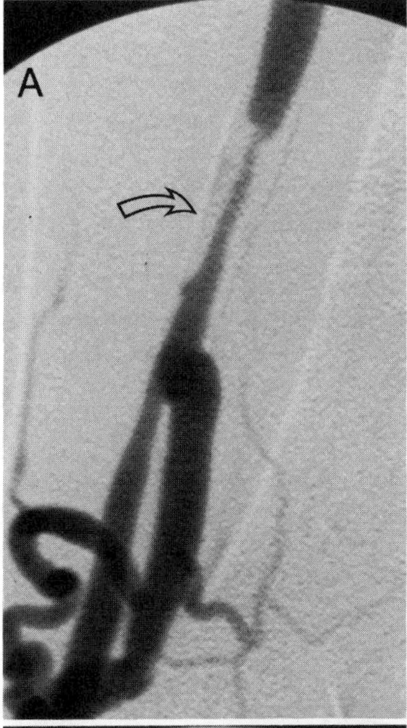

Fig 2–3.—Percutaneous atherectomy inside vascular endoprosthesis. **A,** filiform stenosis *(arrow)* caused by intimal hyperplasia within Wallstent of draining vein of the brachial implant shunt. **B,** Simpson atherectomy catheter within shunt. **C,** after atherectomy and balloon dilatation, fully restored lumen shows smooth cuts and regular wall. (Courtesy of Vorwerk D, Guenther RW: *AJR* 154:617–619, 1990.)

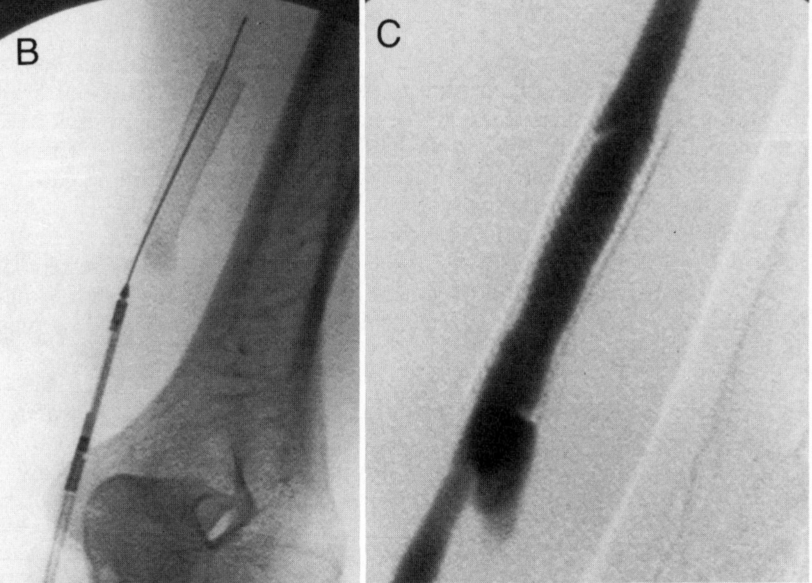

Arterial Stenting

Joffre F, Rousseau H, Puel J (CHU Toulouse Rangueil, Toulouse, France)
J Intervent Radiol 4:155–159, 1989 2–5

A number of techniques have been proposed to improve the results of transluminal angioplasty (PTA), including laser angioplasty and atherectomy procedures that respectively destroy or remove atheroma. An endoprosthesis, however, is expected to restore a near-normal caliber immediately after PTA by preventing medial recoil and smoothing the vascular wall. The endoprosthesis can be considered a true "bypass" that is placed in situ in the vascular wall.

The early failures and rates of restenosis associated with PTA by using a balloon catheter are unrelated to the operator's experience and the materials used. The type of lesion that is dilated is most important. Depending on the site, the long-term patency rate for simple lesions is 80% to 95%. This rate decreases to 35% to 50% when the lesions are complex.

Several different types of prostheses have been studied in animals, including the Nitinol, the self-expandable spiraled and the self-expandable zigzag prostheses. The Palmaz prosthesis involves a stent that can be placed folded onto the balloon of all currently available dilation catheters. Balloon inflation allows the prosthesis to distend to the same diameter as the dilated lesion. The Wallstent prosthesis is a self-expandable device made of 20 metallic spring filaments of 70 μm diameter, which form a tubular wire mesh. It can be stretched longitudinally to a small diameter.

The main reason for using an endoprosthesis seems to be an unsatisfactory post-PTA result. Patients with lesions that are impossible to dilate, immediate recurrence because of a high elastic component, significant intimal lesion with dissection, or residual stenoses of more than 30% with a persisting pressure gradient of more than 20 mm Hg are candidates for the endoprosthesis. In these cases the interventional radiologist may have a clinical failure or an important risk of intermediate term recurrence. The endoprosthesis is justified in such cases to improve the immediate results and long-term prognosis.

Endoprostheses offer many benefits. Therapeutic measures seem to solve the problem of early thrombosis. The major problem is restenosis caused by hyperplasia in the prosthetic area. This technique should not be used in patients in whom anticoagulants are contraindicated or who do not stop smoking.

▶ As indicated, a stent may prevent medial recoil after PTA, but the fundamental problem of myointimal proliferation remains despite the stenting maneuver. Cells, after all, are smaller than interstices of the stent, and arterial injury of whatever kind does produce a myointimal healing response.

Iliac and Femoral Artery Stenoses and Occlusions: Treatment With Intravascular Stents

Günther RW, Vorwerk D, Bohndorf K, Peters I, El-Din A, Messmer B (Aachen Univ of Technology, Germany; Medinvent SA, Lausanne, Switzerland)
Radiology 172:725–730, 1989 2–6

The Wallstent, a flexible, self-expanding metallic intravascular stent, was used to treat 45 patients with atherosclerotic stenosis or occlusion of the iliac or superficial femoral artery. Thirty-seven patients received a stent immediately after inadequate angioplasty, 26 for vascular occlusion. In 7 patients another stenosis developed after angioplasty.

Digital subtraction angiography showed a patent vessel in 40 patients within 2–12 months after stent placement. The mean Doppler ankle/arm index increased from .6 to .9 after stenting and remained at .9 at follow-up. Early thrombotic stent occlusion occurred in 2 cases. Intimal hyperplasia led to late stent stenosis in 3 others and to stent occlusion in 1 patient. Percutaneous recanalization succeeded in 3 patients. Two patients had complications of warfarin therapy.

Stents are especially useful for maintaining patency after angioplasty for iliac or femoral artery occlusions and for the treatment of stenoses caused by eccentric or severely ulcerated plaques. They also can aid the management of complications after angioplasty. Stents should not be used in the popliteal artery or the infrapopliteal segments until the problem of intimal hyperplasia is solved. They should not be placed in arteries with poor peripheral flow because of the risk of early stent thrombosis.

▶ Stents, as a whole, are absolutely ingenious. But, as suggested in this abstract, they should not be accepted in our armamentarium until the problem of intimal hyperplasia is solved.

Percutaneous Implantation of Intravascular Stents Into the Iliac or Femoral Arteries

Guenther RW, Vorwerk D, Bohndorf K, El-Din A, Peters I, Messmer BJ (Rheinisch-Westfälische Technische Hochschule Aachen, Aachen, Germany)
Dtsch Med Wochenschr 114:1517–1523, 1989 2–7

The use of transluminally inserted vascular endoprostheses in the treatment of vascular stenoses and obstructions of the femoral and iliac arteries is gaining acceptance. Data on flexible, self-expanding metallic mesh stent implanted percutaneously in patients in whom angioplasty has been unsuccessful were reviewed.

The study included 59 men and 9 women, aged 40–73 years, who underwent transluminal balloon dilatation of 94 occluded or stenosed iliac or femoral vessel segments, followed by immediate implantation of a flexible, self-expanding mesh stent; 37 patients had arterial occlusions and 31 patients had arterial stenoses. The bridged vessel segments measured 3.5–27 cm in length and 6–12 mm in diameter. Endoprostheses were inserted under fluoroscopic guidance through a 7-F catheter. Three patients had stage IIa atherosclerotic disease, 61 had stage IIb disease, 3 had stage III disease, and 1 had stage IV disease. After the procedure patients were given prophylactic heparin for at least 24 hours, administered at a dose of 1,000 units per hour. Phenprocoumon was used to treat 11 of 28 patients with iliac stents and 13 of 14 patients with femoral stents were treated for at least 6 months with phenprocoumon. All of the other patients were given dipyridamole, 75 mg, and aspirin, 330 mg, daily for maintenance therapy. Doppler ultrasound examinations were performed daily until hospital discharge. Follow-up Doppler examinations were scheduled at 4 weeks, and 6 and 12 months after discharge. Follow-up ranged from 1 to 17 months (average, 6.9 months).

All patients achieved good initial perfusion of the treated vessels. The Doppler ultrasound index increased by an average of .33 to a mean of .9. There were 3 early stent occlusions. Large hematomas at the puncture site developed in 3 other patients, 1 of whom required surgical evacuation of the hematoma. Transient peripheral emboli developed in 2 patients. Stent-induced intimal hyperplasia at the distal end of the prostheses developed in 5 patients 4–10 months after stent placement; 4 were treated successfully by percutaneous techniques.

Percutaneous stent placement is particularly suited to the treatment of arterial stenoses and occlusions that extend over too long a distance to be amenable to angioplasty. The technique is most useful in the treatment of atherosclerotic disease of the iliac artery.

▶ One would predict that stents, if useful, would be best tolerated in the iliac circulation.

Seeding of Intravascular Stents With Genetically Engineered Endothelial Cells

Dichek DA, Neville RF, Zwiebel JA, Freeman SM, Leon MB, Anderson WF (Natl Insts of Health, Bethesda, Md)

Circulation 80:1347–1353, 1989 2–8

Local thrombosis and restenosis caused by intimal proliferation may limit the use of intravascular stents. Stents were seeded with genetically engineered endothelial cells in vitro in an attempt to solve these problems.

Retroviral-mediated gene transfer was used to insert the gene for bacterial β-galactosidase or human tissue-type plasminogen activator (t-PA) in cultured endothelial cells from sheep. The cells were then seeded onto stainless steel stents. They were grown until the stents were covered. Intracellular β-galactosidase expression and high-level t-PA secretion were demonstrated before and after the cells were seeded; 8 stents were then expanded by in vitro balloon inflation. The seeded endothelial layer was observed before and after expansion. Most endothelial cells remained on the stents after the balloon was inflated.

Intravascular stents can be coated with a layer of genetically engineered endothelial cells that can be specifically labeled or made to secrete high levels of a therapeutic protein. After expansion of the stent in vitro, much of the cell layer remains. In vivo implantation of coated stents may permit the introduction of genetically engineered endothelial cells directly into the vascular wall and improvement of stent function through localized delivery of anticoagulant, thrombolytic, or antiproliferative molecules.

▶ This ingenious study sets the stage for local delivery of agents to inhibit myointimal proliferation by using the endothelial cell as a carrier.

Arterial Wall Characteristics Determined by Intravascular Ultrasound Imaging: An In Vitro Study

Gussenhoven EJ, Essed CE, Lancée CT, Mastik F, Frietman P, Van Egmond FC, Reiber J, Bosch H, Van Urk H, Roelandt J, Bom N (Univ Hosp, Dijkzigt; Erasmus Univ, Rotterdam)

J Am Coll Cardiol 14:947–952, 1989 2–9

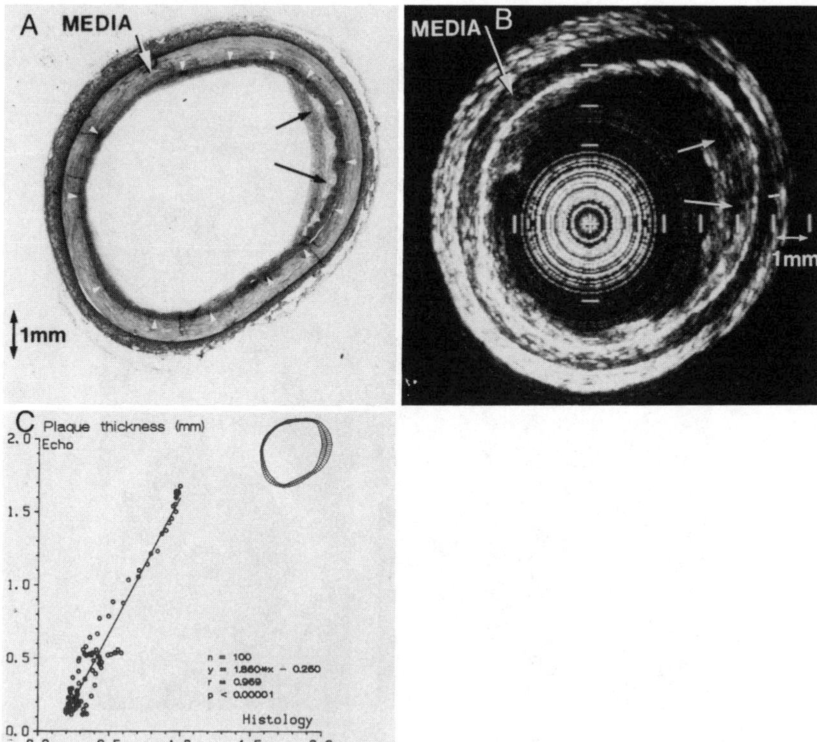

Fig 2–4.—Histologic section (**A**) obtained from a typical iliac artery and corresponding echographic cross-section (**B**). Media appears hypoechoic. An atherosclerotic lesion of fibromuscular nature is recognized with ultrasound as relatively soft echoes attached to the bright echo surface of the intima *(arrows in A)*. Lipid deposits in the histologic section correspond to hypoechoic zone *(arrows)* on the ultrasound study. Plaque thickness (**C**) measured in a clockwise orientation from the histologic section and the ultrasound section are shown in the diagram *(inset)*. Measurements obtained with the 2 techniques are closely related. Verhoeff van Gieson stain; original magnification, ×8, reduced by 20%. (Courtesy of Gussenhoven EJ, Essed CE, Lancée CT, et al: *J Am Coll Cardiol* 14:947–952, 1989.)

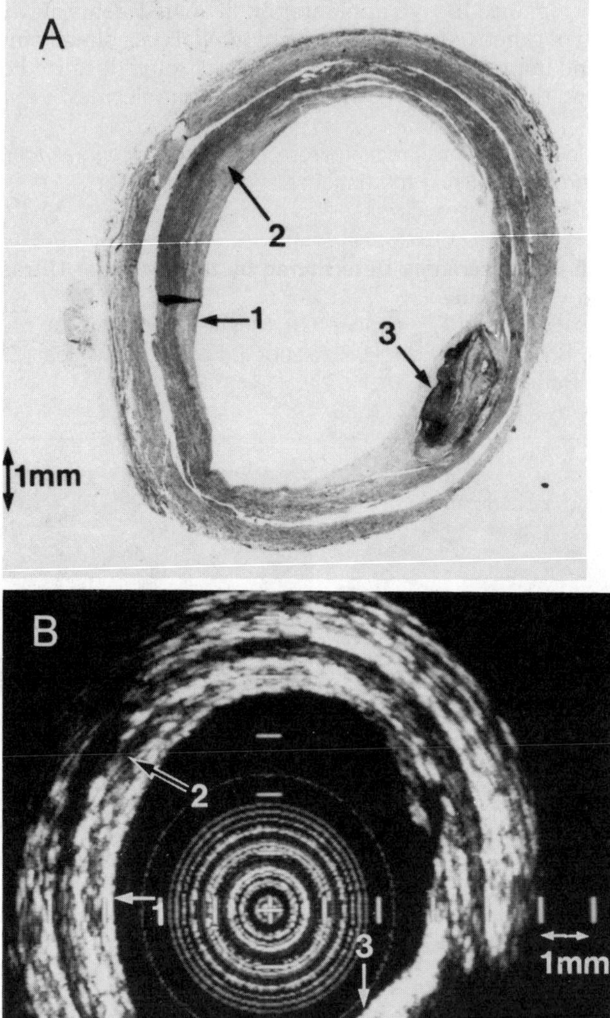

Fig 2–5.—Histologic section (A) and corresponding echographic cross-section (B) obtained from an iliac artery with an advanced atherosclerotic lesion extending along the entire circumference of the vessel. The lesion, predominantly of a fibromuscular nature, was characterized by soft echoes attached to the intimal surface. Microscopically, the boundaries of this plaque presented with dense organized fibrous tissue. Echographically, the structure appears with relative bright echoes *(arrow 1)*. Microscopically, the lipid deposits on the histologic section at the 11 o'clock position correspond to the hypoechoic zone on the ultrasound study *(arrow 2)*. At the 4 o'clock position, a distinct atherosclerotic lesion is characterized by bright echoes *(arrow 3)*. Because of attentuation and reflection on ultrasound caused by calcification in this lesion, no echoes were derived from the intima, media, or adventitia. Hematoxylin-eosin stain; original magnification, ×8. (Courtesy of Gussenhoven EJ, Essed CE, Lancée CT, et al: *J Am Coll Cardiol* 14:947–952, 1989.)

The use of an intravascular 40-MHz ultrasound imaging device in evaluating the arterial wall configuration was assessed in an in vitro study of 11 autopsy specimens of human common carotid and iliac arteries. The cross-sectional ultrasonic images of the arteries were compared with corresponding histologic sections. The system consisted of a single element transducer rotated with a motor mounted on an 8F catheter tip.

Two types of arteries were defined histologically—a muscular artery and an elastic airway. On ultrasound examination, muscular arteries had a hypoechoic tunica media, which on histologic examination was composed of smooth muscle cells (Fig 2–4). The internal and external elastic laminae were clearly defined as bright echoes. In contrast, the media of an elastic artery densely packed with elastin fibers was as hypoechoic as the intima and the adventitia. Fibromuscular plaques, corresponding to soft echoes attached to the intima on ultrasound, were evident in 9 arteries. Of these, 5 had within the plaque a hypoechoic zone that corresponded with the lipid deposits on histologic section (Fig 2–5). The location and thickness of the atherosclerotic plaque measured from the histologic sections correlated well with the data derived from the corresponding ultrasound images.

Intravascular ultrasound imaging can provide cross-sectional images of the arterial wall, including accurate distinction between types of arteries and detection of arterial wall disease. Clinically, this intravascular ultrasound imaging technique has potential application in determining the effects of percutaneous catheter balloon dilation or the suitability of angioplasty.

▶ Just as angioscopy aids the vascular surgeon in the operating room, the intravascular ultrasound image may aid the interventional physician in monitoring the results of his therapy outside the operating room.

Experimental Ultrasonic Angioplasty: Disruption of Atherosclerotic Plaques and Thrombi In Vitro and Arterial Recanalization In Vivo

Rosenschein U, Bernstein JJ, DiSegni E, Kaplinsky E, Bernheim J, Rozenzsajn LA (Meir Gen Hosp, Tel Aviv, Israel; Tel-Aviv Univ; Vasac Ltd, Tel Aviv; Bar-Ilan Univ, Ramat-Gan, Israel)

J Am Coll Cardiol 15:711–717, 1990 2–10

High-energy 20-kHz ultrasound is a possible alternative energy source in angioplasty. Presumably, ultrasound can disrupt plaques and thrombi with a large margin of safety before damaging the arterial wall. An experimental device that guides high-energy ultrasound into the arterial system via a flexible wire attached to a piezoelectric element was examined in 2 bioassay systems: an in vitro system for disrupting atherosclerotic plaque and thrombi, and an in vivo system for recanalizing occluded canine femoral arteries.

In vitro sonication effectively reduced the size of plaques, and disruption took place without damage to the media or adventitia. The plaque debris consisted chiefly of cholesterol monohydrate crystals. Solid thrombus was reduced rapidly in weight by sonication in vitro. In vivo, sonication led to recanalization of all arteries and decreased obstruction from 93% to 18% on average. The treated vessels did not exhibit thermal injury, blast damage, or perforation.

These findings indicate the potential for using ultrasonic angioplasty to disrupt atherosclerotic plaque and thrombus selectively while causing only minimal damage to the arterial wall. Neither precise coaxiality of the ultrasound wire nor power application time was a critical factor.

▶ Siegel and his group in the United States have demonstrated the feasibility of ultrasound as an ablation technique to recanalize occluded arteries in humans (1). In high-intensity ultrasound the effects of cavitation energy are of concern. Further work is needed to establish the role of interventional ultrasound in endovascular technique.

Reference

1. Siegel RJ, et al: *J Am Coll Cardiol* 15:345, 1990.

Percutaneous Ultrasonic Angioplasty: Initial Clinical Experience

Siegel RJ, Cumberland DC, Myler RK, DonMichael TA (Cedars-Sinai Med Ctr, Los Angeles; Northern Gen Hosp, Sheffield, England; San Francisco Heart Inst, Daly City, Calif)

Lancet 2:772–774, 1989 2–11

Previous in vitro and canine in vivo studies have demonstrated the effectiveness of ultrasound energy in treating atherosclerotic arterial occlusions. Percutaneous catheter-delivered ultrasound energy for arterial recanalization was applied in 8 patients with peripheral vascular disease. Four had high-grade stenoses and 4 had total occlusion in a femoral or popliteal artery.

A prototype ultrasound probe was ensheathed in a 7F catheter and advanced to the occlusions under angiographic guidance. The probe had a frequency of 20 kHz and a power output of 20–35 W/cm^2. An angiogram was obtained after the occlusion was crossed and again after the arterial segment was dilated by balloon angioplasty (Fig 2–6).

Three of 4 total occlusions were completely recanalized by the ultrasound probe. In the 4 arterial stenoses residual diameter fell from 77 (14%) to 37 (21%). The final mean residual stenosis in the 7 patients who subsequently underwent balloon angioplasty was 20%. Pedal pulse was restored distal to the arterial lesions. No patient had evidence of arterial emboli, perforation, dissection, or vasospasm.

From this first report, percutaneous ultrasound angioplasty appears to be a safe and effective procedure. The duration of the applied ultrasound energy and the size of the probe tip govern the size of the lumen after

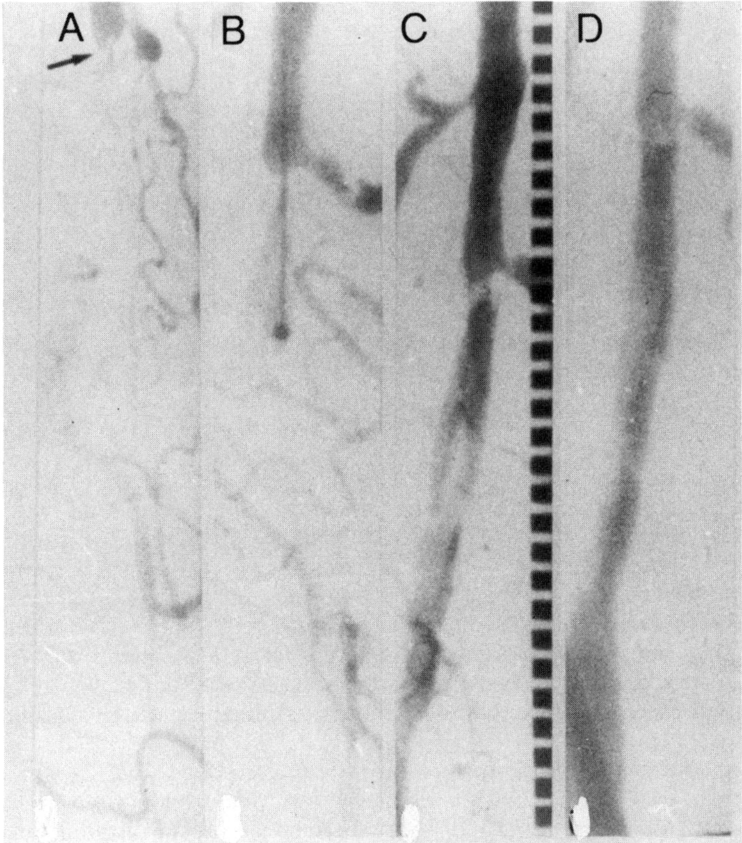

Fig 2–6.—Angiograms of man aged 73 years at ultrasound angioplasty. **A,** total occlusion of superficial femoral artery; **B,** ball-tipped ultrasound probe initiating arterial recanalization; **C,** probe traversed lesion, producing arterial lumen with minor filling defects, suggesting residual thrombus; and **D,** definitive lumen produced after balloon angioplasty. (Courtesy of Siegel RJ, Cumberland DC, Myler RK, et al: *Lancet* 2:772–774, 1989.)

treatment. The effects of the probe appear to be primarily mechanical. Some ultrasonic effects may also result from the generation of bubbles in tissues, fluids, and cells.

▶ It is remarkable to see how quickly experimental observations are taken to clinical utility.

Application of a New Phased-Array Ultrasound Imaging Catheter in the Assessment of Vascular Dimensions: In Vivo Comparison to Cineangiography

Nissen SE, Grines CL, Gurley JC, Sublett K, Haynie D, Diaz C, Booth DC, DeMaria AN (Univ of Kentucky; VA Med Ctr, Lexington)

Circulation 81:660–666, 1990 2–12

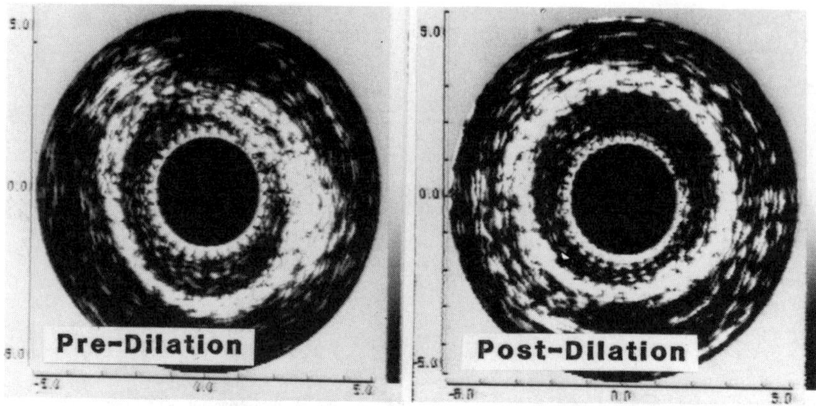

Fig 2–7.—Representative intravascular ultrasound of a vascular site before and after balloon angioplasty. (Courtesy of Nissen SE, Grines CL, Gurley JC, et al: *Circulation* 81:660–666, 1990.)

Although tomographic imaging using ultrasound techniques has advanced the evaluation of vascular anatomy, it remains difficult to visualize small vessels within the thorax and abdomen. Technical developments have permitted fabrication of a small (1.83 mm), phased-array, intravascular ultrasonic imaging catheter capable of continuous real-time, cross-sectional imaging of blood vessels. Diameter and cross-sectional area measurements of peripheral vessels obtained by an ultrasound catheter were compared with those obtained by direct cineangiography.

Experiments were performed in 8 mongrel dogs and 2 minipigs. Stenoses were created with a tissue ligature or by balloon dilation. At the vascular sites subjected to balloon dilation, ultrasound images were acquired both before and after balloon inflation (Fig 2–7). The ultrasound device used was a 32-element array, 5.5F (1.83 mm) intravascular ultrasound catheter system. The catheter incorporates a central lumen that accommodates a .014-in. steerable angioplasty guidewire to facilitate safe positioning. The mean value for measurements of vessel diameter was 5.6 mm by cineangiography and 5.7 mm by intravascular ultrasound. The mean cross-sectional area by angiography was 28.8 mm^2 and by ultrasound, 29.6 mm^2. The percent diameter reduction produced by the stenoses averaged 48.4% by cineangiography and 40.1% by ultrasound.

Images were obtained successfully in all animals with the ultrasound catheter. Catheter orientation in the vessel determined image quality; the best images were those obtained with the catheter located centrally in the vessel and positioned orthogonally with reference to the vessel long axis. Intravascular ultrasound is a promising technique that yields accurate and reproducible results.

▶ A variety of improvements in intravascular ultrasound technology are predictable. Therefore, it is imperative to know the differences between phased ray and 360-degree rotational devices. These are going to be used by us to guide minimally invasive therapy.

Percutaneous Intravascular US as Adjunct to Catheter-Based Interventions: Preliminary Experience in Patients With Peripheral Vascular Disease

Isner JM, Rosenfield K, Losordo DW, Kelly S, Palefski P, Langevin RE, Razvi S, Pastore JO, Kosowsky BD (St Elizabeth's Hosp, Boston)

Radiology 175:61–70, 1990 2–13

High-resolution images of the vessel wall and lumen can be obtained by introducing catheter-based ultrasound transducers into the vascular system. To determine the potential advantages and current liabilities of percutaneous intravascular ultrasound as an adjunct to transluminal vascular recanalization, 17 patients undergoing percutaneous transluminal angioplasty (PTA) were studied.

Of the patients, 10 had PTA alone, 2 had PTA with implantation of an endovascular stent, 2 had atherectomy alone, and 3 had laser angioplasty with PTA and/or atherectomy. A 6.6F braided, polyethylene catheter enclosing a rotary drive shaft with a single-element, 20 MHz transducer at the distal tip was used. The arteries that were treated and examined included the common iliac, the external iliac, the superficial femoral, and a vein graft-arterial anastomosis.

Ultrasonography consistently demonstrated the normal organization of the arterial wall into 3 layers with no or minimal reduction in luminal patency (Fig 2–8). Plaque cracks were clearly delineated with intravascular ultrasound in all 14 patients in whom PTA was used alone or as an adjunct, and dissections were noted in 11 (78%). Plaque-arterial wall disruption was less marked in arteries treated with mechanical atherectomy. The results of laser angioplasty depended on the adjunctive treatment used. Serial intravascular ultrasound documented effacement of PTA-induced plaque cracks and/or dissections after stent implantation. It also aided in the quantitative evaluation of luminal cross-sectional areas after the procedures.

These findings demonstrate the potential utility of intravascular ultrasound as an adjunct to conventional angiography in patients undergoing percutaneous revascularization. Intravascular ultrasound, however, also has some important limitations. Available devices are unable to discriminate boundaries between the 3 layers of the arterial wall at sites of severe narrowing by atherosclerotic plaque; also, the design of these devices allows only side viewing. The current library of images is sufficiently limited that the relationship of any given intravascular ultrasonic finding to long-term outcome of a given intervention is unknown.

▶ As intravascular ultrasound moves from the laboratory to the clinic, limitations of the technique become apparent. Certainly, exquisite images can be obtained, and it is the detail within these images that suggests that atherectomy

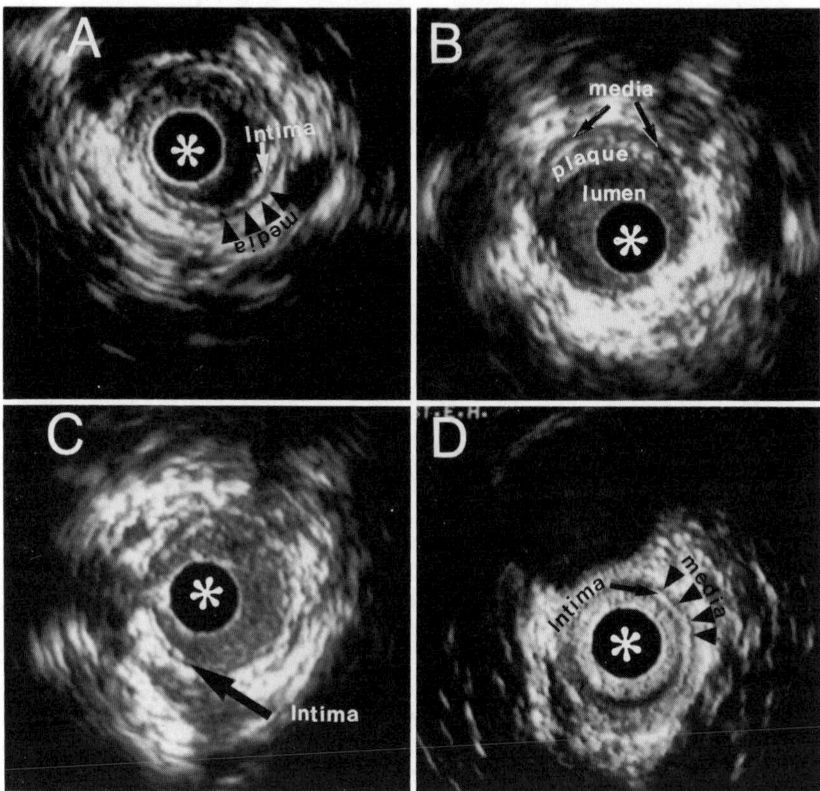

Fig 2–8.—Variable persistence of 3-layered appearance of arterial wall with varying degrees of atherosclerotic involvement. The intravascular ultrasound probe is indicated by an *asterisk*. **A,** 3-layered appearance is preserved in nearly circumferential manner at a site of near-normal luminal caliber. Intima is seen as the innermost echo-intense line; the media is represented by an anechoic ring immediately peripheral to intima, and the adventitia is represented by an echogenic ring encircling media. **B,** quarter moon of atherosclerotic plaque is cleanly demarcated from underlying, well-preserved media. **C,** the 3-layered appearance of arterial wall is focally preserved at site of moderate atherosclerotic narrowing. **D,** media can be appreciated only along eccentric arc of artery severely narrowed by atherosclerotic plaque. Relatively thick, echogenic layers circumferential to US catheter is artifactual "ring-down" resulting from the acoustic pathway between the rotating transducer element and fixed mirror. (Courtesy of Isner JM, Rosenfield K, Losordo DW, et al: *Radiology* 175:61–70, 1990.)

produces less visible arterial trauma than PTA. Whether or not this is important to the ultimate myointimal hyperplastic response remains to be determined.

Intravascular High Frequency Two-Dimensional Ultrasound Detection of Arterial Dissection and Intimal Flaps

Pandian NG, Kreis A, Brockway B, Sacharoff A, Caro R (Tufts Univ; New England Med Ctr Hosps, Boston)
Am J Cardiol 65:1278–1280, 1990 2–14

The anatomy of arterial lesions is important prognostically and therapeutically. There is a need for more detailed morphological information

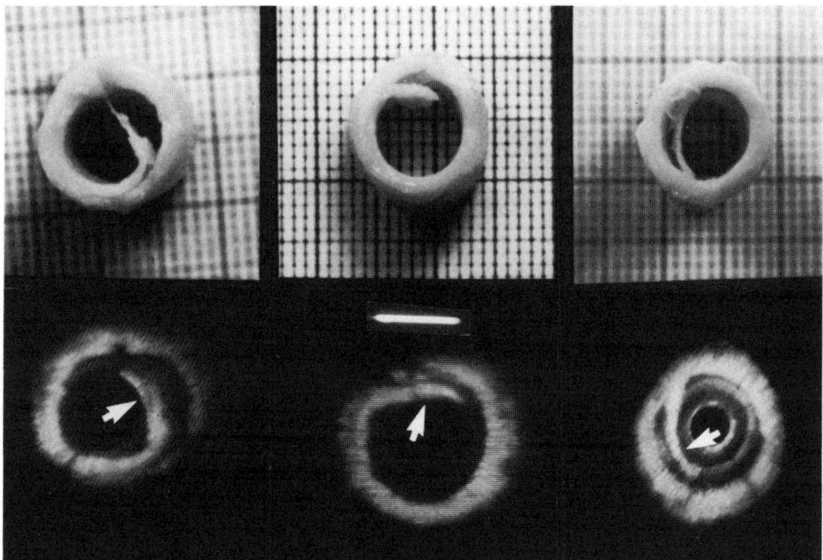

Fig 2–9.—In vitro intravascular ultrasound images and anatomical photographs of 3 arterial segments. The *white line* seen in the ultrasound image is a 5-mm calibration mark. A linear echo protruding into the lumen is the flap *(arrows)*. (Courtesy of Pandian NG, Kreis A, Brockway B, et al: *Am J Cardiol* 65:1278–1280, 1990.)

on arterial anatomy than can be derived from contrast angiography. Whether intravascular ultrasound imaging is of value in detecting arterial dissection and delineation of flaps from the arterial wall was assessed in experimental dissection and in raised intimal flaps in 15 normal arterial segments from dogs and rabbits.

Intravascular ultrasound yielded high-resolution, 2-dimensional images of all arteries. The site of dissection and the presence of the intimal flap were identified correctly in all segments. There was a linear echo separating from the vessel wall and protruding into the lumen in the postdissection image of all vessels (Fig 2–9). The shape of the intimal flap in the ultrasound images was comparable to that of the anatomical photographs in all arterial segments, except for 1 in which introduction of the ultrasound catheter displaced the flap. The flap length measured from ultrasound images highly correlated with anatomical data. In vivo studies also yielded promising results.

Intravascular high-frequency ultrasound can detect arterial dissection and intimal flaps in both in vitro and in vivo settings. This ability enhances the potential of intravascular imaging to provide detailed data on anomalies of the arterial wall.

▶ Now that intravascular ultrasound can detect intimal flaps and dissection, it is clear that therapeutic decisions regarding stenting or other manipulations are going to be monitored by such observations.

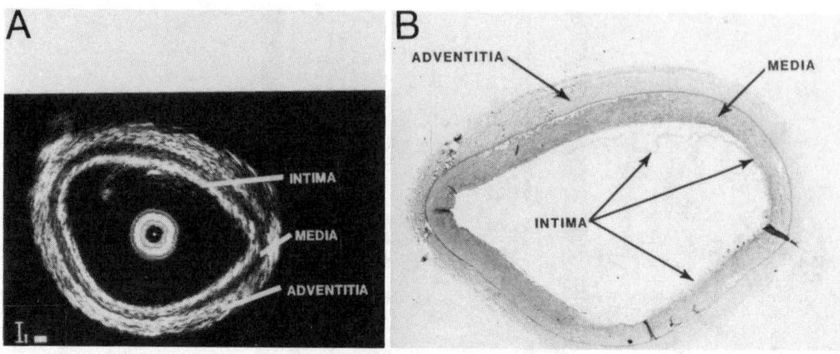

Fig 2–10.—**A,** intravascular ultrasound image of normal human carotid artery showing characteristic 3-layer appearance. Muscular medial layer of artery is relatively echo-lucent and provides a reference point in the arterial cross-section separating intima from adventitia. Intima is seen extending from the lumen-tissue interface to echo-lucent media. Adventitita consists of all echoes originating peripherally to media. **B,** histologic section corresponding to ultrasound image showing thin intima *(open arrows)*, which is partially removed from media. Dense echoes on ultrasound image overestimate intimal thickness. Media *(filled arrows)* appears thicker on histologic section than on ultrasound image. (Courtesy of Mallery JA, Tobis JM, Griffith J, et al: *Am Heart J* 119:1392–1400, 1990.)

Assessment of Normal and Atherosclerotic Arterial Wall Thickness With an Intravascular Ultrasound Imaging Catheter

Mallery JA, Tobis JM, Griffith J, Gessert J, McRae M, Moussabeck O, Bessen M, Moriuchi M, Henry WL (Univ of California, Irvine; VA Hosp, Long Beach; Intertherapy Inc, Orange, Calif)

Am Heart J 119:1392–1400, 1990 2–15

Arterial wall thickness may be estimated by placing a miniaturized ultrasound transducer on the end of a catheter. A prototype ultrasound imaging catheter was assessed by examining 59 segments of 14 human arteries. The 20-MHz transducer was oriented so that the beam was parallel to the long axis of the catheter. The catheter had a diameter of 1.2 mm and was mounted in a precision positioning device.

The muscular media was seen in all specimens as a zone of relative echolucency (Fig 2–10). Eccentric intimal plaque (Fig 2–11) and segmental calcification were seen in diseased arteries. Intimal thickness, as measured by ultrasound, correlated closely with histologic measurements.

Intra-arterial ultrasound imaging is a feasible means of measuring wall thickness, thereby providing an idea of the extent of atheromatous involvement. This method could prove helpful in determining the severity of coronary, carotid, and peripheral arterial disease.

▶ Intravascular ultrasound allows cross-sectional examination in an artery. The technique can see beyond the surface. Media not visualized by angioscopy can now be examined by this technique.

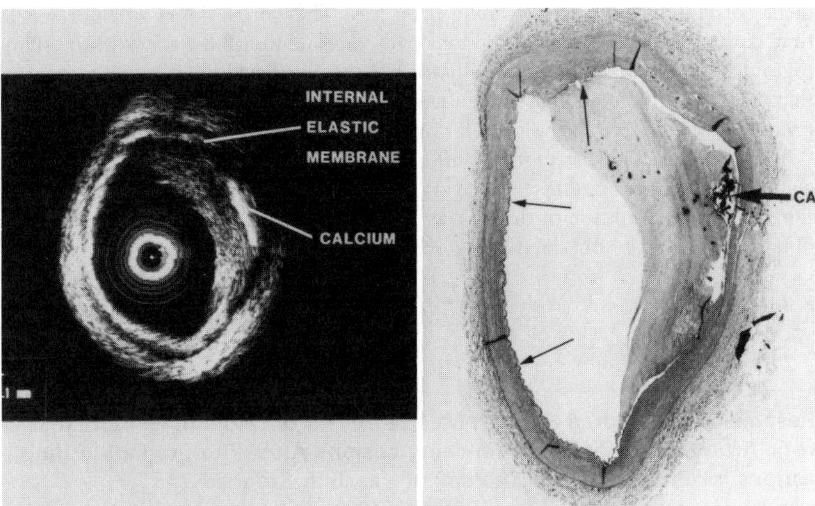

Fig 2–11.—Ultrasound image showing diseased human carotid artery. Eccentric intimal plaque contains small region of calcification at its base, which causes shadowing *(open arrow)*. Echo-lucent media is seen circumferentially. Echogenic line believed to arise from internal elastic lamina is seen extending behind plaque *(filled arrows)*. (Courtesy of Mallery JA, Tobis JM, Griffith J, et al: *Am Heart J* 119:1392–1400, 1990.)

Fluorescein Angiography and Distal Arterial Pressure in Patients With Arterial Disease of the Legs

Wallin L, Lund F, Westling H (Univ Hosp, Lund, Sweden)

Clin Physiol 9:467–480, 1989 2–16

Measurement of arterial pressures in the ankle and the big toe is commonly used to assess blood circulation in the legs. Dynamic fluorescein angiography (FA) has been used to evaluate the circulation in many parts of the body, including the feet of patients with arterial disease. Reportedly, FA is at least as accurate as ankle pressure for predicting the healing of foot ulcers or assessing the need for amputation. To assess the relationship between arterial ankle pressure values and various FA values, FA was performed in 119 patients, most of whom had advanced arterial disease of the legs.

Technique.—Before the FA examination patients were given 30 mL of alcohol solution to insure maximum cutaneous vasodilatation. After rapid injection of fluorescein dye into a cubital vein, sequential photographs of the foot soles were taken at the big toe, foot pad, and heel. Fluorescence optical densities were plotted against the times of fluorescence appearance. The initial slope was defined as the rate of density increase during the first 10 seconds after appearance. The relationship between the different FA variables and arterial ankle and big toe pressures was analyzed.

Fluorescence appearance times correlated inversely with arterial ankle pressures. The initial slopes of the fluorescence-time curves at all 3 sites of measurement correlated with arterial ankle pressures. The initial slopes of fluoresence-time curves of the big toe and the foot pad correlated with big toe pressure. Photographs that were inspected visually for fluoresence distribution patterns showed that 11 foot soles had markedly uneven distribution patterns of fluorescence, probably attributable to the vascular anatomy of the foot.

The differences in distribution patterns will be addressed in future studies for clinical significance. Fluorescein angiography is a useful technique for evaluating the circulatory condition of the foot, either when neither ankle nor toe pressure is obtainable, or when obtained ankle pressure values appear to be falsely high.

▶ Although it seems unlikely that this technique will ever be useful, one never knows.

Responses of Cultured Smooth Muscle Cells From Human Nonatherosclerotic Arteries and Primary Stenosing Lesions After Photoradiation: Implications for Photodynamic Therapy of Vascular Stenoses

Dartsch PC, Ischinger T, Betz E (Univ of Tübingen, Germany; Kliniküm Bogenhaüsen, Munich, Germany)

J Am Coll Cardiol 15:1545–1550, 1990 2–17

Hematoporphyrin derivative and its purified products, dihematoporphyrinester and ether (DHE), are photosensitizers used mainly to localize tumors through laser-induced fluoresence. Hematoporphyrin derivative also accumulates in atherosclerotic plaque, and the possibility of photodynamic therapy has been demonstrated in rabbits and swine.

The effects of ultraviolet radiation of DHE-labeled cell cultures were examined by using cultured smooth muscle cells obtained from both nonatherosclerotic human arteries and primary stenosing lesions. Both the carotid and superficial femoral arteries were sampled. Cells labeled for 24 hours were exposed to ultraviolet light at 365 nm at energy densities of 30–1,200 mJ/cm^2.

Eighty percent of smooth muscle cells from nonatherosclerotic vessels remained viable and adherent 24 hours after photoradiation, compared with 20% of cells from atherosclerotic plaques. Microtubules were depolymerized by radiation exposure, and actin filaments were disrupted. Vimentin filaments were unchanged.

Photoradiation of atherosclerotic plaque by using DHE is a possible approach to treating vascular stenoses because smooth muscle cell migration and proliferation from the media into the subendothelial space are key early events in atherogenesis. Photodynamic therapy could be helpful in treating new restenoses and also as an adjunctive measure for lowering the rate of restenosis after recanalization of advanced and frequently calcified primary stenoses.

▶ This form of study represents a new approach to recurrent stenosis caused by intima hyperplasia. The use of photoactive substances to inhibit smooth muscle cells and fibroblasts has been reported. The therapeutic potential of this technique includes the prevention of keloid formation or ablation of atheroma (1). The selective uptake of a photosensitive substance by cells appears to be the key element in avoiding wall injury.

Reference

1. Neave V, et al: *Neurosurgery* 23:307, 1988.

3 Nonsurgical Treatment

Lumbar Sympathectomy in the Elderly Subject: Surgery or Phenolization? A Prospective Study of Early Results

Becquemin J-P, Kassab M, Bellouard A, Brugière P, Mellière D (Hôpital Henri-Mondor, Créteil, France)

J Mal Vasc 14:327–333, 1989 3–1

There is much controversy over the use of lumbar sympathectomy in the treatment of severe ischemia or arterial occlusion of the lower extremities. Improvement is usually only marginal, and the benefits do not last much longer than approximately 12 weeks. In France, lumbar sympathectomy is reserved for patients with severe arterial ischemia or occlusion who are not candidates for bypass surgery. Phenol sympathectomy under CT guidance is less invasive than surgical sympathectomy and would be the preferred treatment if mortality and morbidity were comparable with those obtained with surgical sympathectomy. The results of surgical lumbar sympathectomy and percutaneous phenol sympathetic ablation were compared in patients with advanced vascular disease of the lower extremities.

During a 6-year period, 446 lumbar sympathectomies were performed in 428 patients, 227 of whom were younger than 70 years of age. Surgical sympathectomy via the retroperitoneal route, performed with the use of general anesthesia, involved excision of the second, third, fourth, and fifth lumbar ganglions. In patients younger than 70 years of age who required bilateral procedures, at least 1 second ganglion was preserved. The duration of hospitalization ranged from 10 to 15 days. Phenol sympatholysis under CT guidance involved injection of a 6.7% phenol solution at L3 and L4. This procedure required no anesthesia and only 24–48 hours of hospitalization. Bilateral procedures were done 8 days apart.

Mortality rates were 4.7% for surgery and 2.5% for chemolysis in patients younger than 70 years of age, and 12% for surgery and 10% for chemolysis in patients older than 70 years. The differences in mortality between the 2 techniques were not significant, but the differences between the 2 age groups were significant. Amputation rates were also similar with either technique. Complication rates were 7.4% for surgery but none for phenol ablation in patients younger than 70, and 10% for surgery and 8% for phenol in patients older than 70. Complication rates were independent of disease stage. Lumbar sympathectomy failed in 87 patients, and they subsequently underwent revascularization procedures. The overall early failure rate of lumbar sympathectomy was 40%.

Chemical lumbar sympathectomy and surgical sympathectomy are equally effective, but phenol sympathectomy requires much shorter hospitalization and results in lower mortality. However, when severe ischemia and femoropopliteal obstruction are present, surgical bypass remains the treatment of choice, as the results in terms of limb salvage are superior to those with lumbar sympathectomy.

▶ The question is asked: Lumbar sympathectomy in the elderly subject—surgery or recanalization?

The answer is: Neither! The detailed results of this study show why. Look at the mortality and morbidity figures.

Isn't it amazing that 428 patients could be found who were not candidates for bypass surgery?

Percutaneous Video Angioscopy in Peripheral Vascular Disease

Rees MR, Gehani AA, Ashley S, Davies GA (Killingbeck Regional Cardiothoracic Ctr, Leeds, England)

Clin Radiol 40:347–351, 1989 3–2

Angioscopy has been suggested as a complementary technique to angiography in the assessment and treatment of peripheral vascular disease. Angioscopic findings and angiographic results were compared in the same patients.

Angioscopy was used to study 2 iliac arteries and 10 superficial femoral arteries in 10 patients before intervention. Eleven arteries underwent angioplasty, with 1 failure. Arteries in which angioplasty was successful underwent repeat angioscopy. All patients also underwent angiography.

In 10 arteries, clear blood-free views of the whole length of the artery were obtained. Two arteries were partially visualized. In all arteries, clinically significant findings were detected by angioscopy that were not seen on angiography. These included thrombus in the artery and vascular sheath, intimal flaps, and fractured atheroma. Angioscopic findings helped to evaluate the effects of angioplasty in various types of occlusions.

Percutaneous angioscopy is a procedure complementary to angiography that may yield additional diagnostic information. After angioplasty, angioscopy is also useful in evaluating results.

▶ It seems unlikely that percutaneous angioscopy in its present incarnation will achieve any real utility.

The Use of Carbon Dioxide Gas to Displace Flowing Blood During Angioscopy

Silverman SH, Mladinich CJ, Hawkins IF Jr, Abela GS, Seeger JM (Univ of Florida; VA Med Ctr, Gainesville)

J Vasc Surg 10:313–317, 1989 3–3

Carbon dioxide (CO_2) gas is a safe and effective arterial contrast agent that images arteries by displacing blood. The use of CO_2 gas to displace blood during angioscopy may improve intraoperative angioscopy and allow percutaneous angioscopy.

Forty-six angioscopic studies were carried out in the femoral arteries of 4 dogs without inflow occlusion. The ability of CO_2 gas to clear flowing blood was compared with that of a high-pressure infusion of saline. Either a 1.4-mm or a 2-mm (outer diameter) angioscope was used.

Carbon dioxide gas successfully displaced flowing blood in 20 of 25 attempts (80%), but only 3 of 21 attempts with infusion of saline (14%) were effective. The image remained clear for 9 seconds on average after infusion of CO_2 gas ceased, but with infusion of saline, the image remained clear only as long as the infusion continued. Motion picture images had better contrast and depth of field when CO_2 gas was used.

Infusion of CO_2 gas at angioscopy can clear the field of flowing blood and precludes the need for inflow occlusion. This technique should permit percutaneous angioscopy.

▶ Carbon dioxide has been used to displace blood in performance of arteriography. Therefore, with the new delivery systems, it is clear that there may be real utility of this agent in clearing arteries for angioscopy. Perhaps percutaneous angioscopy will be enhanced by this technique. At present, it seems that intravascular ultrasound is much more efficient in monitoring minimally interventional therapy.

Percutaneous Aspiration of a Thromboembolus

Dorros G, Jamnadas P, Lewin RF, Sachdev N (St Luke's Med Ctr, Milwaukee)

Cathet Cardiovasc Diagn 17:202–206, 1989 3–4

Thromboembolization is a complication that occurs in 1% to 5% of patients who undergo percutaneous catheter treatment for peripheral vascular disease. Thrombotic debris, which appears radiographically as radiolucent intraluminal densities, impedes flow and endangers the limb. Percutaneous aspiration of a thromboembolus (PAT) was successfully performed in 12 of 13 patients.

Before PAT, 10 patients had no flow and 2 had impaired flow. Distal embolization had developed in 10 patients, in situ thrombosis in 4, and both complications in 2 patients. Debris was aspirated with a custom-made 8F Teflon-coated sheath inserted in the superficial femoral and proximal below-the-knee arteries. Urokinase was administered intra-arterially in 9 patients for distal embolization in below-the-knee arteries. The PAT procedure was repeated as needed to achieve good antegrade arterial flow, confirmed by angiography.

In 12 patients PAT was successful in removing large amounts of thromboembolic debris and restoring patency of the affected vessel. In 5 patients the procedure was repeated within 24 hours. No further complications occurred in 7 patients, who were discharged within 48 hours. Two patients had below-, rather than above-the-knee, amputation after PAT; another had a transmetatarsal amputation but was spared below-the-knee amputation. One patient died of a myocardial infarction unrelated to PAT.

Limb-threatening embolic or thrombotic episodes have frequently been treated with thromboembolectomy. Surgery, however, may result in significant morbidity and mortality. This catheter technique avoids surgery and is reliable in removing debris and restoring blood flow; it may be used in conjunction with balloon angioplasty or thrombolytic therapy.

▶ As thromboembolic complications are common and unwanted during performance of minimal intervention, it is pleasant to note that percutaneous aspiration of such debris can be accomplished, thus providing an adjunct to lytic therapy.

Endoscopic Intravascular Surgery Removes Intraluminal Flaps, Dissections, and Thrombus

White GH, White RA, Kopchok GE, Colman PD, Wilson SE (Harbor-UCLA Med Ctr, Torrance, Calif; Univ of California, Los Angeles)

J Vasc Surg 11:280–288, 1990 3–5

Endoscopy of the vascular system has become an increasingly important procedure since its evolution from an experimental procedure to a definitive therapeutic device for selected arterial lesions. The usefulness of angioscopically guided intravascular instrumentation was examined in 73 patients undergoing thrombectomy or embolectomy, 11 patients with vascular trauma, and 32 during laser angioplasty and balloon dilation.

After balloon-catheter thromboembolectomy, retained thrombus was observed in 88% of patients, varying from a thin layer of mural thrombus to large amounts of adherent thrombus. Flexible biopsy forceps were used in 13 patients (18%) to remove occlusive thrombi tightly adherent to the arterial wall and in 4 more to remove underlying intimal flaps. In patients with vascular trauma, traumatic intimal defects were caused by iatrogenic cannulation injuries in 5 patients and by external trauma in 4. Management consisted of thrombectomy and complete or partial intravascular removal with long flexible biopsy forceps (Fig 3–1) of an intimal flap in 6 patients or a dissection plane in 3. The remaining 2 patients with traumatic intimal defects warranted immediate bypass grafting because of the severity of the defects. Angioscopic inspection after laser thermal angioplasty revealed wall charring and obvious thermal damage in 28 patients (87%) and plaque cracking, intimal flaps, and fragmentation in 26 arteries (81%). In most patients these defects were underestimated on intraoperative angiograms. Large flaps and thrombus were removed endoscopically in 3 patients.

Angioscopic examination reveals the extent of intimal injury after angioplasty, trauma, and thrombectomy, and provides insight into the

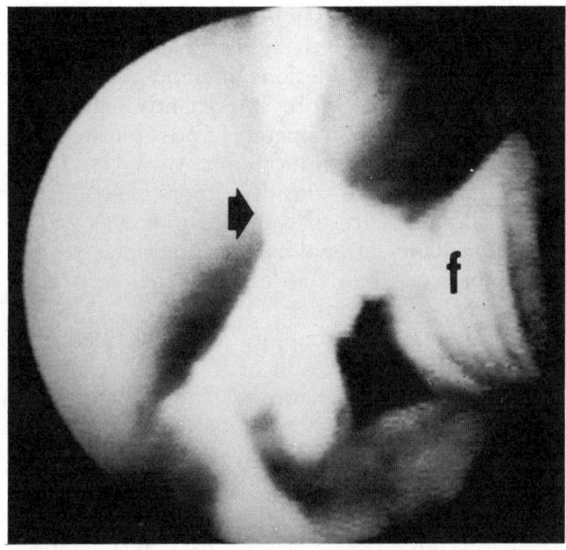

Fig 3–1.—Flexible biopsy forceps *(f)* used to remove an intimal flap *(arrow)* from wall of the common iliac artery with angioscopic guidance. (Courtesy of White GH, White RA, Kopchok GE, et al: *J Vasc Surg* 11:280–288, 1990.)

mechanisms and effect of instrumentation. Adherent thrombus after embolectomy by balloon catheter and intimal flaps caused by vascular surgery are common and, in selected patients, can be removed successfully with endoscopic intravascular manipulation.

▶ Increasing utility of angioscopy as an adjunct to direct vascular surgery is to be anticipated. Development of new instrumentation will aid this greatly.

Peripheral Laser-Assisted Balloon Angioplasty: Initial Multicenter Experience in 219 Peripheral Arteries

Sanborn TA, Cumberland DC, Greenfield AJ, Motarjeme A, Schwarten DE, Leachman DR, Ferris EJ, Myler RK, McCowan TC, Tatpati D, Ginsburg R, White RI (Boston Univ)

Arch Surg 124:1099–1103, 1989 3–6

Results of initial studies in peripheral arteries suggest that laser thermal angioplasty may be a safe and effective adjunct or alternative to conventional balloon angioplasty. Data were reviewed on a multicenter study of peripheral laser-assisted balloon angioplasty with an argon laser-heated, metallic-capped fiberoptic in 219 peripheral arteries in 208 patients. All but 8 procedures were performed through percutaneous arterial puncture of the ipsilateral femoral artery; the other 8 were performed through a cutdown. Success was defined based on symptomatology, angiographic results, and measurements of the Doppler ankle-arm index.

Angiographic and clinical success was achieved in 155 of 219 procedures. For lesions considered possible to treat by conventional balloon angioplasty, as determined subjectively by the angiographer, clinical success was achieved in 116 of 149 lesions, including 39 of 41 stenoses and 77 of 108 total occlusions. More importantly, clinical success was achieved in 39 of 70 lesions considered impossible to treat by conventional means. The overall perforation rate with this laser device was 4.1%, and only 2.1% in lesions considered possible to be treated by conventional means. The incidence of complications was equal to or better than that reported for conventional balloon angioplasty, improved as the operator gained experience, and was less than that reported for argon laser angioplasty with bare fiberoptics.

Laser thermal angioplasty with an argon laser-heated, metallic-capped fiberoptic allows rapid recanalization of lesions that are difficult or impossible to treat by conventional means. The technique can be learned easily by physicians skilled in interventional techniques and can be performed as safely as conventional balloon angioplasty.

▶ A number of centers participating in this trial have presented their own work, but this combination of their results appears even less impressive. In Robert Hobson's commentary, he pointed out that in the 70 lesions that were impossible to treat by conventional balloon angioplasty, success was achieved only in 39 (56%). Further, no data were presented in the article to suggest that lower restenosis rates would be achieved by the combined technique than by PTA alone. Sustained clinical benefit is the objective of all interventions for arterial occlusive disease. This fact should be emphasized.

Percutaneous Excimer-Laser and Excimer-Laser-Assisted Angioplasty of the Lower Extremities: Results of Initial Clinical Trial

Litvack F, Grundfest WS, Adler L, Hickey AE, Segalowitz J, Hestrin LB, Mohr FW, Goldenberg T, Laudenslager JS, Forrester JS (Cedars-Sinai Med Ctr, Los Angeles; Univ of California, Los Angeles)

Radiology 172:331–335, 1989 3–7

The 308-nm excimer laser vaporizes atheroma with minimal heat generation and little tissue injury even when the material is densely calcified. The instrument acts through photochemical desorption of constituent products. Angioplasty was performed percutaneously using the excimer laser in 30 patients with symptomatic peripheral vascular disease. A balloon was also used in all but 2 cases. Most patients were pretreated with aspirin and heparin was given intravenously.

The laser was immediately successful in 77% of 31 femoropopliteal stenoses and occlusions. Six of 7 occlusions less than 5 cm long were successfully opened, as were 7 of 8 occlusions measuring 6–10 cm, and 3 of 4 occlusions measuring 11–15 cm. Failure to open a total occlusion was because of the inability to maintain coaxial position and subintimal passage of the fiber. The rate of restenosis after a mean follow-up of 9 months was 29%.

Balloon angioplasty with the excimer laser is feasible for percutaneous treatment of vascular disease in the lower extremity. The success of the excimer laser warrants a randomized test comparing the excimer laser-balloon system with other methods such as the hot-tip laser, conventional balloon angioplasty, and bypass surgery.

▶ The excimer laser has been heralded as having great promise, and this present report is welcome. It is, after all, the first description of laser angioplasty performed with this device. However, the conclusions of this study are limited by the small number of patients and by the developmental nature of the instrumentation. Recent analysis of the Northwestern experience has been disappointing; 7 of 15 patients (47%) remain patent with a mean follow-up of 5 months.

Randomized Trial of Laser-Assisted Passage Through Occluded Femoro-Popliteal Arteries

Jeans WD, Murphy P, Hughes AO, Horrocks M, Baird RN (Univ of Bristol; Bristol Royal Infirmary, England)

Br J Radiol 63:19–21, 1990 3–8

The failure of balloon angioplasty in treatment of lower limb ischemia occurs most often in the initial attempt and in the first few months after treatment. To improve the initial success rate, bare optical fibers heated by laser energy have been applied directly to the atheromatous lesion. Although this technique improves the passage rate, it is also associated with a high incidence of vessel perforation. Metal-tipped optical fibers heated by laser energy were compared with conventional guidewires and catheters for their ability to gain passage through an occluded femoropopliteal artery.

Of 50 patients with an occluded femoropopliteal artery who were scheduled to undergo balloon angioplasty, 25 (mean age, 69 years) were randomly assigned to attempted passage of the occlusion with a laser-heated, metal-tipped optical fiber and 25 (mean age, 71 years) were assigned to the conventional guidewire and catheter technique. End points were successful passage through the occlusion and the outcome 1 month after passage.

Successful passage through the occlusion followed by balloon dilatation was obtained in 18 laser-treated vessels and 20 control vessels. The difference was not statistically significant. One month after balloon angioplasty, 13 laser-treated arteries and 13 guidewire-treated arteries remained patent. These findings indicate that laser-heated, metal-tipped optical fibers are no better than conventional guidewires and catheters in obtaining passage through an occluded vessel. Although metal-capped optical fibers reduced the incidence of perforation when compared with bare fibers, the incidence of perforation was still twice that with the conventional guidewire and catheter technique. The laser installation and the metal-tipped optical fibers are considerably more expensive than the guidewires used in conventional methods.

▶ All laser users need to be reminded of the editorial entitled "Indiscriminate use of laser angioplasty" by a group of distinguished vascular surgeons and interventional radiologists (1).

Reference

1. Editorial: *Radiology* 172:945, 1989.

Peripheral Laser Angioplasty With Pulsed Dye Laser and Ball-Tipped Optical Fibres

Murray A, Wood RFM, Mitchell DC, Edwards DH, Grasty M, Basu R (St Bartholomew's Hosp, London)

Lancet 2:1471–1474, 1989 3–9

Balloon angioplasty can now achieve cumulative patency rates of more than 80% at 5 years in stenotic iliac vessels, but it is usually less successful in the narrower femoropopliteal segment, for which the 5-year cumulative patency rates are about 70%. Laser angioplasty is under assessment for the treatment of both peripheral and coronary artery disease. Early results indicate that this technique may be suitable for recanalizing segments of artery not amenable to treatment by balloon angioplasty. The early results were assessed after laser angioplasty with the pulsed dye laser and a novel, atraumatic ball-tipped optical fiber.

The series consisted of 24 patients with occlusive femoropopliteal vascular disease in 26 limbs. All had critical ischemia or severe disabling claudication that warranted operative intervention. Four patients had distal gangrene. The mean length of the femoropopliteal occlusions was 21 cm and ranged from 3 to 49 cm. The delivery device consisted of the laser fiber loaded retrogradely into a standard 6-mm balloon angioplasty catheter, which was introduced through a common femoral artery cutdown.

Technical success was observed after 23 of the 26 laser angioplasties in which a mean energy of 250 joules was used. Recanalization failed in the other 3 limbs. Clinical success was seen in 19 limbs, with striking improvement in symptoms. After 3 of the technically successful procedures, thrombosis occurred within 48 hours, and 1 technically successful recanalization did not bring about clinical improvement. Eighteen patients with clinically successful recanalizations in 19 limbs have now been followed for a median of 7 months (Fig 3–2). Three patients, aged 76–83 years, died of myocardial infarction; all 3 had severe cardiac disease before operation. The laser-treated vessels were patent at autopsy. Late thrombosis occurred in another 2 patients. Thus 13 patients had 14

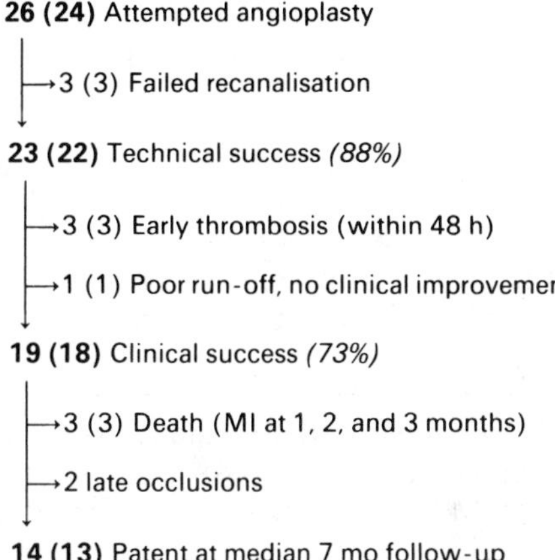

Fig 3–2.—Flow chart summary of results. Number of limbs (number of patients). (Courtesy of Murray A, Wood RFM, Mitchell DC, et al: *Lancet* 2:1471–1474, 1989.)

patent vessels after 7 months of follow-up. All 13 patients were well and symptom free at the time of this report.

▶ It seems that the pulsed-dye laser adds very little to the minimal interventional armamentarium.

Cholesterol Embolization After Treatment With Tissue Plasminogen Activator
Shapiro LS (Albany, NY)
N Engl J Med 2:1270, 1989 3–10

Cholesterol embolization has been associated with angiography, aortic surgery, anticoagulant therapy, and intravenous streptokinase therapy. Cholesterol embolization syndrome developed in a patient after he received recombinant tissue plasminogen activator (r-tPA) intravenously.

Man, 52, with a history of hypertension, type II diabetes mellitus, and heavy smoking, had ECG evidence of myocardial ischemia. He received an infusion of 100 mg of tPA during a 3-hour period, after which heparin was administered intravenously for 24 hours. Chest pain resolved rapidly and the creatine kinase value remained normal, but sharp midepigastric pain developed a week later, with purplish mottling of the lower trunk and legs. Leukocytosis was observed and the amylase level was twice the upper normal limit. Gastrointestinal assessment revealed mild gastritis and duodenitis. Recurrent pain in the abdomen and testicular pain a week later preceded cyanosis of the left fifth toe. The creatine kinase level at this time was 420 units per L. Gastrocnemius biopsy revealed cholesterol emboli in muscular arteries and no evidence of vasculitis. Episodic skin rashes and abdominal pain continued until the patient died 1 year later of myocardial infarction. Autopsy revealed severe, diffuse atherosclerosis of the aorta.

It appears that treatment with tPA may place patients with severe atherosclerosis at an increased risk of cholesterol embolization.

▶ As tPA treatment becomes utilized increasingly, recognition of the distal atheromatous microembolization syndrome is important. Therapy for this must be instituted quickly to minimize permanent tissue damage.

Blue Toe Syndrome: Treatment With Percutaneous Atherectomy

Dolmatch BL, Rholl KS, Moskowitz LB, Dake MD, van Breda A, Kaplan JO, Katzen BT (Baptist Hosp, Miami; Alexandria Hosp, Alexandria, Va)

Radiology 172:799–804, 1989 3–11

"Blue toe syndrome" refers to digital ischemia resulting from microembolic occlusion of small vessels of the feet and toes. Percutaneous transluminal angioplasty has been advocated for its treatment because the syndrome may be related to the degree of stenoses caused by an ulcerated plaque. Others believe that the syndrome may be caused by cholesterol embolism from a proximal lesion, and dilation of this segment may increase the risk of cholesterol embolism despite improved flow to the lesion. Because of these uncertainties, a different method for treating patients with blue toe syndrome percutaneously was developed. Percutaneous transluminal atherectomy was performed in the treatment of embologenic superficial femoral artery lesions in 7 patients.

Stenoses ranged from 1.2 to 2.4 cm in length and the percentage of stenosis ranged from 90% to 99%, except for 1 patient with 75% stenosis. All 7 patients had prompt healing of the ischemic toes, and none required surgical revascularization or amputation. One patient had recurrent stenosis at the atherectomy site and underwent repeat atherectomy with a larger device. Histologically, fibrinoplatelet aggregates were seen in 4 patients, organizing thrombus in 5, and cholesterol deposits in 2. A common finding was fibrous plaque in 6 patients and intimal hyperplasia in smooth muscle in 5.

Percutaneous atherectomy is effective in the treatment of embologenic superficial femoral artery stenoses in patients with ipsilateral blue toe syndrome. Emboli arise from adherent fibrinoplatelet aggregates or thrombus and less often from cholesterol-rich atheromatous plaque. Whereas the underlying stenosis can be treated with percutaneous transluminal angioplasty, percutaneous atherectomy offers the advantage of nonsurgical removal of embologenic material and provides material for histologic study.

▶ Treatment of ulcerative atheromas, which produce distal atheromatous embolization, is generally rewarding. The effects of surgical elimination of the lesion from the arterial tree are often dramatic. This report of atherectomy treatment needs confirmation by other centers before atherectomy in treatment of this particular lesion can be accepted universally.

The Effect of Plaque Composition on Laser Recanalization

Kaelin LD, Werts SG, Smith S, Abela GS, Seeger JM (Univ of Florida; VA Med Ctr, Gainesville)

J Surg Res 48:363–367, 1990 3–12

Atherosclerotic arteries may be recanalized using metal-capped laser fibers activated by a continuous-wave laser source. Occluding plaque and thrombus are ablated thermally. In 16 patients with symptomatic occlusions in the mid or distal superficial femoral artery, B-mode ultrasonography was performed before attempted argon laser recanalization. Lesions were classified as soft or dense on the basis of their echogenicity or as calcified (echoreflective).

Recanalization succeeded in 11 patients, including 8 of the 12 who had claudication and 3 of 4 with rest pain. Vessels occluded by soft plaque were recanalized significantly more often than those containing dense or calcified plaque. Subintimal probe passage and perforation occurred only in the latter cases. In general, recanalized occlusions were shorter than lesions that could not be recanalized.

Plaque composition appears to be a useful predictor of the outcome of attempted arterial recanalization using a thermal laser probe. Patients with soft occlusions are ideal candidates. Those with dense or calcified occlusions are unlikely to do well unless the occlusion is short. These patients may do better if treated with the excimer laser or if subjected to arterial bypass surgery.

▶ It may be that careful selection of patients for laser angioplasty may improve the results.

Intra-Arterial Low-Dose Streptokinase Infusion for Superior Mesenteric Artery Embolus

Hillers TK, Ginsberg JS, Panju A, Gately J, Gill G, Waterfall WE (McMaster Univ, Hamilton, Ont)

Can Med Assoc J 142:1087–1088, 1990 3–13

Usually, acute superior mesenteric artery embolism is treated by embolectomy with local papaverine infusion. Streptokinase infusion was used successfully to lyse a superior mesenteric embolus.

Man, 71, had increasing discomfort in the chest and epigastrium for 2 weeks; more recently, nausea, vomiting, and bloody stools occurred. He had a history of angina, hypertension, chronic atrial fibrillation, peptic ulcer and alcohol abuse. An irregular pulse was noted. Abdominal angiography showed an embolus in the distal superior mesenteric artery. Streptokinase was infused at a rate of 10,000 units per hour at a point 4 cm proximal to the obstruction. Distal small bowel obstruction was somewhat improved after 12 hours, and at 36 hours the clot was smaller. After 60 hours of treatment the embolus had lysed and symptoms had resolved. Coagulation factors were unchanged. Heparin and warfarin were given and the patient was discharged.

In each case the clinician has to decide whether there is enough time to lyse the clot by streptokinase infusion or whether immediate embolectomy is necessary. This is the fourth patient so treated to be reported in the English literature.

▶ One cannot help but be amazed by this case report: first, by the fact that an embolus could be dissolved by lytic therapy, and, second, that lytic therapy did not provoke massive gastrointestinal bleeding in a patient who was having bloody stools on admission. The known consequences of revascularization of ischemic bowel are mucosal slough and intraluminal bleeding, yet that seemed not to have occurred in this patient. Other reports of use of lytic agents in treatment of mesenteric embolus have described local infusion of low-dose streptokinase and topical infusion of streptokinase. As the first of these was in 1979 and the present report is only the fourth, one can see that this is not becoming a popular form of treatment.

4 Nonatherosclerotic Conditions

Stenotic Intimal Thickening of the External Iliac Artery in Competition Cyclists

Rousselet M-C, Saint-Andre J-P, L'Hoste P, Enon B, Megret A, Chevalier J-M (Angers, France)

Hum Pathol 21:524–529, 1990 4–1

Stenotic intimal thickening of the external iliac artery that can produce transient ischemia during violent effort has been described in competitive cyclists. Between 1985 and 1989, 23 professional or top-class competitive amateur cyclists (mean age, 29) were seen with this disorder. Annual training ranged from 8,000 to 25,000 km. Competitive riding had begun at a mean age of 17 years.

None of the patients had identifiable vascular risk factors. Symptoms, usually claudication of a lower extremity, began at a mean age of 26 years. Pain at first occurred during a sprint or when riding up a steep slope. Some patients had a systolic murmur in the iliac fossa with the thigh flexed on the pelvis. Ankle systolic pressure was significantly lowered compared with the opposite limb. A narrowed segment of external iliac artery was seen on arteriography.

The artery was elongated and exhibited abnormal loops with the thigh flexed. Wall thickening was caused by translucent intimal material that extended for 2–6 cm. On microscopy, intimal thickening usually involved half or two thirds of the circumference of the vessel. Moderately cellular loose connective tissue was present. Ultrastructural study showed features of synthetic smooth muscle cells.

This lesion differs from both atherosclerosis and intimal fibrodysplasia, although it might possibly dispose to atherosclerosis. The lesion may result from abnormal local hemodynamic conditions.

▶ It is important for vascular surgeons to recognize this lesion. Just as popliteal artery entrapment and popliteal artery cyst cause precocious claudication in an exercising patient, this lesion affects a particular class of exercisers. As cycling becomes more accepted in the United States, this lesion will be seen predictably more often. It is interesting to speculate on its cause.

Bilateral Compartment Syndrome After a Long Gynecologic Operation in the Lithotomy Position

Adler LM, Loughlin JS, Morin CJ, Haning RV Jr (Women and Infants' Hosp; Miriam Hosp; Brown Univ, Providence, RI)

Am J Obstet Gynecol 162:1271–1272, 1990 4–2

Compartment syndrome is characterized by an acute increase in pressure in a limited anatomical space, compromising both circulation and neurologic function of structures contained in that space. This syndrome is seen most often after trauma or vascular procedures, but it can also complicate prolonged gynecologic surgery in the lithotomy position. Compartment syndrome occurred in a patient after a tubal anastomosis in a prolonged lithotomy position.

Woman, 30, underwent tubal anastomosis after previously having tubal ligation. She was given a general endotracheal anesthetic and placed in the lithotomy position. The patient was left in this position for the 6 hours it took to complete lysis of adhesions and bilateral isthmic-ampullary anastomoses. She complained of severe cramping in both lower legs, which were tense and firm, 2 hours after the operation. She reported numbness, burning, and difficulty in moving her legs 12 hours postoperatively. A left footdrop and reduced sensation over both feet were noted. Compartment syndrome was diagnosed by a consulting vascular surgeon. The patient was treated conservatively by positioning the lower legs at heart level, and bicarbonate drip was initiated to prevent renal injury. Physical therapy was started 6 days postoperatively. The left-sided footdrop and hypesthesia persisted, but she had only mild hypoesthesia on the right side; at 6-week follow-up visit, these symptoms persisted.

Complications of compartment syndrome include permanent neuromuscular dysfunction, skin necrosis, and myoglobinuric renal failure. The incidence of compartment failure may be decreased by avoiding prolonged lithotomy positioning. Attention to postoperative symptoms and timely intervention are crucial in minimizing complications.

▶ As vascular surgeons will be called in consultation in a condition such as this, it is important to recognize it swiftly and treat it effectively to prevent permanent neuromuscular damage.

Scintigraphic Patterns of the Reflex Sympathetic Dystrophy Syndrome of the Lower Extremities

Intenzo C, Kim S, Millin J, Park C (Thomas Jefferson Univ, Philadelphia)
Clin Nucl Med 14:657–661, 1989 4–3

Radiographic and scintigraphic studies may help to confirm a diagnosis of reflex sympathetic dystrophy syndrome (RSDS). Thirty-two patients clinically suspected of having RSDS of the lower extremity had scintigraphy with 20 mCi of ^{99m}Tc-MDP administered intravenously. Anterior blood pool images were recorded from the pelvis to the feet, and delayed imaging was performed 3–4 hours later. Eight patients had stage I, 21 had stage II, and 3 had stage III RSDS.

Of 23 patients with scintigraphic images positive for RSDS, 18 had a good response to nerve block or sympathectomy. Three others improved after a dorsal column stimulator was inserted. Scans were considered

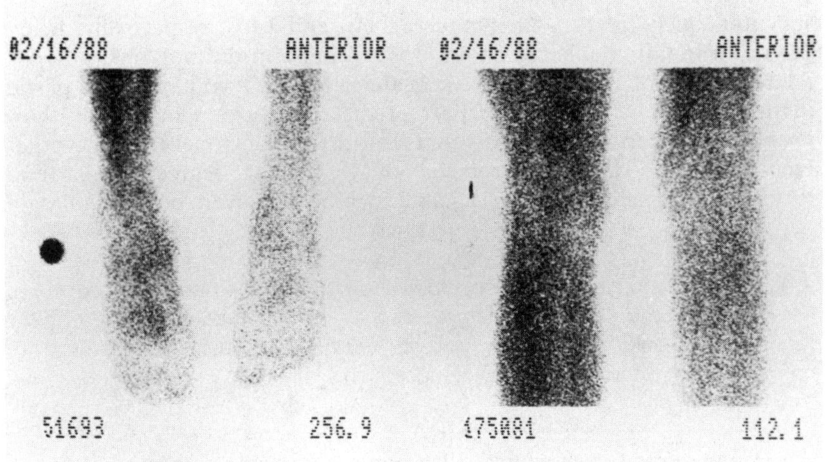

Fig 4–1.—Anterior blood pool images of feet and legs of a 25-year-old man who sustained an injury to his left foot demonstrate decreased vascularity to the left lower extremity (**L**). **R**, right lower extremity. (Courtesy of Intenzo C, Kim S, Millin J, et al: *Clin Nucl Med* 14:657–661, 1989.)

positive if periarticular activity was increased or decreased relative to the contralateral, asymptomatic lower extremity (Fig 4–1). Of 9 patients with normal scintigrams, 8 also were relieved by nerve block or sympathectomy. Two of 8 patients with stage I RSDS had increased periarticular activity in the affected limb. All 3 with stage III RSDS also had increased periarticular activity.

Bone scintigraphy had a sensitivity of 72% for the diagnosis of RSDS. It is more likely to be positive in the later clinical stages of disease.

▶ Reflex sympathetic dystrophy is difficult to diagnose and treat. Objective criteria that will assist both in the diagnosis and in therapy are welcome.

Low Incidence of Thrombocytopenia With Porcine Mucosal Heparin: A Prospective Multicenter Study

Rao AK, White GC, Sherman L, Colman R, Lan G, Ball AP (Temple Univ; Univ of North Carolina, Chapel Hill; Washington Univ; Natl Heart, Lung, and Blood Inst, Bethesda, Md)

Arch Intern Med 149:1285–1288, 1989 4–4

Sudden severe thrombocytopenia has occurred in patients given porcine intestinal mucosal or bovine lung heparin, sometimes in association with arterial thrombosis. The incidence of thrombocytopenia was determined in 193 patients who received porcine intestinal mucosal heparin for at least 5 days, either intravenously or subcutaneously.

No patient had a platelet count of less than 100×10^9/L or heparin-related thrombosis. Eight patients had counts between 100 and 140 × 10^9/L during treatment. The mean lowest platelet counts in intravenously and subcutaneously treated patients were 11% and 14%, respectively, below the mean initial counts. The total dose of heparin did not generally correlate significantly with the lowest platelet count. Two patients at participating centers who were not part of the study group proper did have problems—arterial thrombosis in 1 and thrombocytopenia in the other. Heparin-related thrombocytopenia of significant degree and arterial thrombosis appear to be infrequent in patients given porcine mucosal heparin.

▶ The heparin-induced thrombocytopenia syndrome has been referred to earlier in this volume. Its importance to vascular surgeons is emphasized by this report. One would hope that porcine-derived heparin would decrease the frequency of this often devastating complication.

Thrombocytopenia Associated With Heparin-Coated Catheters in Patients With Heparin-Associated Antiplatelet Antibodies

Laster JL, Nichols WK, Silver D (Univ of Missouri-Columbia Health Sciences Ctr, Columbia)

Arch Intern Med 149:2285–2287, 1989 4–5

Heparin-induced thrombocytopenia is a recognized complication of heparin administration. Data on a patient who had thrombocytopenia associated with the presence of a heparin-coated pulmonary artery catheter and those of 11 other similar patients were reviewed.

All 12 patients had heparin-associated antiplatelet antibodies and demonstrated marked thrombocytopenia while undergoing hemodynamic monitoring with heparin-coated pulmonary artery catheters. The thrombocytopenia persisted for as long as the heparin-coated catheters were in place, even when all other sources of heparin were discontinued. The platelet counts returned to normal levels when the heparin-coated catheters were removed. All patients had previous heparin exposure or were receiving heparin at the time of insertion of the heparin-coated catheters.

Because of the widespread use of heparin-coated catheters, especially in unstable or critically ill patients, it is mandatory that platelet counts be monitored closely in patients having these devices in place. Patients with heparin-associated antiplatelet antibodies should not receive heparin or heparin-coated catheters. A non-heparin-coated catheter can be used should these patients require a pulmonary artery catheter. To reduce the risk of thromboembolic complications, inhibition of platelet function with aspirin is advocated in all patients in whom heparin-associated antiplatelet antibodies develop.

▶ Although heparin-coated catheters have been reported in the past to cause heparin-induced thrombocytopenia, nevertheless, this abstract was selected to reemphasize the fact that miniscule amounts of heparin such as used in heparin-coated catheters can trigger the onset of what can be a disasterous series of events.

Rupture of a Non-Aneurysmal *Salmonella* Infected Aorta

Cook AM, Christopoulos D (Hull Royal Infirmary, Hull, England)

Clin Radiol 40:605–606, 1989 4–6

Salmonella infection of the aorta is rare, and its clinical diagnosis is often difficult. Computed tomography remains the diagnostic procedure of choice, and the diagnosis depends largely on demonstrating an aneurysm. A retroperitoneal collection developed in a patient with *Salmonella* bacteremia, as a result of infection and subsequent rupture of the abdominal aorta.

Man, 65, with *Salmonella* bacteremia, reported severe bilateral groin and leg pain and paresis. Abdominal ultrasound showed large bilateral retroperitoneal fluid collections, suggesting retroperitoneal abscesses. The aorta had a calcified wall, which was of normal caliber. Laparotomy revealed a 1.1-cm hole in the posterior aortic wall and a collection of blood clots in the retroperitoneal space. Histologic examination of the aortic wall showed fibrosis and calcified atheroma with a dense polymorph infiltrate. Culture of the retroperitoneal blood clot yielded *Salmonella typhimurium*.

The very unusual feature in this patient with *Salmonella* aortitis was the direct rupture without preceding aneurysm formation. Although the weakened aortic wall usually undergoes aneurysmal dilatation, a fibrotic reaction can occur, maintaining a normal-sized lumen. The diagnosis of a ruptured nonaneurysmal aorta should be considered in a man older than 50 years with *Salmonella* bacteremia and retroperitoneal collections seen on CT.

▶ *Salmonella* arteritis is particularly dangerous because of the tremendously destructive nature of its effect on the arterial wall.

A Ten-Year Experience With Bacterial Aortitis

Oz MC, Brener BJ, Buda JA, Todd G, Brenner RW, Goldenkranz RJ, McNicholas KW, Lemole GM, Lozner JS (Columbia-Presbyterian Med Ctr, New York; Newark Beth Israel Med Ctr, NJ; Overlook Hosp, Summit, NJ; Med Ctr of Delaware, Wilmington)

J Vasc Surg 10:439–449, 1989 4–7

Bacterial aortitis is associated with high morbidity and mortality. Although the diagnosis and treatment of bacterial aortitis have improved during the past decade, there remains much controversy over the optimal clinical approach. The case reports of 21 patients who were treated for bacterial aortitis during a 10-year period at 4 institutions were reviewed. The series included 13 men and 8 women, aged 45–85 years.

Most of the patients had the common clinical features of fever leukocytosis, back pain, and a pulsatile abdominal mass, but none of the clinical signs was pathognomonic. The radiographic appearance (e.g., unusual aortic nodularity, gas in the aortic wall, or unusual lobulation of an aneurysm) were good diagnostic clues. Fifty percent of the patients had positive preoperative blood cultures in the presence of an aortic abnormality. *Salmonella* and *Staphylococcus* were the most commonly identified pathogens. In situ graft repair was done when the infected aorta could be removed entirely or when the thoracic or suprarenal aorta was involved. Axillofemoral bypass grafting was used in patients with extensive infection.

Nine patients underwent in situ repair, 11 patients had extra-anatomical bypass grafting combined with aortic ligation, and 1 had aneurysmorrhaphy. Two of the 9 patients with in situ repairs and 6 of the 11 with extra-anatomical bypass died of disease-related causes. Most patients were maintained on long-term antibiotics, and none of the survivors had graft infections. As the data for these 21 patients were collected from 4 institutions, there was no single treatment protocol. The choice of surgical procedures was based on surgeon bias rather than on objective findings.

▶ Modern vascular surgery is plagued with recurrent problems of major artery infections. *Salmonella,* in particular, is virulent, and there is no agreed-upon therapeutic strategy that is uniformly efficacious.

The History of Temporal Arteritis or Ten Centuries of Fascinating Adventure

Henriet J-P, Marin J, Gosselin J, Hamel-Desnos C, Ducrocq M, Brard G, Maiza D, Courtheoux P, Evrard C, Théron J (Centre Hospitalier Universitaire, Caen, France)

J Mal Vasc 14:93–97, 1989 4–8

Although temporal arteritis has generated a voluminous body of literature, its precise etiology remains elusive. Two case reports of temporal arteritis published in 1932 are considered the first definitive descriptions of temporal arteritis. In reality, however, the syndrome was first described much earlier.

The oldest report on record is a brief description suggestive of temporal arteritis, written between 940 and 1010 by the ophthalmologist Ali Ibn Isa from Baghdad, which was not translated into English until 1936. In 1890 a patient with inflamed and swollen temporal arteries was described. In a 1930 paper on intracranial aneurysms, a patient was reported with extremely severe temporal pain that developed after several weeks of a flulike syndrome. The clinical characteristics and histology of temporal arteritis were first fully described in 1934 and 1936 by Horton. The first report of blindness caused by temporal arteritis appeared in 1938.

Except for a patient with temporal arteritis reported by Paviot in 1934, the French have made only modest contributions to the literature. In 1936 Chavany first described the pillow sign, and in 1948 he was also the first to prescribe steroid therapy and report its results. Also, the French were the first to use bilateral carotid arteriography in the diagnosis of temporal arteritis. Several French-designed types of ultrasound equipment that use Doppler velocimetry for the diagnosis and follow-up of patients with temporal arteritis are now used worldwide. Nevertheless, 10 centuries after Alib Ibn Isa first described temporal arteritis, this disease remains an enigma.

A Population-Based Case-Control Study of Temporal Arteritis: Evidence for an Association Between Temporal Arteritis and Degenerative Vascular Disease?

Machado EBV, Gabriel SE, Beard CM, Michet CJ, O'Fallon WM, Ballard DJ (Mayo Clinic and Found, Rochester, Minn)

Int J Epidemiol 18:836–841, 1989 4–9

Giant cell, or temporal, arteritis (TA) is a vasculitis of unknown origin that affects large and medium-sized vessels in persons older than 50 years. Its epidemiology has not been established definitively. A population-based case-control analysis of TA used data from the Rochester Epidemiology Program Project.

From 1950 to 1985, 88 patients with newly diagnosed, biopsy-proved TA were identified in Olmsted County, Minnesota. Each patient was matched to 4 community controls on the basis of sex, age, and duration of community medical record. Odds ratios were determined for marital status, education, Quetelet index, pregnancy, age at menopause, thyroid disease, diabetes, smoking, hypertension, angina, myocardial infarction, peripheral vascular disease, and stroke.

The odds ratio for smoking was statistically significant. Elevated odds ratios were not significant for angina, myocardial infarction, or peripheral vascular disease. Arteriosclerosis and TA may share a common etiologic pathway. Alternatively, histopathologic misclassification of TA biopsy specimens may explain the observed associations. Multicenter collaboration is needed to define more precisely the epidemiology of TA.

▸ Vascular surgeons are involved in providing the biopsy specimens to the internist for confirmation of diagnosis. Therefore, it is well for us to have access to the literature on the various aspects of this syndrome. These articles provide a current summary for us.

Duplex and Color Doppler Sonographic Evaluation of Vasculogenic Impotence

Quam JP, King BF, James EM, Lewis RW, Brakke DM, Ilstrup DM, Parulkar BG, Hattery RR (Mayo Clinic Found, Rochester, Minn)

AJR 153:1141–1147, 1989 4–10

Vascular disease is a potentially curable cause of erectile dysfunction. Because accurate diagnosis is crucial, the role of conventional duplex sonography with spectral analysis and color Doppler imaging was studied in 180 patients with suspected vasculogenic impotence. Mean peak systolic and end-diastolic velocities of the cavernosal arteries were measured before and after intracavernosal injections of papaverine. Sixty-one patients were also examined with dynamic cavernosography and cavernosometry, and 12 were studied with selective internal pudendal and penile arteriography.

All 5 patients with abnormal arteriographic findings had abnormal mean peak systolic velocities (≤25 cm/sec), whereas 6 of 7 patients with normal findings had mean peak systolic velocities (>25 cm/sec) after injection of papaverine. This comparison yielded a sensitivity of 100%, specificity of 85.7%, and overall accuracy of 91.7%. On the basis of the receiver-operating-characteristic curve, a mean end-diastolic velocity in the cavernosal arteries of ≥5 cm/sec was indicative of excessive venous leakage on cavernosometry, yielding a sensitivity of 90% and specificity of 56%.

Penile duplex sonography with spectral analysis and color Doppler imaging is a promising noninvasive screening method for evaluating patients with suspected vasculogenic impotence. The addition of color Dop-

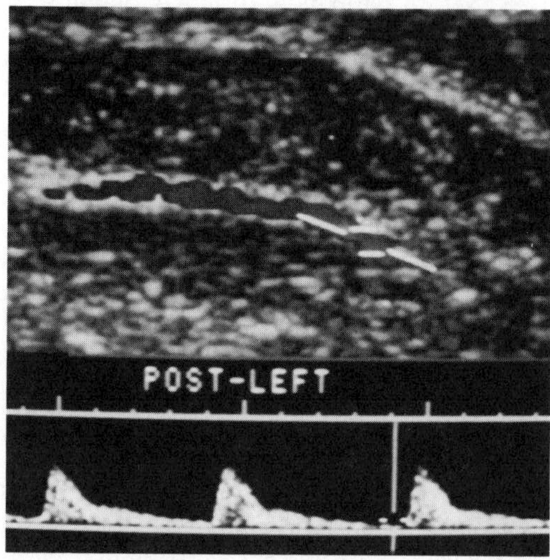

Fig 4–2.—Longitudinal duplex Doppler sonogram obtained at base of penis shows use of color flow to identify cavernosal artery correctly and to align angle-correction cursor with axis of flow accurately. (Courtesy of Quam JP, King BF, James EM, et al: *AJR* 153:1141–1147, 1989.)

pler sonography allows easier identification of cavernosal arteries and more accurate correction of the Doppler angle, resulting in more rapid and accurate acquisition of data (Fig 4–2).

▶ Increasingly sophisticated and less invasive means of diagnosing vasculogenic impotence are now available. Although few vascular surgeons are concerned with the surgical aspects of treatment of this condition, it is an area of fruitful investigation and rewarding surgical relief.

Outcome of Vascular Microsurgery for Erectile Dysfunction of Vascular Origin

Biedermann H (I. Universitätsklinik für Chirurgie, Innsbruck, Austria)

Wien Klin Wochenschr 101:723–728, 1989 4–11

Patients with erectile dysfunction caused by abnormal drainage of the cavernous bodies can benefit from microsurgical vascular reconstruction. Between 1984 and 1989, 71 men aged 20–65 years who had erectile dysfunction of arterial and venous origin underwent 66 microsurgical vascular reconstructions and 5 operations to reduce venous outflow from the corpora cavernosa.

Ten patients had congenital vascular abnormalities and 61 patients had acquired vascular deficiencies, of which 4 were caused by trauma, 48 by atherosclerosis, and 9 exclusively by venous obstruction. Thirty-seven patients had arterial as well as venous obstructions. All patients underwent preoperative Doppler ultrasound and angiographic evaluations. Follow-up ranged from 6 to 65 months (average, 35 months). Fifty-four patients underwent follow-up angiography, usually 1 month after operation.

Of 56 assessable patients, 46 were able to resume adequate to normal sexual intercourse, including 5 of the 7 diabetic patients. Only 10 patients were either minimally improved or their condition had remained unchanged. None of the patients reported deterioration when their condition was compared with preoperative sexual function. In addition to the usual complications of delayed wound healing and postoperative hemorrhage in 1 instance attributable to anticoagulant therapy, hypervascularization syndrome occurred in 16.7% of the 50 patients who had undergone primary or revision Virag I procedures. However, all patients except 1 were treated successfully with banding, and in some cases by additional venous ligatures. In addition, 43% of the 21 patients who underwent Virag I reconstruction in which the inferior epigastric artery was used and 14.8% of 27 patients who had a Virag I reconstruction in which a venous graft was used experienced occlusions of the reconstruction. Eighteen patients underwent revision operations.

Microsurgical reconstruction should be attempted in all patients with erectile dysfunction of vascular origin before life-long self-injection with papaverine or implantation of a penile prosthesis is considered.

▶ This paper describes heterogeneous operative experience in patients with erectile dysfunction of varying etiologies, among them, venous leakage and traumatic interruptions of the pudendal artery.

The follow-up among the 71 men was 78%. Of these, 46 (82%) of those contacted are characterized as having "adequate to normal sexual intercourse." Complications included a 16.7% incidence of glans hypervascularization with deep dorsal vein arterialization. The incidence of thrombosis was deep dorsal vein reconstruction was 43% for the inferior epigastric artery and 14.8% using a venous graft. Eighteen patients (25%) required a reoperation.

The unusual aspect of this report was reoperation for revision. We have abandoned the use of the Virag I operation because of the problem of glans hypervascularization; we now perform a modification in which the vein is ligated proximally and distally. Our experience with late thrombosis is the same; however, when this occurs we would not recommend another microvascular operation. Current thinking is also contrary to the author's conclusion that microsurgical reconstruction should be attempted in *all* patients with erectile dysfunction of vascular origin. The trend is to use self-injection programs or medical therapy, which can be quite successful.

I would agree with the view that microvascular penile surgery can be offered to patients who refuse prostheses. Once a microvascular reconstruction fails, or if there is a need for prompt restoration of sexual function, prosthetics offer a secure choice.—Ralph G. DePalma, M.D., Professor and Chairman, Department of Surgery, The George Washington Medical Center, Washington, D.C.

5 Claudication

Conservative Drug Treatment in Patients With Moderately Severe Chronic Occlusive Peripheral Arterial Disease

Lindgärde F, Jelnes R, Björkman H, Adielsson G, Kjellström T, Palmquist I, Stavenow L (Malmö Gen Hosp, Lund, Sweden; Gentofte Hosp, Copenhagen; Central Hosp, Växjö, Sweden)

Circulation 80:1549–1556, 1989 5–1

The use of vasoactive drugs in the treatment of chronic occlusive arterial disease is controversial. To determine who would benefit from such drugs, the use of pentoxifylline was compared with placebo in a multicenter study of 150 patients who had moderately severe chronic occlusive peripheral arterial disease. For 4–6 weeks all patients received placebo; they then were randomized to receive pentoxifylline, 400 mg, or placebo for a 6-month double-blind observation period.

Patients who took pentoxifylline had significantly better minimum percentage improvement in absolute claudication distance for weeks 16–24. Analysis of background variables to find a target population for whom trial results were most important identified a baseline ankle-arm pressure ratio of .8 or less and duration of disease for more than 1 year. For patients with these characteristics, pentoxifylline yielded significantly superior results over those of placebo for all end point and all summary measures.

Patients who have had chronic occlusive peripheral arterial disease for less than 1 year or an ankle-arm pressure greater than .8 will benefit by avoidance of risk factors and initiation of physical training. For the target population with severe hemodynamic impairment and a longer history, the use of pentoxifylline should bring clinically successful results.

▶ Surgeons know that the greater the indications for surgery, the better the results. This study brings out the fact that, paradoxically, the less the indications, the better the results of rheologic therapy in patients with claudication.

Walking Ability and Ankle Systolic Pressures: Observations in Patients With Intermittent Claudication in a Short-Term Walking Exercise Program

Carter SA, Hamel ER, Paterson JM, Snow CJ, Mymin D (Univ of Manitoba; St Boniface Gen Hosp, Winnipeg, Man)

J Vasc Surg 10:642–649, 1989 5–2

Walking exercise improves walking distance in patients with intermittent claudication, but the effects of the training on practical walking ability or on limb hemodynamics are not well known. Practical walking ability and limb hemodynamics were assessed in 56 patients with intermittent claudication in an exercise program. The patients walked 3 times a week for 1 hour.

After at least 3 months of training the patients' average maximal walking distance on the treadmill increased significantly from .59 to 1 km. In addition, 84% of patients could walk freely, without much discomfort, more than 2 km/hr at a time. The increased walking distance was significant in patients with obstruction of the femoropopliteal and aortoiliac artery with or without coronary disease, and in patients taking β blockers. Ankle pressures did not increase significantly, but returned to resting levels more quickly after training; brachial-ankle pressure differences decreased.

Walking has little effect on circulatory parameters, except for reducing postexercise hyperemia, so other factors are involved in walking ability. Whatever the mechanisms responsible, walking exercise can improve the practical walking ability of patients with claudication who are not candidates for arterial reconstruction.

▶ It seems that the results of an exercise program are even better than the results of drug therapy.

A Double-Blind Trial of Dextran-Haemodilution vs. Placebo in Claudicants

Ernst E, Kollar L, Matrai A (Med Hochschule, Hannover, Germany; Univ of Peçs, Hungary)

J Intern Med 227:19–24, 1990 5–3

Hemodilution is effective treatment in peripheral occlusive arterial disease but there are few data to support this clinical efficacy. To determine if dextran hemodilution is effective in intermittent claudication, 20 men with intermittent claudication were randomly assigned to 1 of 2 treatment groups: 11 patients in group 1 received isovolemic hemodilution with dextran 40, 500 mL per session, for 3 weeks, followed by a washout period, and then placebo therapy for 3 weeks; the sequence was reversed in 9 patients in group 2. On angiography, long arterial obstructions with ample visible collaterals were observed. In addition to measurement of pain-free and maximal walking distance on a treadmill ergometer, plethysmographic blood flow, Doppler pressures, hematocrit, blood and plasma viscosity, and fibrinogen were measured.

During hemodilution the walking distance increased significantly by about 50%, paralleled by a decline in hematocrit and blood viscosities. All other variables remained unchanged. Hemodilution was well tolerated. No significant changes occurred during placebo therapy.

These findings support those of previous studies on the safety and efficacy of dextran-hemodilution in selected patients with peripheral occlusive arterial disease. Its clinical efficacy is comparable to that of hydroxyethyl starch 200. Potential responders to dextran-hemodilution can be identified with conventional angiogram before therapy, particularly those with long arterial obstructions and good collateralization.

▶ Repeatedly, various methods of decreasing blood viscosity have been found to be briefly efficacious in increasing claudication distance. There seems to be no reason to continue such studies.

Is Percutaneous Transluminal Angioplasty Better Than Exercise for Claudication? Preliminary Results From a Prospective Randomised Trial

Creasy TS, McMillan PJ, Fletcher EWL, Collin J, Morris PJ (John Radcliffe Hosp, Oxford, England)

Eur J Vasc Surg 4:135–140, 1990 5–4

Patients with claudication of a lower extremity whose symptoms are not severe enough to justify reconstructive arterial surgery frequently undergo percutaneous transluminal angioplasty (PTA). Regular graduated exercise therapy can also improve symptoms in patients with intermittent claudication. These 2 treatments were compared in a randomized study of 36 patients (mean age, 63 years). Twenty patients had PTA and 16 undertook a program of exercise therapy. Assessment included measurement of resting ankle brachial pressure indices (ABPI) and claudicating and maximum walking distances on a treadmill up to a 10-degree incline.

The mean resting ABPI increased significantly in the PTA group at 3, 6, and 9 months. This increase was not seen at any follow-up period in the exercise group (Fig 5–1). The PTA group had a significant increase in claudicating distance at 3 months but not at the other review periods. In contrast, patients who exercised showed significant increases in mean claudicating distance at 6, 9, 12, and 15 months (Fig 5–2). The mean maximum walking distance increased only at 3 months in the PTA group, and this increase was not significant. Exercise, however, resulted

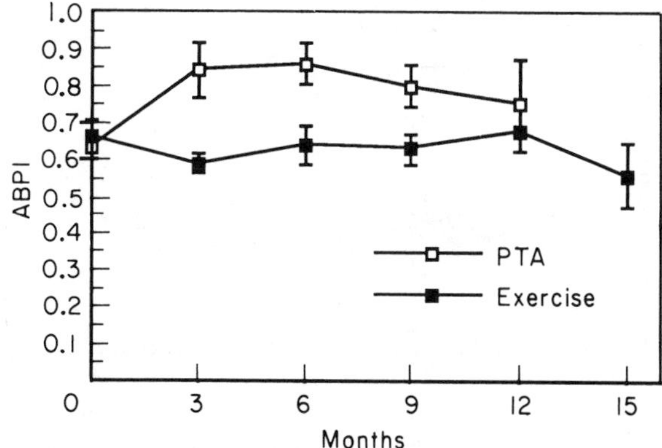

Fig 5–1.—Mean resting ABPI in 2 study groups plotted against time with standard error bars. (Courtesy of Creasy TS, McMillan PJ, Fletcher EWL, et al: *Eur J Vasc Surg* 4:135–140, 1990.)

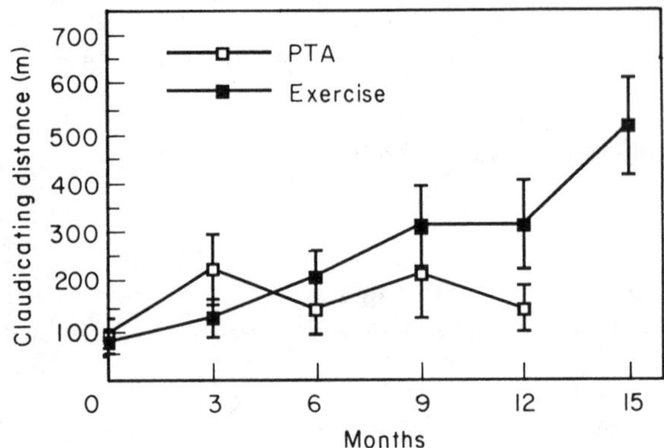

Fig 5–2.—Mean claudicating distance in 2 study groups plotted against time with standard error bars. (Courtesy of Creasy TS, McMillan PJ, Fletcher EWL, et al: *Eur J Vasc Surg* 4:135–140, 1990.)

in significant increases in mean maximum walking distance at 6, 9, 12, and 15 months (Fig 5–3).

Although the mean resting ABPI were not improved with exercise training, patients in this group had significant and progressive increases in both claudicating and maximum walking distances. Thus patients suitable for PTA can obtain better long-term improvement with systematic exercise. Relapse is more common with PTA because of the local nature of the treatment.

▶ The American trial that compared PTA with bypass has been reported. Its conclusions could be paraphrased in simplest terms by saying that PTA was effective and less expensive in the short term, but that long-term follow-up of patients showed that recurrence of the lesions after PTA nullified the initial benefits, both hemodynamically and economically.

The study reported above is much more valuable, because an exercise pro-

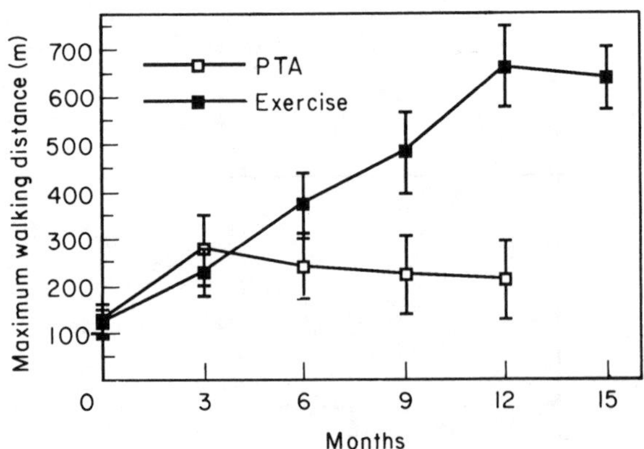

Fig 5–3.—Mean maximum walking distance in 2 study groups plotted against time with standard error bars. (Courtesy of Creasy TS, McMillan PJ, Fletcher EWL, et al: *Eur J Vasc Surg* 4:135–140, 1990.)

gram is more liable to be considered when physicians entertain the thought of doing PTA. There are actually too few patients in the present study to draw any firm conclusions. However, these preliminary results suggest that PTA improves hemodynamics without increasing walking distance and exercise programs increase walking distance without improving ankle brachial index. From the outcomes reported in this collection of abstracts published in this YEAR BOOK, it appears that both an exercise program and the PTA are superior to pentoxifylline.

Benefit of Exercise Conditioning for Patients With Peripheral Arterial Disease

Hiatt WR, Regensteiner JG, Hargarten ME, Wolfel EE, Brass EP (Univ of Colorado)

Circulation 81:602–609, 1990 5–5

Exercise training improves walking ability in patients with atherosclerotic peripheral arterial disease of the lower extremities. A controlled, prospective study was undertaken to assess the changes in exercise performance for patients with peripheral arterial disease and to study the possible mechanisms associated with improvement. Nineteen men with disabling intermittent claudication were randomly assigned to treated and control groups. The exercise training program consisted of supervised treadmill walking for 1 hour daily, 3 days per week, for 12 weeks, with progressive increases in speed and grade as tolerated. Patients were evaluated before and after 12 weeks of training by graded treadmill testing performed to maximal toleration of claudication pain.

After 12 weeks of training, significant increases in peak walking times (123%), peak oxygen consumption (30%), and pain-free walking time (165%) were noted in treated patients. In contrast, peak oxygen consumption did not change in controls, although peak walking time increased by 20% after 12 weeks. Maximal calf blood flow increased significantly after training, but there was no correlation between peak walking time and change in blood flow. A 26% reduction in the resting plasma short-chain acylcarnitine concentration in the treated patients correlated significantly with the improvement in peak walking time, whereas no such changes occurred in the controls.

A 12-week exercise training program for patients with peripheral arterial disease increases peak exercise performance, delays the onset and progression of claudication pain, and improves community-based walking ability. Improvement in exercise performance correlates with improved skeletal muscle oxidative metabolism but not with a change in blood flow. A supervised exercise rehabilitation program is an important treatment option for patients with peripheral arterial disease.

▶ Our colleagues in cardiac vascular surgery allow their patients to pursue exercise programs after surgery. In reviewing the results of exercise programs in patients with claudication, the inescapable conclusion is that patients with peripheral arterial disease would profit by a 12-week exercise program as outlined in this abstract. Perhaps, an exercise rehabilitation program much similar to the cardiac rehabilitation program should be an integral part of treatment for claudication.

Is It Possible to Reduce the Risk of Cardiovascular Events in Subjects Suffering From Intermittent Claudication of the Lower Limbs?

Boissel JP, Peyrieux JC, Destors JM (Hôp Neuro-Cardiologique, Lyon, France)

Thromb Haemost 62:681–685, 1989 5–6

Patients with intermittent claudication of the lower limbs are at high risk for thrombotic cardiovascular events. Because platelets are involved in both thrombosis and atherosclerosis, it was hypothesized that platelet antiaggregating agents may reduce the incidence of cardiovascular events. To test this hypothesis, a meta-analysis of randomized, double-blind, placebo-controlled trials involving ticlopidine, a pure antiplatelet agent, was undertaken. Four trials involving 611 patients were studied. Follow–up ranged from 6 to 12 months.

There was a highly significant reduction, from 9% to 3%, in the incidence of fatal or nonfatal cardiovascular events with ticlopidine as compared with placebo. This included reduction in the incidence of fatal and nonfatal myocardial infarction, strokes, transient ischemic attacks, and aggravation of lower limb arterial disease. Side effects that warranted withdrawal from treatment were 2.4 times more common in patients treated with ticlopidine than in those who received a placebo.

Platelet antiaggregating agents can reduce the risk of thromboatherosclerotic events in patients with intermittent claudication of the lower limbs. The hypothesis that platelets are involved in the etiology of thrombosis in atherosclerosis is supported.

▶ If the conclusion drawn from the previous abstract is that exercise programs are of benefit in patients with claudication, the corollary would be that antiplatelet therapy is similarly of benefit, the former to improve quality of life by increasing claudication distance, the latter by extending duration of such comfortable life.

Prevention of Myocardial Infarction and Stroke in Patients With Intermittent Claudication; Effects of Ticlopidine: Results From STIMS, the Swedish Ticlopidine Multicentre Study

Janzon L, Bergqvist D, Boberg J, Boberg M, Eriksson I, Lindgärde F, Persson G (Malmö Gen Hosp; Univ of Lund, Malmö, Academic Hosp; Univ of Uppsala, Sweden)

J Intern Med 227:301–308, 1990 5–7

The Swedish Ticlopidine Multicenter Study (STIMS) was a double-blind, placebo-controlled trial intended to show whether the platelet antiaggregatory drug ticlopidine can reduce the risks of stroke and myocardial infarction in patients with intermittent claudication. Nearly 700 patients were followed for 5 years or until an end point was reached. End points included stroke, myocardial infarction, and transient ischemic attacks. The dose of ticlopidine was 250 mg twice daily.

Overall mortality was 29% lower in ticlopidine-treated patients. End points were lowered by 10% in the ticlopidine group; the effect was explained by decreased mortality from ischemic heart disease. Side effects were more frequent with ticlopidine than in the placebo group; diarrhea was most frequent. One ticlopidine-treated patient had temporary pancytopenia. Bleeding problems occurred in 16 ticlopidine-treated and 9 placebo patients.

Ticlopidine is associated with reduced mortality from ischemic heart and cerebrovascular disease in patients with intermittent claudication. Side effects are fairly frequent, but there are few serious, permanent adverse effects.

▶ This abstract confirms the preliminary information reported in the previous abstract, Abstract 5–6.

6 Preoperative Consideration

Forefoot Transcutaneous Oxygen Tension at Different Leg Positions in Patients With Peripheral Vascular Disease

Larsen JF, Jensen BV, Christensen KS, Egeblad K (Aalborg Sygehus, Aalborg, Denmark)

Eur J Vasc Surg 4:185–189, 1990 6–1

Measurement of transcutaneous oxygen tension ($TcPo_2$), a noninvasive method of assessing the severity of peripheral vascular disease (PVD), does not always distinguish patients with moderate PVD from healthy subjects. Measurements have been obtained during exercise, after temporary ischemia, and at various leg positions.

In an attempt to increase the accuracy of measurements of $TcPo_2$, measurements were obtained at rest in the forefoot in the sitting and supine positions for 128 patients (150 legs) with 4 different stages of PVD: ischemic pain only during exercise, ischemic rest pain but without chronic ulceration, ischemic rest pain with ulceration, diabetics with rest pain and ulceration. A control group contained 18 healthy subjects (36 legs).

Measurements of $TcPo_2$ obtained at the forefoot of patients in the sitting and supine positions made it possible to differentiate controls from the patient group. Measurements could also identify patients with different degrees of PVD. In the supine position the median $TcPo_2$ was 12 mm Hg in patients with severe PVD, 50 mm Hg in patients with moderate PVD, and 60 mm Hg in controls. Severe ischemia is suggested by a $TcPo_2$ of less than 40 mm Hg at the forefoot in the supine position. Supine measurements of $TcPo_2$ and toe systolic pressure are equally accurate in discriminating between the various stages of PVD.

The overlap values of $TcPo_2$ obtained in patients with different stages of PVD reflects the continuous spectrum of the disease, not the accuracy of the methods. Measurement of $TcPo_2$ is easy to perform, noninvasive, and causes the patient no discomfort.

▶ Measurement of transcutaneous oxygen is indeed noninvasive, easy, and causes the patient no discomfort, but so is obtaining Doppler ankle pressures and toe pressures. The latter technique is also quicker to perform, easier for the technician, and cheaper for the institution.

A Prospective Comparison of Intra-Arterial Digital Subtraction and Conventional Angiography Prior to Lower Extremity Revascularization

Friedman SG, Moccio CG (North Shore Univ Hosp; Cornell Univ, Manhasset, NY)

J Cardiovasc Surg 30:462–466, 1989 6–2

Although intra-arterial digital subtraction angiography (IADSA) is considered a useful adjunct to conventional angiography before lower limb revascularization, it is not clear whether it should be the sole examination. A prospective comparison study of the 2 techniques was undertaken in 60 patients scheduled for lower extremity revascularization. The 30 patients having each procedure were demographically and clinically similar.

All conventional angiograms gave an accurate picture of the severity and distribution of disease. Five IADSA procedures were difficult because of attempted anastomosis to ill-suited vessels. The severity of disease had been underestimated in these 5 cases. Two of the patients had disease at the iliac level and 3 had disease at the popliteal level.

Intra-arterial digital subtraction angiography should not replace conventional angiography in the evaluation of patients with peripheral vascular disease. It may, however, be added when distal runoff vessels are not visualized with conventional imaging. The IADSA technique is most problematic in the assessment of larger vessels, because its lack of detail and resolution can produce misleading findings.

▶ It seems that each additional diagnostic technique is only additive to previous techniques and not a replacement. If this is true, then the cost of evaluation of patients must increase sequentially with every improved method of diagnosis. Perhaps this cycle will be broken when magnetic resonance arteriography becomes universally available. That method might produce total body arteriography in a single examination performed without injection of contrast media. An intriguing possibility.

Sequential Analysis of Staphylococcal Colonization of Body Surfaces of Patients Undergoing Vascular Surgery

Levy MF, Schmitt DD, Edmiston CE, Bandyk DF, Krepel CJ, Seabrook GR, Towne JB (Med College of Wisconsin, Milwaukee)

J Clin Microbiol 28:664–669, 1990 6–3

Slime production by coagulase-negative staphylococci enhances their adherence and persistence on vascular prosthetic grafts. Slime production and antimicrobial resistance were studied by culturing abdominal and inguinal skin sites in 41 consecutive patients hospitalized for lower extremity revascularization.

A total of 330 staphylococcal species were recovered from 21 patients who underwent revascularization; 49% were *Staphylococcus epidermidis*, 22% were *Staphylococcus haemolyticus*, and 20% were *Staphylococ-*

cus hominis. Slime-producing coagulase-negative staphylococci were recovered at admission from 81% of patients, at surgery from 48%, and 5 days after surgery from only 38%.

From admission to day 5 after operation, all *S. epidermidis* isolates showed increasing multiple resistance to gentamicin, clindamycin, trimethoprim-sulfamethoxazole, erythromycin, and methicillin. *Staphylococcus haemolyticus* also acquired multiple drug resistance. Susceptibility to vancomycin and ciprofloxacin was shown by all coagulase-negative staphylococcal isolates.

The presence of slime-producing coagulase-negative staphylococci in patients undergoing revascularization is a risk factor for infection of vascular grafts. Antimicrobial prophylaxis, which may preferentially select strains that exhibit microbial resistance, provides an independent risk factor for such infection.

▶ The Milwaukee group has educated all of us to the frequency of contamination of arterial anastomoses with *S. epidermidis.* The results of this study are frightening indeed.

Combining Clinical and Thallium Data Optimizes Preoperative Assessment of Cardiac Risk Before Major Vascular Surgery

Eagle KA, Coley CM, Newell JB, Brewster DC, Darling RC, Strauss HW, Guiney TE, Boucher CA (Massachusetts Gen Hosp, Boston)

Ann Intern Med 110:859–866, 1989 6–4

Preoperative cardiac evaluation of patients undergoing major surgery is important in identifying high-risk patients in whom special monitoring or treatment may help to improve outcomes. This evaluation is especially important in patients considered for major vascular surgery, whose prevalence of severe underlying coronary disease is about 33% and whose cardiac ischemic events account for more than 50% of postoperative deaths. The results of preoperative screening and short-term outcomes of 200 patients undergoing nonemergent vascular surgery were evaluated. The ability of clinical features and dipyridamole-thallium imaging to predict postoperative ischemic events was compared.

Of the 200 patients studied, 30 had 1 or more postoperative ischemic events. Six patients died of cardiac causes. Acute nonfatal myocardial infarction occurred in 4.5%, unstable angina pectoris in 8.5%, and acute ischemia-related pulmonary edema in 4.5%. Of all patients with postoperative ischemic events, including all 6 who died, 83% had thallium redistribution on preoperative dipyridamole-thallium imaging. The univariate correlates of the postoperative end points of cardiac death or myocardial infarction included a history of angina, congestive heart failure, and diabetes mellitus. Gallop of S_3 on evaluation and pathologic Q wave on ECG were correlated with postoperative ischemic outcomes.

Two of 4 dipyridamole-thallium test variables correlated with ischemic events—ischemic ECG changes during dipyridamole infusion and thallium redistribution. Of the 64 patients with none of the 4 clinical variables—Q wave on ECG, age more than 70 years, history of angina, history of ventricular ectopic activity necessitating treatment, and diabetes mellitus requiring treatment—only 2 patients had postoperative cardiac ischemic events. None of these patients died. Ten of the 20 patients with 3 or more of these variables had postoperative ischemic events.

Preoperative dipyridamole-thallium imaging is most useful in stratifying patients determined to be at intermediate risk by clinical examination. Thallium redistribution correlates with substantial change in probability of events in patients with 1 or 2 clinical predictors. However, for almost 50% of patients, thallium imaging may be unnecessary because of very high or low cardiac risk according to clinical assessment.

▶ This study suggests that the clinical examination may be quite valuable. It certainly is less expensive.

Eliminating Homologous Blood Transfusions During Abdominal Aortic Aneurysm Repair

Pittman RD, Inahara T (St Vincent Hosp and Med Ctr, Portland, Ore)
Am J Surg 159:522–524, 1990 6–5

Increased use of autologous predonation and intraoperative salvage are needed to eliminate homologous blood transfusions during abdominal aortic aneurysm (AAA) repair. The transfusion histories of 100 consecutive patients undergoing elective AAA repairs were reviewed to determine the quantity of predonated blood needed to avoid the use of homologous blood.

A total of 445 units of blood were transfused. The number of units required was directly proportional to the size of the aneurysm; 166 (37%) units of blood were homologous and 279 (63%) were autologous. Of the autologous units, 255 (91%) were from intraoperative salvage and 24 (9%) were predonated. Stratification of transfusions by size showed that for aneurysms no more than 7 cm in size, 132 units of homologous blood and 21 of predonated blood were transfused. For aneurysms larger than 7 cm, 34 units of homologous blood and 3 of predonated blood were transfused.

Predonation of blood before surgery of a minimum 2 units for patients with smaller aneurysms combined with intraoperative salvage should eliminate the need for homologous blood transfusions associated with elective AAA repair. For larger aneurysms, 3 units per patient would be needed.

▶ The conclusions of this study can prove to be quite valuable in selected patients.

Frequency and Significance of Early Postoperative Silent Myocardial Ischemia in Patients Having Peripheral Vascular Surgery

Ouyang P, Gerstenblith G, Furman WR, Golueke PJ, Gottlieb SO (Francis Scott Key Med Ctr, Baltimore)

Am J Cardiol 64:1113–1116, 1989 6–6

Coronary disease causes most perioperative complications after peripheral vascular surgery. To determine the frequency of silent perioperative myocardial ischemia and its relation to postoperative clinical ischemia, 24 patients with stable coronary disease were monitored continuously by ECG before, during, and after peripheral revascularization.

Perioperative silent ischemia was detected in 63% of patients; it was postoperative in 100% of these patients, but preoperative in only 13%. The patients with perioperative silent ischemia did not differ from those without silent ischemia in clinical characteristics, perioperative medication for angina, or postoperative hemodynamic instability. However, 53% of those with silent ischemia later had clinical ischemic events in the hospital, compared with 11% of those without silent ischemic events, which is a significant difference.

Silent myocardial ischemia is frequent in the early period after peripheral vascular surgery and is significantly associated with clinical ischemic events in the later postoperative period. Use of computerized equipment might permit immediate recognition of transient myocardial ischemia and the use of anti-ischemic therapy.

7 Thoracic Aorta

Familial Aortic Dissecting Aneurysm

Nicod P, Bloor C, Godfrey M, Hollister D, Pyeritz RE, Dittrich H, Polikar R, Peterson KL (Univ of California, San Diego; Shriners Hosp for Crippled Children, Portland, Ore; Johns Hopkins Med Insts)

J Am Coll Cardiol 13:811–819, 1989 7–1

Nine members in 2 generations of a single family had aortic or arterial dilatation or a dissecting aortic aneurysm when young. The family has been followed since 1977. None of the patients had Marfan's syndrome or a history of systemic hypertension.

Three family members died of ruptured aortic dissecting aneurysm and acute hemopericardium before age 25 years. Another died suddenly at age 40, a few years after repair of aortic aneurysmal dilatation. One subject is alive after repair of a dissecting ascending aortic aneurysm at age 18. Examination of the aortic wall showed a loss of elastic fibers and deposition of mucopolysaccharide-like material in the arterial media. In addition, cystic medial changes were present. Collagen from cultured fibroblasts appeared normal on gel electrophoretic analysis, and results of immunofluorescence studies also were normal.

A genetic disorder transmitted by autosomal-dominant inheritance is likely in this family. The findings suggest that dissecting aortic aneurysms may be determined genetically. Possibly, the disease is an unclassified heritable disorder of connective tissue with manifestations confined largely to the arterial media.

▶ It appears that the most likely explanation for the findings described in this abstract is an autosomal-dominant inheritance of the defect.

Dissecting Aneurysm: A Clinicopathologic and Histopathologic Study of 111 Autopsied Cases

Nakashima Y, Kurozumi T, Sueishi K, Tanaka K (Kyushu Univ, Fukuoka, Japan)

Hum Pathol 21:291–296, 1990 7–2

The pathogenesis of a dissecting aneurysm remains uncertain. Although cystic medial necrosis (CMN) has been considered a pathognomonic finding, recent studies show that it is not frequently present. The autopsy findings in 111 patients seen in 1975–1985 were reviewed.

Hemorrhage caused by aneurysmal rupture was the chief cause of death; it occurred most commonly in the acute phase. Accompanying disease or an obvious cause of aneurysm other than hypertension was found in 16 patients. Hypertension was present in nearly 75% of the other pa-

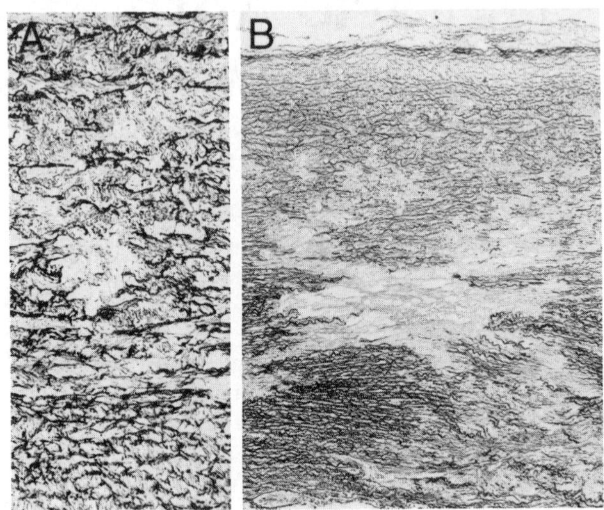

Fig 7–1.—Cystic medial necrosis. **A,** large CMN found in the ascending aorta of type I dissection in a 69-year-old woman. (Elastica van-Gieson's stain; original magnification, ×29.) **B,** small CMN found in the descending aorta of a type III dissection in a 45-year-old man. (Elastica van-Gieson's stain; original magnification, ×114.) (Courtesy of Nakashima Y, Kurozumi T, Sueishi K, et al: *Hum Pathol* 21:291–296, 1990.)

tients. An intimal tear was found in 99 patients. Cystic medial necrosis was present in 9 of 11 patients with Marfan's syndrome and in 19 of the remaining 100 patients (Fig 7–1). Laminar medial necrosis (LMN) (Fig 7–2) was present in 39% of all patients, and was comparably frequent in

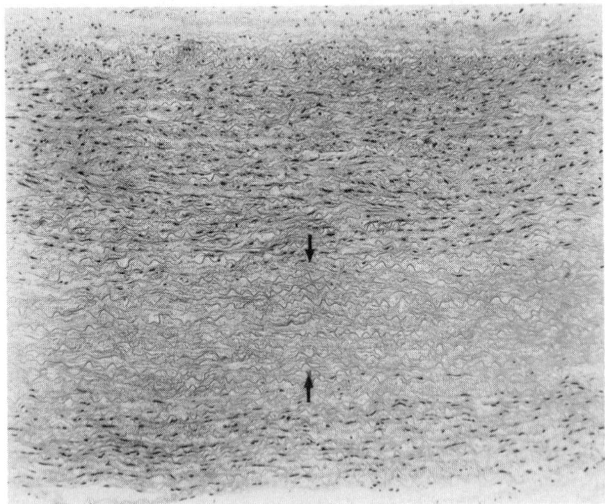

Fig 7–2.—Laminar medial necrosis. Laminar loss of smooth muscle cells found in the ascending aorta of a 34-year-old woman with type I dissection and Marfan's syndrome *(between arrows)*. A false lumen was present at the lowest part, and several layers of well-preserved medial laminae were found between LMN and the false lumen. (Hematoxylin-eosin; original magnification, ×71.) (Courtesy of Nakashima Y, Kurozumi T, Sueishi K, et al: *Hum Pathol* 21:291–296, 1990).

those with and those without Marfan's syndrome. Atherosclerosis often involved the media and disrupted elastic fibers, but the dissection did not occur in this part of the vessel.

Dissecting aneurysms in most patients remain of uncertain origin. Cystic medial necrosis is not prominent in patients who do not have Marfan's syndrome, and laminar medial necrosis is considered to be a secondary ischemic change consequent to dissection. Dissection appeared to be caused directly by atherosclerotic disease in only a few patients.

▶ It seems there are more questions than answers in the study of pathologic specimens of dissecting aneurysms. Questions that require answers include these; What is the relationship of the atherosclerotic process to the dissection? What is the influence of hypertension on dissection? How is CMN related to dissection? What is the pathogenesis of laminar medial necrosis? Do alterations occur in the chemical composition of collagen, or do biochemical changes occur in elastin?

Medial Smooth-Muscle Cell Lesions and Dissection of the Aorta and Muscular Arteries

Hartman JD, Eftychiadis AS (Albert Einstein Med Ctr, Philadelphia)
Arch Pathol Lab Med 114:50–61, 1990 7–3

No specific lesion has ever been documented as the predisposing cause of arterial dissections. The morphological features of lesions that appeared to cause medial hemorrhages, some of which progressed to dissection, were reviewed.

In 1 patient had dissections of the aortic, coronary, renal, and common iliac arteries associated with pregnancy. Myxomatous cystic changes, fibrosis and collagen degeneration, elastin fragmentation, vacuolar degeneration, and coagulation necrosis in areas of smooth-muscle cell proliferation were associated with hemorrhage. In 3 other patients with lesions not related to pregnancy but to hypertension or strenuous exercise, these changes usually were identified, often in the plane of dissection of muscular and aortic arteries (Fig 7–3). In these patients the dissections appeared to result from smooth-muscle cell activity, which involved systemic vasculopathy in patterns that seemed to result from medial smooth-muscle cell metabolism.

The histologic changes related to dissections appear to result from metabolism of medial smooth-muscle cells acting as a multifunctional mesenchyma. Variable penetrance of a gene that controls such metabolism could predispose to dissection in patients subjected to such other variables as pregnancy, hypertension, or strenuous physical activity.

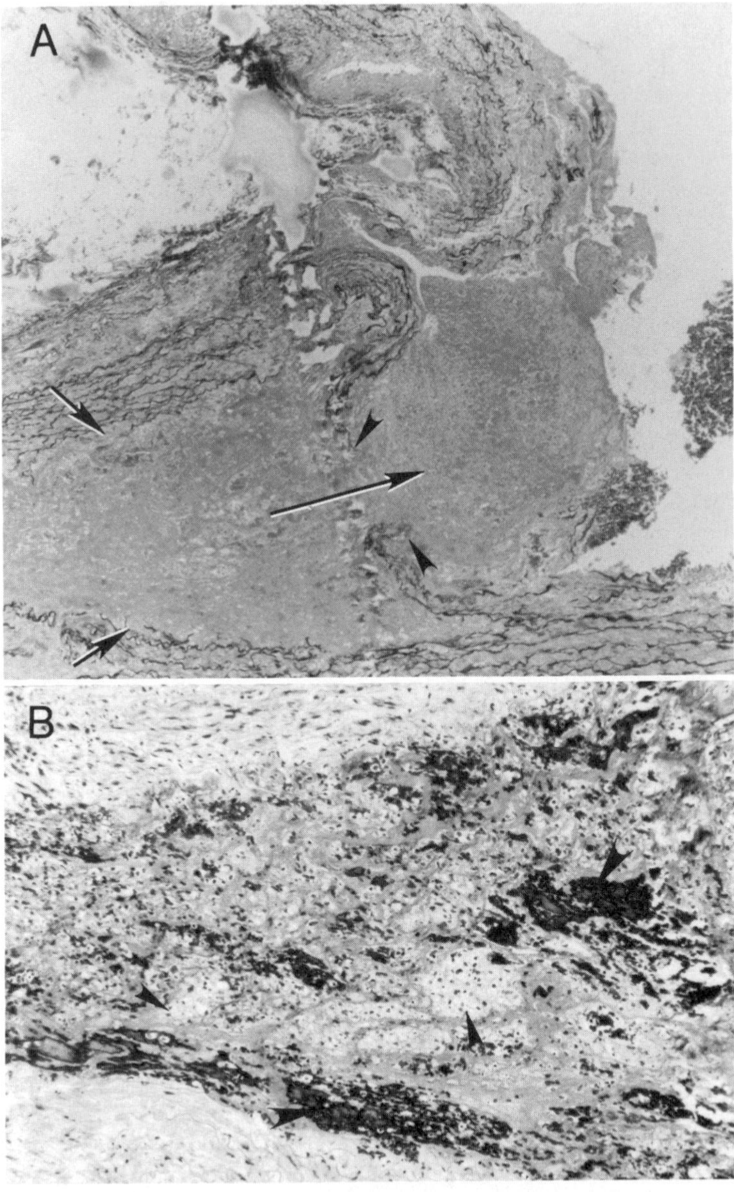

Fig 7–3.—Possible origin of aortic dissection. **A,** ascending aorta. Configuration of fragmented arterial media *(arrowsheads)* suggests direction of hemorrhage *(long arrow)* into dissection channel from origin of hemorrhage (between *short arrows*) (Verhoeff's elastic; original magnification, ×7). **B,** higher power of area between *short arrows* showing pools of blood coagulum *(large arrowheads)* in area of degenerate collagen with smooth-muscle cells showing vacuolar degeneration *(small arrowhead)*. Blood coagulum stains differently than cytoplasm of necrotic smooth-muscle cells (Goldner trichrome; ×35). (Courtesy of Hartman JD, Eftychiadis AS: *Arch Pathol Lab Med* 114:50–61, 1990.)

▶ This fascinatingly complete article appears to identify a combination of specific lesions in the media of arteries even remote from the planes of dissection. These lesions include smooth-muscle cell proliferation, fibroplasia, coagulation necrosis, and vacuolar degeneration.

Fenestration Revisited: A Safe and Effective Procedure for Descending Aortic Dissection

Elefteriades JA, Hammond GL, Gusberg RJ, Kopf GS, Baldwin JC (Yale Univ)
Arch Surg 125:786–790, 1990 7–4

Aortic fenestration is far from a new procedure, but in recent years it has not been widely used. This procedure was performed in 10 men and 2 women aged 41–88 years with descending aortic dissection with organ ischemia, i.e., lower extremity ischemia, renal ischemia, or paraplegia. In this operation the infrarenal abdominal aorta is completely transected, as much dissected intima as possible is removed, and the aorta is reapproximated after first suturing the intimal and adventitial layers in the lower segment (Fig 7–4).

All 12 patients survived the operation and 7 were alive after a mean follow-up of nearly 7 years. Organ perfusion returned immediately in all

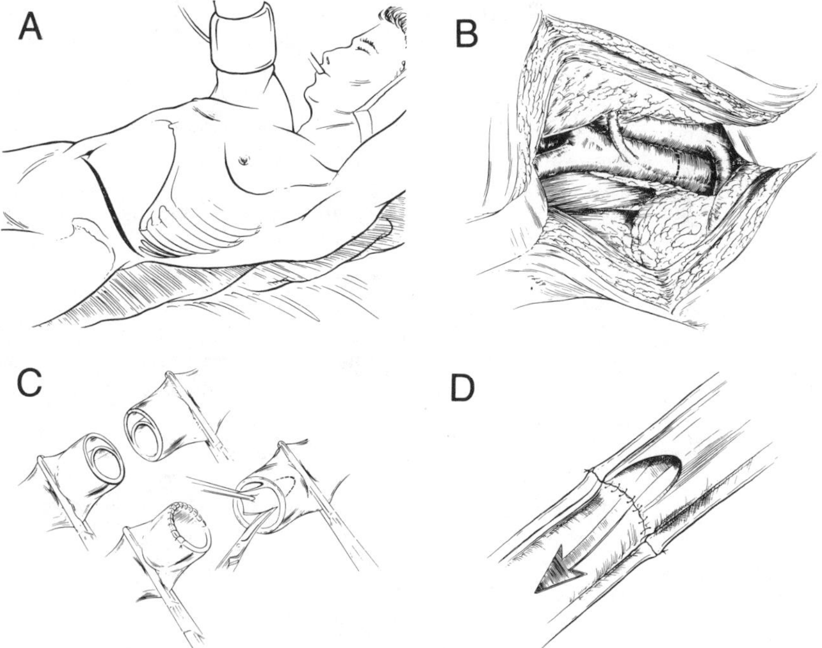

Fig 7–4.—Schema of fenestration procedure. Incision (**A**), exposure of aorta; (**B**), transection of aorta with double lumen visible and resection of intima proximally (**C**), and suturing of adventitial aorta above to reconstituted distal aorta below (**D**). (Courtesy of Elefteriades JA, Hammond GL, Gusberg RJ, et al: *Arch Surg* 125:786–790, 1990.)

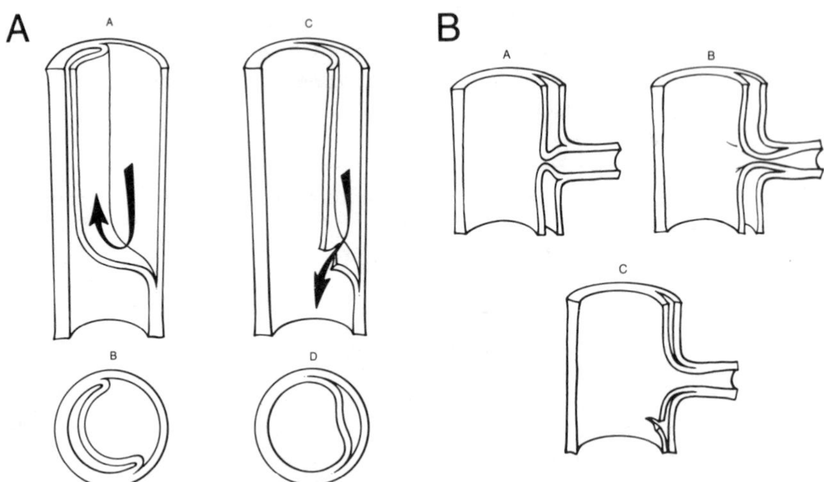

Fig 7–5.—**A,** schema showing aortic occlusion by tense lumen and ameliorization by reentry. **B,** schema showing branch vessel occlusion by tense false lumen and ameliorization by reentry. (Courtesy of Elefteriades JA, Hammond GL, Gusberg RJ, et al: *Arch Surg* 125:786–790, 1990.)

patients but 1. There were no deaths from late rupture, and no surviving patient has had aortic or ischemic problems. The pathophysiology of aortic and branch vessel occlusion (Fig 7–5) makes it plausible that decompression of the false lumen by fenestration may reduce the obstruction caused by a tense false lumen.

Aortic fenestration is a safe and clinically effective procedure. It is best done at the level of the abdominal aorta as soon as there is evidence of organ ischemia. Long-term survival is acceptable. At present, fenestration is not recommended for acute dissection with rupture or impending rupture, or for chronic aortic dissection if aortic enlargement mandates surgery.

▶ For those of us who were disappointed with experience in fenestration of the aorta in the treatment of dissection, this is a somewhat nostalgic report. It should be emphasized that fenestration of the aorta is not to be used in treatment of the acute process, because fenestration does not prevent rupture of the dissection into the pericardium or externally.

Outcome of 290 Patients With Aortic Dissection: A 12-Year Multicentre Experience

Chirillo F, Marchiori MC, Andriolo L, Razzolini R, Mazzucco A, Gallucci V, Chioin R (Universita' di Padova, Italy)

Eur Heart J 11:311–319, 1990 7–5

There are at least 2,000 new cases of spontaneous aortic dissection per year in the United States. The availability of more accurate diagnostic methods and the refinement of surgical procedures have dramatically changed the prognosis in these patients. The clinical, hemodynamic, and angiographic data collected by questionnaire from 11 catheterization laboratories in northern Italy were reviewed retrospectively.

During an 12-year study period, 290 patients had an angiographic diagnosis of aortic dissection, including 217 (mean age, 55 years) who had dissection involving the ascending aorta and 73 (mean age, 61 years) who had distal dissection. Emergency catheterization was performed in 199 patients, and elective aortography was done in 91. Shock, tamponade, acute myocardial infarction, renal failure, or heart failure occurred in 68 of the 199 patients who underwent emergency aortography and in 11 of the 91 who had elective catheterization.

Nine patients were lost to follow-up, 23 died before any therapy could be given, 39 were not operated on, and 219 underwent emergency operation (Fig 7–6). Of latter 219 patients, 101 died within 30 days after operation and 118 were discharged alive. Fourteen of the 118 patients who were discharged after operation died subsequently, 5 were lost to follow-up, and 99 were still alive. Ten of the patients not operated on were still alive, 25 died, and 4 were lost to follow-up. Only 2 of the 39 patients who were not operated on were referred for medical treatment; the other 37 could not undergo surgery because of their overall poor condition. Most survivors were symptom free, but all were monitored at regular intervals and took drugs to control hypertension and reduce inotropism.

During the 12-year period there was a significant increase in the number of diagnosed cases, a significant increase in the number of operations, and a significant decline in operative mortality. Acute myocardial infarction, persistent shock, and persistent CNS deficit were significant inde-

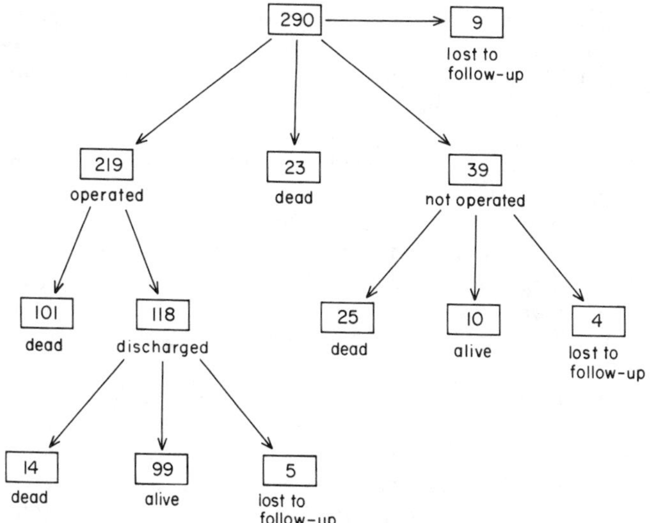

Fig 7–6.—Outcome of 290 patients with aortic dissection diagnosed over a 12-year period. (Courtesy of Chirillo F, Marchiori MC, Andriolo L, et al: *Eur Heart J* 11:311–319, 1990.)

pendent predictors of operative mortality in patients with dissection involving the ascending aorta. Persistent shock was the only independent predictor of operative mortality in those with distal aortic dissection. The overall late mortality related to aortic dissection in patients who underwent surgical treatment was 8.8%.

▶ It is somewhat surprising that the overall late mortality related to aortic dissection was so low in this collected group of patients.

Thoracic Aortic Aneurysms After Acute Type A Aortic Dissection: Necessity for Follow-Up

Heinemann M, Laas J, Karck M, Borst HG (Hannover Med School, Hannover, West Germany)

Am Thoracic Surg 49:580–584, 1990 7–6

Acute type A aortic dissection requires emergency surgical intervention to prevent death by rupture of the ascending aorta. However, emergency operation is limited to the area of highest risk, i.e., the proximal portion of the aorta. In most patients the remainder of the aorta is left dissected, which often leads to further complications that require reoperation. Dilatation with ultimate rupture of the distal aorta is the most common cause of late death in the survivors. Scrupulous long-term follow-up by CT and digital subtraction angiography to detect changes in the residual aorta are therefore mandatory.

During a 10-year period, 86 patients (mean age, 48 years) underwent emergency operation on the ascending aorta for acute type A aortic dissection. Of the patients, 23 had reconstruction of the ascending aorta with or without aortic valve reconstruction, 33 had the ascending aorta replaced by a tubular prosthetic graft with or without aortic valve reconstruction, and 30 had aortic valve replacement by a composite graft or by separate replacement of the valve and the ascending aorta. The native aortic valve was retained in 56 patients.

A total of 64 patients survived the operation, none of whom died of late aortic complications. Follow-up data were available for 58 patients. After a mean follow-up of 3 years, dilatation of the distal aorta, which ranged from 6 to 10.5 cm in diameter, developed in 10 of these patients. Six patients underwent replacement of the descending aorta within 1–21 months after primary aortic dissection repair; 2 of these required third-stage thoracoabdominal replacement. One of 2 patients for whom replacement of the descending aorta was scheduled died before operation. Another patient refused reoperation. Two patients underwent aortic arch replacement, and another was scheduled to undergo aortic arch replacement as a fourth-stage procedure. None of the 10 patients reoperated on died. In all, 12 of the 58 patients for whom follow-up data were available either underwent, or were scheduled to undergo, 17 reoperations—14 for aneurysm formation in the thoracic aorta and 3 because of complications at the primary site.

Patients who survive emergency operation for acute type A aortic dissection are at considerable risk of dying of late complications, notably aneurysm formation with aortic rupture. As follow-up of these patients by cardiologists is often not systematic, it is suggested that follow-up be directed by the cardiovascular surgeon, as timely reoperation sharply reduces postoperative mortality from aortic rupture.

▶ In this report from Hannover, the mortality of aortic replacement is seen to decrease from 20% to near 0, and the aggressive postoperative follow-up has shown that extensive dilation of the distal aorta occurs with great frequency and must be monitored carefully.

Assessment of Transesophageal Doppler Echography in Dissecting Aortic Aneurysm

Hashimoto S, Kumada T, Osakada G, Kubo S, Tokunaga S, Tamaki S, Yamazato A, Nishimura K, Ban T, Kawai C (Takeda Hosp; Kyoto Univ, Japan)

J Am Coll Cardiol 14:1253–1262, 1989 7–7

The mortality rate in patients with untreated dissecting aortic aneurysm may be as high as 90% within 3 months. Diagnostic methods include angiography, echocardiography, x-ray CT, and nuclear magnetic resonance imaging. Of these methods, only echocardiography can be performed noninvasively at bedside; however, clear images are often unobtainable because of interference from thoracic tissues.

To improve diagnostic imaging, the technique of 2-dimensional echography was developed. Both transesophageal and conventional echography were carried out in 22 patients with dissecting aortic aneurysm; 17 patients also underwent angiography and 8 underwent x-ray CT. Four patients had both angiography and CT, and 12 patients underwent surgery. The methods were compared in the ascending aorta, aortic arch, thoracic descending aorta, and upper abdominal aorta. The angiographic findings were used as the standard for comparison.

The rate of correct detection of an intimal flap was 100% in all 4 segments in patients assessed by the transesophageal approach, a much better rate than that achieved by conventional echography. The rate of detection of entry sites (Fig 7–7) was also 100% with the transesophageal approach, compared with 42% with the conventional approach. The site of entry could not be detected by x-ray CT in all patients. The transesophageal approach clearly revealed the presence of thrombus, pericardial hemorrhage, and aortic regurgitation. Transesophageal Doppler echography is a rapid, accurate diagnostic method for suspected dissecting aortic aneurysm. The procedure permits prompt evaluation and initiation of appropriate treatment.

▶ Transesophageal echography of the thoracic aorta has arrived.

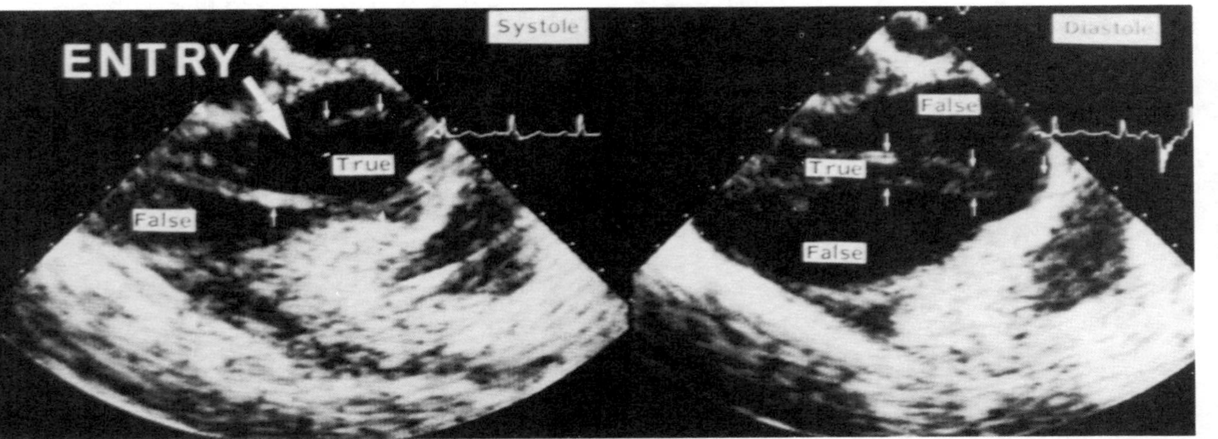

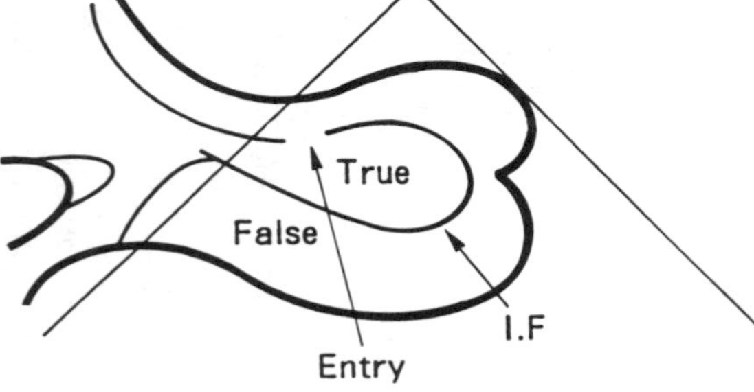

Fig 7–7.—Upper panel, systolic and diastolic images of the ascending aorta obtained by transesophageal Doppler echography (longitudinal scanning probe). **Lower panel,** schematic drawing of the upper left panel. *Small arrows* indicate the intimal flap *(IF)*. The entry was identified as the defect of the intimal flap appearing in systole *(large arrow)*. In diastole, the true lumen was compressed by the false lumen. (Courtesy of Hashimoto S, Kumada T, Osakada G, et al: *J Am Coll Cardiol* 14:1253–1262, 1989.)

Ambulatory Follow-Up of Aortic Dissection by Transesophageal Two-Dimensional and Color-Coded Doppler Echocardiography

Mohr-Kahaly S, Erbel R, Rennollet H, Wittlich N, Drexler M, Oelert H, Meyer J
(Johannes Gutenberg Univ, Mainz, Germany)

Circulation 80:24–33, 1989 7–8

The role of angiography in the diagnosis of acute aortic dissection has recently been questioned as less invasive methods such as echocardiogra-

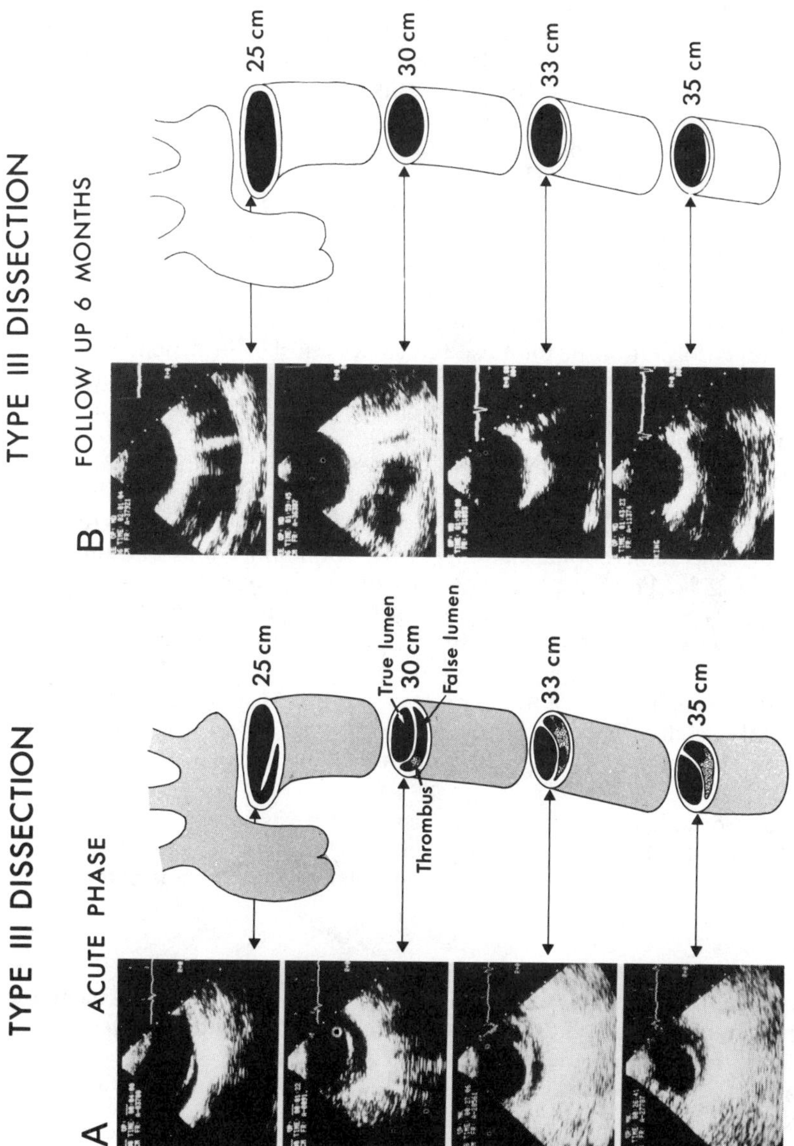

Fig 7–8.—Transesophageal echocardiographic study during acute phase and follow-up in a patient with complete obliteration of the false lumen caused by thrombus formation. (Courtesy of Mohr-Kahaly S, Erbel R, Rennollet H, et al: *Circulation* 80:24–33, 1989.)

phy, CT, and digital subtraction angiography (DSA) have shown increased clinical reliability. Although echocardiography is considered the method of choice, it is less reliable in patients with obesity, pulmonary emphysema, or thorax deformation. To determine whether transesophageal, M-mode, 2-dimensional, and color-coded Doppler echocardiography is more reliable than conventional transthoracic echocardiography for follow-up in patients with aortic dissection, studies were made in 13 men and 5 women aged 23–76 years.

Five patients had type I, 1 had type II, and 12 had type III aortic dissections. All patients were followed by conventional transthoracic and transesophageal 2-dimensional and color-coded Doppler echocardiography performed at 1, 6, and 12 months after the initial diagnosis and once-yearly thereafter. Seven patients were operated on and 11 patients with type III dissections were treated medically with β-blocking agents and calcium antagonists. The mean follow-up period was 15 months.

At the last transesophageal follow-up examination, the false lumen persisted in 5 of the 7 patients operated on and in 9 of the 11 who were treated medically. In 2 patients who were operated on the dissected part of the aorta had been resected, and in 2 medically treated patients progressive and complete obliteration of the false lumen occurred (Fig 7–8). Thrombus formation in the false lumen was absent in 4 patients, localized in 4, and progressive in 6. In 14 patients, flow was seen within the false lumen in 2 distinct patterns: a laminar biphasic flow, and a slowly circulating flow.

Transthoracic echocardiography showed persisting intimal tears in 4 patients, but transesophageal color-coded Doppler showed an additional 1–3 intimal tears in the descending aorta of 10 patients. Flow across the aperture was bidirectional in 75% of the communications and unidirectional in 25%. Transesophageal echocardiography also provided accurate information concerning complications, including extension of the dissection in 1 patient and aortic regurgitation in 3 others. The transesophageal approach was superior to conventional echocardiography, especially in the descending thoracic aorta. Transesophageal, M-mode, 2-dimensional, and color-coded Doppler echocardiography is an ideal, well-tolerated noninvasive method for the detection and follow-up of aortic dissection.

▶ The color-coded Doppler transesophageal echo has revealed additional intimal tears in the descending thoracic aorta not visualized by other techniques and has shown the beat-to-beat direction of flow within the true and false lumens.

Surgical Treatment of Aneurysm and/or Dissection of the Ascending Aorta, Transverse Aortic Arch, and Ascending Aorta and Transverse Aortic Arch: Factors Influencing Survival in 717 Patients

Crawford ES, Svensson LG, Coselli JS, Safi HJ, Hess KR (Baylor College of Medicine, Houston)

J Thorac Cardiovasc Surg 98:659–674, 1989 7–9

To be successful, treatment of disease of the ascending aorta and arch may need to include extensive graft replacement up to and including the entire aorta. A 9-year experience in the treatment of 717 patients with aneurysm or dissection involving the ascending aorta and transverse aortic arch was analyzed.

The study population consisted of 445 males and 272 females aged 10–88 years (median age, 61 years). Causes of aortic disease included trauma in 6, infection in 20, aortitis in 46, acute dissection in 72, chronic dissection in 189, and medial degeneration in 384 patients. Patients with long-standing disease and older patients often had atherosclerosis superimposed on the basic mural lesions. Of 717 patients, 150 had undergone 173 previous cardiac or aortic operations. Concurrent distal aneurysmal disease was present or developed in 37% of the patients, and it was most prevalent in patients with aortic arch involvement. Aneurysm symptoms were absent or mild in 593 and severe in 124 patients. Atriofemoral cannulation was used in 597 patients. Treatment included ascending aorta or aortic arch reconstruction, or both, by composite valve graft in 281, separate valve graft in 117, graft only in 256, and other procedures in 63 patients.

The 30-day survival rate was 91%. Independent determinants predictive of early death were increasing age, severe aneurysm symptoms, diabetes, previous proximal aortic operation, need for cardiac support, postoperative tracheostomy, postoperative heart dysfunction, and stroke. Survival among 319 patients with none of the 4 preoperative factors was 97%. Survival decreased to 74% among patients with 2 or more of these factors. The entire aorta was replaced in 53 patients, near-total aorta in 35, the entire thoracic artery in 78, and the total aorta except for the arch in 27.

The 5-year survival rate was 66%, and the 7-year survival rate was 57%. Independent predictors of death were severe aneurysm symptoms, preoperative angina, extent of proximal replacement, associated residual distal aneurysm, balloon pump, renal dysfunction, cardiac dysfunction, and stroke. The 5-year survival rate varied with the incidence of the 4 preoperative variables and age present in a single patient: 78% in 413 who had up to 1 variable, 57% in 193 with 2 or 3 variables, and 39% in 111 with 3 or 4 variables. The introduction of profound hypothermic circulatory arrest, composite valve grafting, and other technical improvements has led to more favorable results in the treatment of ascending aorta and arch disease.

▶ This abstract is provided to readers as a ready reference to the original publication. This and the discussion that followed the presentation at the annual meeting of the American Association for Thoracic Surgery is a virtual textbook on the subject.

Diffuse Aneurysmal Disease (Chronic Aortic Dissection, Marfan, and Mega Aorta Syndromes) and Multiple Aneurysm: Treatment by Subtotal and Total Aortic Replacement Emphasizing the Elephant Trunk Operation

Crawford ES, Coselli JS, Svensson LG, Safi HJ, Hess KR (Baylor College of Medicine, Houston; Methodist Hosp, Houston)

Ann Surg 211:521–537, 1990 7–10

Graft replacement therapy can significantly prolong the life expectancy of patients with aortic aneurysm. Complications of residual aortic aneurysmal disease or the development of additional aortic aneurysms are important predictors of late death. Data on 4,170 patients with aneurysmal disease of either dissection or medial degenerative origin were reviewed.

Multiple segment involvement was or became present in 1,262 patients; (30%); 463 (67%) of 694 patients with dissection; and 799 (23%) of 3,476 patients without dissection. Regardless of cause, multiple involvement varied with the location of the presenting involved segment, including the ascending aorta in 38%, ascending and arch in 70%, descending thoracic aorta in 73%, and the abdominal aorta in 26%. Detailed study was limited to 81 patients with ascending and ascending and aortic arch replacement for aneurysm. These patients were divided into 3 groups; 524 with no distal disease (group 1), 135 with distal disease treated by subtotal replacement or total replacement (group 2), and 152 with untreated distal disease (group 3). The 5-year survival rate from the time of first surgery including operative deaths was 75% in group 1,

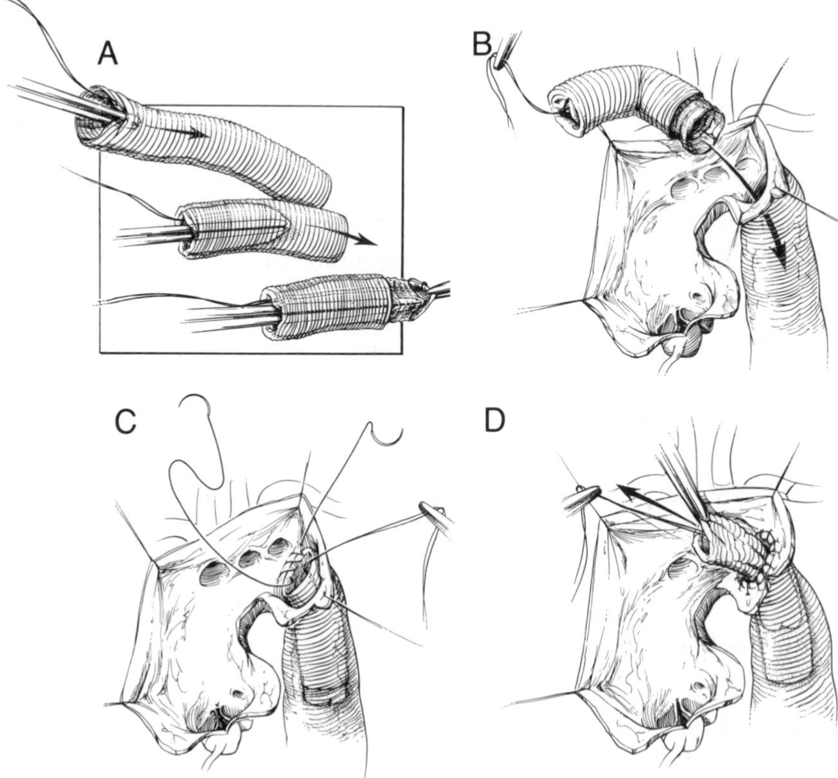

Fig 7–9.—A Dacron graft is inverted on itself (**B**) and inserted into the distal aorta. **C**, the inverted end of the graft is sutured to the aorta beyond the origin of the left subclavian artery. **D**, the inverted end of the graft is withdrawn.

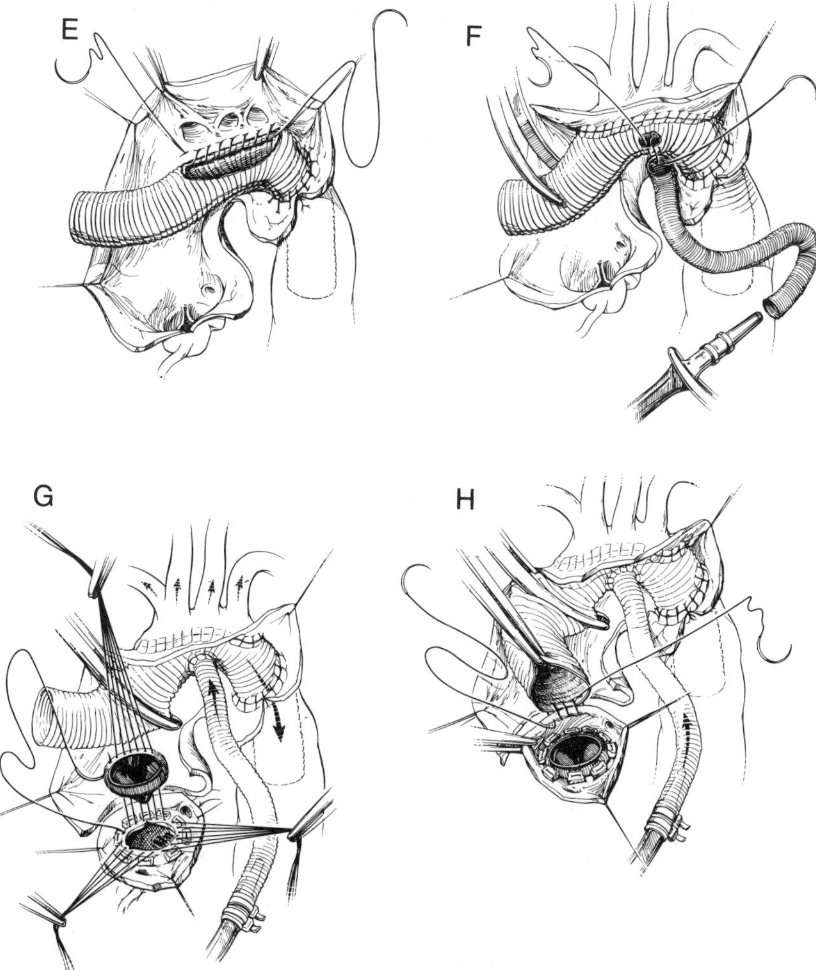

(**Fig 7–9,** *cont'd*).—**E,** an opening is made in the side of the graft and sutured around the origin of the brachiocephalic vessels. **F,** a small tube is attached to the side of aortic graft. **G,** after removing air from distal aorta, antegrade perfusion is performed to prevent cerebral emboli. The aortic valve is replaced (**H**), and the proximal end of the graft is sutured to the proximal aorta near the origins of the coronary arteries. (Courtesy of Crawford ES, Coselli JS, Svensson LG, et al: *Ann Surg* 211:521–537, 1990.)

65% in group 2, and 39% in group 3. Causes of death in group 3 were aneurysmal rupture and/or associated disease.

Initial total aortic study and regular postoperative monitoring with CT is recommended to detect extensive or recurrent disease. Aggressive replacement is indicated in all but those with associated disease that contraindicates surgery (Fig 7–9).

▶ This abstract and the preceding one (Abstract 7–9) are complementary, but the article abstracted here contains many accurate references to history and contains a wealth of information in the figures and other illustrative material.

Preliminary Report of Localization of Spinal Cord Blood Supply by Hydrogen During Aortic Operations

Svensson LG, Patel V, Coselli JS, Crawford ES (Baylor College of Medicine, Houston; Methodist Hosp, Houston)

Ann Thorac Surg 49:528–536, 1990 7–11

Failure to reattach the spinal cord blood supply is 1 cause of paraplegia after surgery on the aorta (Fig 7–10). A rapid new method of identifying cord vessels intraoperatively was evaluated. Using the hydrogen-induced current impulse (HICI) technique, the surgeon can determine which segmental vessels can safely be oversewn and which should be rejoined to the aortic graft.

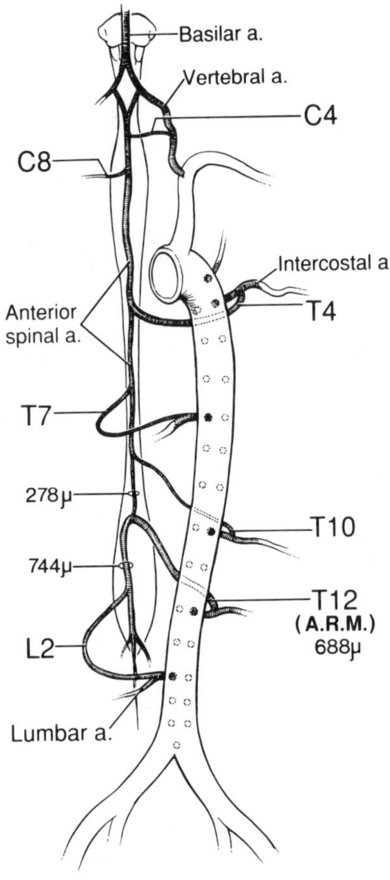

Fig 7–10.—Statistical composite of spinal cord blood supply in primates. The sites of the radicular arteries reflect the most common levels of origin and arrangements found on anatomical dissections. The sizes of the arteries are those of nonhuman primates. The equivalent sizes in humans are the following: arteria radicularis magna (ARM), 871 μm; anterior spinal artery above the ARM, 231 μm; and anterior spinal artery below the ARM, 941 μm. (Courtesy of Svensson LG, Klepp P, Hinder RA: *S Afr J Surg* 24:32–34, 1986. From Svensson LG, Patel V, Coselli JS, et al: *Ann Thorac Surg* 49:528–536, 1990.)

Procedure.—A catheter containing platinum and stainless steel electrodes was inserted intrathecally in pigs, and saline solution saturated with hydrogen was injected sequentially into arterial ostia from T-15 to L-4. The current impulses generated were recorded by the conditioned platinum electrode.

Impulses were detected in all animals immediately after injection of hydrogen solution. Of 28 segmental arteries shown at autopsy to supply the spinal cord, 89% were correctly localized by the HICI technique. All vessels larger than 180 μm in diameter were located. The 3 radicular arteries not identified were at least 3 vertebral levels further away from the platinum electrode.

In this porcine model the radicular arteries supplying the spinal cord are accurately and rapidly localized by the HICI method. The entire spinal cord from the lower thoracic segments caudally can be perfused by these radicular arteries. It appears feasible to use this method to identify arteries that, when reattached during aortic replacement, will preserve spinal function.

▶ In the patients at highest risk, aortic replacement is still associated with a devastating incidence of paraplegia. This is true despite CSF drainage and attachment of all intercostals available. Svensson's continuing interest in this subject and the opportunity to apply this technique with Dr. E.S. Crawford will ultimately provide a useful adjunct that will reduce the incidence of paraplegia.

Cerebrospinal Fluid Drainage and Steroids Provide Better Spinal Cord Protection During Aortic Cross-Clamping Than Does Either Treatment Alone

Woloszyn TT, Marini CP, Coons MS, Nathan IM, Basu S, Acinapura AJ, Cunningham JN (Maimonides Med Ctr; State Univ of New York, Brooklyn)

Ann Thorac Surg 49:78–83, 1990 7–12

It is postulated that the increase in CSF pressure during infusion of sodium nitroprusside (SNP) to control central hypertension during aortic operations may be related to a loss of compliance of the spinal canal secondary to edema of the spinal cord. In addition, CSF drainage is ineffective in reducing the increase in CSF pressure caused by SNP. Because steroids can increase the warm ischemic time of the spinal cord by acting as free radical scavengers and membrane stabilizers and have antiedema effects, a study was undertaken to determine whether steroids could enhance the effects of CSF drainage on spinal cord perfusion pressure and postoperative paraplegia in a canine model in which SNP and partial exsanguination were used to control proximal hypertension.

Dogs were randomized into 3 groups: group 1 acted as control; group 2 was given methyl prednisolone, 30 mg/kg, intravenously 30 minutes before and 4 hours after aortic cross-clamping; in group 3, CSF drainage was performed in addition to steroid therapy. During aortic cross-clamping, blood pressure proximal to the clamp decreased significantly in each group, but did not differ significantly between groups. Similarly, the mean distal pressure decreased after aortic cross-clamping and did not differ between groups. The CSF pressure did not change significantly between groups 1 and 2 but was significantly reduced in group 3. This difference was maintained throughout the aortic cross-clamping interval. The spinal cord perfusion pressure was significantly greater in group 3 compared with groups 1 and 2, but did not differ between the latter groups.

Neurologic outcome, in terms of the incidence of paraplegia, in group 3 was significantly better than in group 1 but did not differ significantly with group 2. In addition, postoperative paraplegia occurred in 2 of 9 animals with positive spinal cord perfusion pressure compared with 7 of 9 animals with negative spinal cord perfusion pressure. Loss of somatosensory evoked potentials occurred significantly earlier in groups 1 and 2 than in group 3, but did not differ significantly between groups 1 and 2. These findings suggest that steroids plus CSF drainage provide spinal cord protection during aortic cross-clamping, whereas steroids alone are ineffective.

▶ The Maimonides research group confirms the previous observations of Blaisdell and Cooley (1) that CSF drainage alone is relatively ineffective.

Reference

1. Blaisdell FW, Cooley DA: *Surgery* 51:351, 1962.

Detection of Dissection of the Aortic Intima and Media After Angioplasty of Coarctation of the Aorta: An Angiographic, Computer Tomographic, and Echocardiographic Comparative Study

Erbel R, Bednarczyk I, Pop T, Todt M, Henrichs KJ, Brunier A, Thelen M, Meyer J (Johannes Gutenberg Univ, Mainz, Germany)

Circulation 81:805–814, 1990 7–13

Percutaneous angioplasty is an effective approach to coarctation of the thoracic aorta, but aneurysm formation related to cystic medial necrosis is a possible complication. Transesophageal echocardiography was used to monitor angioplasty in 8 patients with discrete postductal coarctation not previously operated on or, in 1 case, with postoperative recoarctation. Echocardiography was performed under lidocaine spray anesthesia during balloon angioplasty.

Dilatation was successful in 7 of the 8 patients but failed in the patient who had previously had surgical correction. No aneurysm formation was seen. The diameter of the coarctation site increased significantly, followed by luminal narrowing in some cases in the subsequent 6 months. One patient with persistent pain had medial dissection (Fig 7–11) as well as a thickened aortic wall and an entry tear. The dissection healed spontaneously. Color Doppler echocardiography, done in 5 cases, showed turbulent flow distal to the coarctation that persisted after angioplasty.

Balloon angioplasty can be used effectively to treat coarctation in

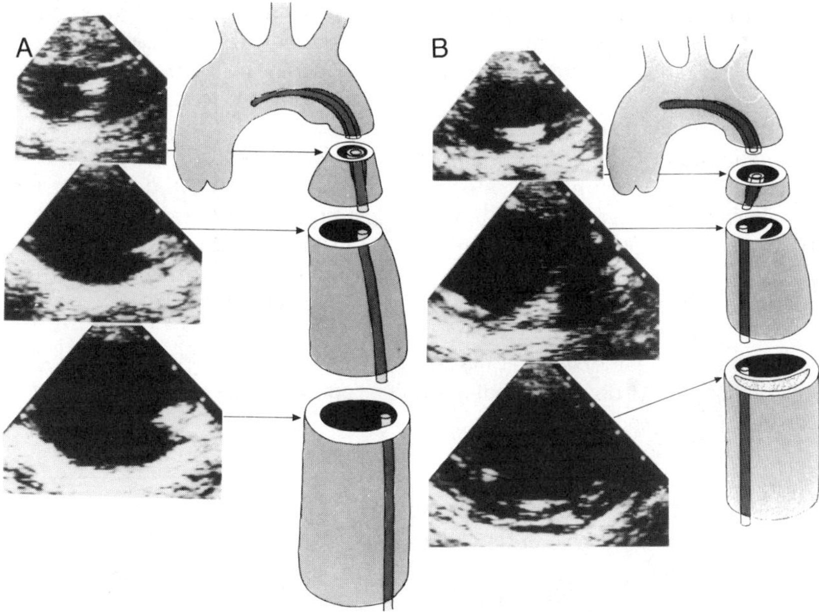

Fig 7–11.—Transesophageal 2-dimensional echocardiographic imaging of aorta before (**A**) and after (**B**) angioplasty of coarctation of aorta that demonstrates medial dissection over 15 cm distally with spontaneous healing after 6 months. (Courtesy of Erbel R, Bednarczyk I, Pop T, et al: *Circulation* 81:805–814, 1990.)

adults younger than 50 years of age. Aortic dissection can be detected by transesophageal echocardiography when this procedure is used to monitor angioplasty.

▶ This report provides nice information on the natural history of a balloon-dilated coarctation and documents by transesophageal color Doppler images the dissections identified.

Aortic Aneurysm After Patch Aortoplasty Repair of Coarctation: A Prospective Analysis of Prevalence, Screening Tests, and Risks
Bromberg BI, Beekman RH, Rocchini AP, Snider AR, Bank ER, Heidelberger K, Rosenthal A (Univ of Michigan)
J Am Coll Cardiol 14:734–741, 1989 7–14

Twenty-nine children who underwent prosthetic patch repair of aortic coarctation at least a year previously were studied prospectively for formation of aneurysm. The mean age at surgery was 6 years, and at the time of evaluation, 11½ years. Thirteen patients had systolic hypertension and 5 were taking antihypertensive medication. Five patients had a residual arm/leg systolic gradient exceeding 20 mm Hg.

Seven patients (24%) had an aneurysm, 6 of whom had had repair with a Dacron patch. One of the children with an aneurysm was hypertensive and 1 had a residual coarctation gradient above 20 mm Hg. Although no clinical factors correlated with aneurysm formation, previous coarctation resection appeared to have a protective effect. Only 1 patient with an aneurysm had a polytetrafluorethylene nontextile patch.

Aortic aneurysms are frequent after patch aortoplasty for coarctation in childhood. A compliance mismatch is probably not the dominant factor, because polytetrafluoroethylene is less compliant than Dacron. Local tissue reaction to the patch may be a more significant factor. Resection of ductal tissue before patch aortoplasty may protect against aneurysm formation. The chest radiograph is a sensitive screening measure.

▶ Although the authors stress the need for follow-up of children with repair of coarctation, they do not mention transesophageal echocardiography as a means of achieving such follow-up.

Aneurysm of the Descending Thoracic Aorta in a Young Woman

Locufier JL, Bosschaerts Th, Barthel J, Delwarte D, Barroy JP (Univ Hosp Saint-Pierre, Brussels)

J Cardiovasc Surg 30:499–502, 1989 7–15

It is rare to diagnose a thoracic aortic aneurysm in an otherwise healthy young woman.

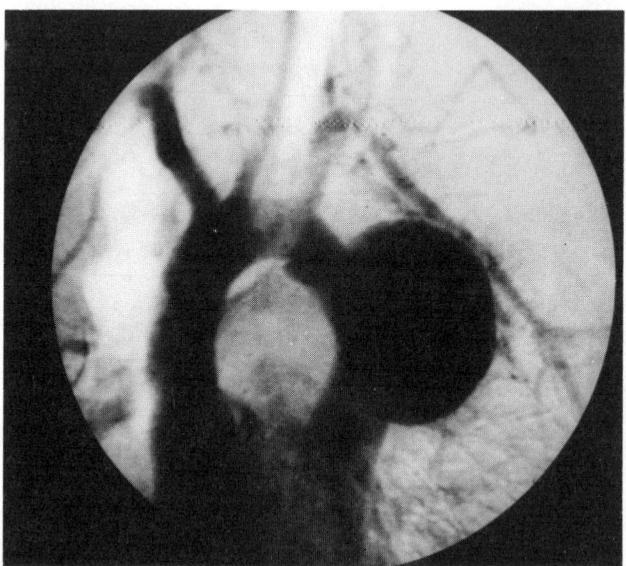

Fig 7–12.—Preoperative aortography shows the saccular aneurysm originating 2 cm distal to the left subclavian artery. (Courtesy of Locufier JL, Bosschaerts Th, Barthel J, et al: *J Cardiovasc Surg* 30:499–502, 1989.)

Woman, 22, delivered an infant after a pregnancy complicated by an episode of preeclampsia. A routine x-ray film obtained the day after delivery revealed a left upper paramediastinal mass that was not present on the prepartum examination. A systolic murmur was noted, and CT and magnetic resonance studies confirmed a saccular aneurysm. Digital angiography showed the aneurysm starting about 2 cm distal to the origin of the left subclavian artery (Fig 7–12). The aneurysmal mass was isolated and opened, revealing a transverse tear of the thoracic aorta, sparing only the adventitia, 3 cm distal to the left subclavian origin. The ectasia was resected and a simple transverse closure carried out, with reinforcement of the suture line with a sleeve of fascia lata. Angiography a year later showed an intact repair.

An aneurysmal process may progress in pregnant women as stress on the weakened arterial wall increases. Nevertheless, aneurysm formation during pregnancy is rare.

▶ The explanation of increased total circulating blood volume, acceleration of cardiac rhythm, and increased stroke volume and cardiac output, combined with hormonal changes during pregnancy, provide too simplistic an explanation for the arterial dysplasias that accompany pregnancy.

Thoracoabdominal Aortic Aneurysm

Weimann S, Gschnitzer F (Universitätsklinik für Chirurgie, Innsbruck, Austria)

Chirurg 61:163–167, 1990 7–16

In contrast to the routine repair of strictly abdominal aortic aneurysms, the surgical treatment of thoracoabdominal aortic aneurysms (TAAA) presents a challenge to the vascular surgeon. In 1965 a bypass technique was developed by DeBakey, but the perioperative mortality was 26%. In the same year Crawford introduced the first in-graft technique of direct revascularization of the widened arterial segment. The technique has since been standardized and has been used with good early and late results.

Crawford classified TAAAs into 3 anatomical categories based on aneurysm site and size. Type I aneurysms are found between the distal aortic arch and the celiac trunk, type II aneurysms comprise the entire AAA from the distal aortic arch to the aortic bifurcation, and type III aneurysms originate at the distal branching of the descending aorta, also comprising the entire length of the AAA. Type I TAAAs can be repaired via a thoracic access, whereas type II and type III TAAAs always require a thoracolaparotomy. The classification is important in that there is a direct association between the postoperative paraplegia rate and extent of the TAAA.

Previous reviews of large patient samples have shown that type I TAAA occurs in 14% of cases, type II in 57%, and type III in 29%. There has been a significant increase in the incidence of TAAA among women in recent years. Because arteriosclerosis is the underlying disease mechanism for TAAA, many patients with TAAA often have significant other risk factors, (e.g., coronary heart disease, chronic obstructive lung disease, and chronic renal insufficiency with abnormal creatinine values).

Thoracoabdominal aortic aneurysms represent approximately 10% of all AAAs. The reported incidence of TAAAs that rupture is 15% to 30%. The natural course of TAAA is characterized by a high mortality. In large reviews, 76% of the patients had died by 2 years after diagnosis, 35% of a ruptured TAAA. The rupture rate for TAAAs is similar to those for pure thoracic or pure abdominal aortic aneurysms.

Most TAAAs are asymptomatic for many years. Rupture causes symptoms, including chest pain and abdominal pain radiating to the back. Large TAAAs may mimic lumbar spinal symptoms, often leading the patient to an orthopedic or neurologic surgeon. Other symptoms are breathing difficulties caused by airway compression, hematemesis and dysphagia caused by erosion and compression of the esophagus or duodenum, and neurologic symptoms resulting from nerve compression.

The main advantages of the Crawford in-graft technique over the De Bakey bypass technique are a shorter operation time and thus less blood loss, as well as fewer anastomoses and consequently less risk of technical failure.

▶ This article provides a nice summary of data regarding thoracoabdominal aneurysms.

Traumatic Rupture of the Thoracic Aorta: A Clinicopathological Study

Søndenaa K, Tveit B, Kordt KF, Fossdal JE, Pedersen P-H (Rogaland Central County Hosp, Stavanger, Norway)

Acta Chir Scand 156:137–143, 1990 7–17

The incidence of traumatic rupture of the thoracic aorta is probably underestimated as most patients die before arrival at the hospital and autopsy is often not performed. A retrospective review was performed to determine the incidence of traumatic rupture of the thoracic aorta.

During a 6-year study period, 18 males aged 7–72 years and 9 females aged 16–83 years sustained traumatic rupture of the thoracic aorta. Eighteen patients died instantaneously, but 2 of them died of fatal head injuries. One patient had vital signs after the accident but died during transport to the hospital. Five patients were treated but died in the hospital. All 5 had extensive injuries other than the aortic rupture, and in 4 of them the aortic injuries were not diagnosed before death. The remaining 3 patients survived. Twenty of the 27 patients were injured in automobile accidents.

Two of the 3 survivors underwent direct cross-clamping of the aorta

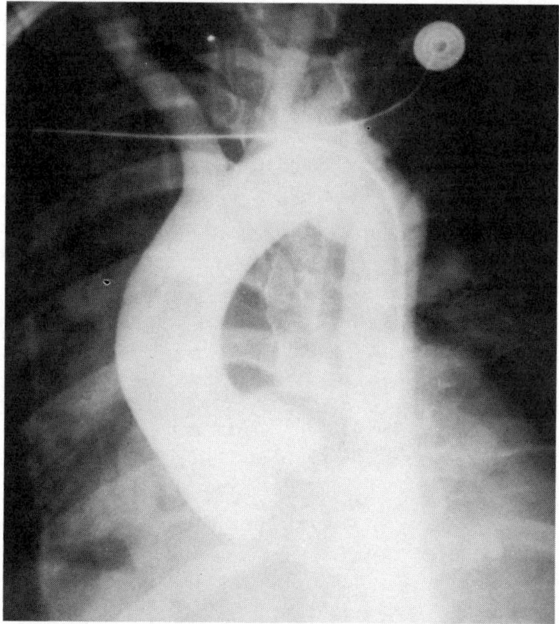

Fig 7–13.—Aortography shows aortic rupture just distal to the left subclavian artery. (Courtesy of Søndenaa K, Tveit B, Kordt KF, et al: *Acta Chir Scand* 156:137–143, 1990.)

with Dacron interposition grafting soon after admission. The third survivor received a Gott shunt and Dacron interposition graft the day after the accident. The chest radiograph demonstrated rib fractures and lung contusions on the right side, and widening of the mediastinum with deviation of the trachea to the right (Fig 7–13). This patient survived with paraplegia.

Most patients who died at the scene could not have been salvaged in any event (Fig 7–14). A chest radiograph in survivors suspected of traumatic injury of the thoracic aorta is mandatory, and it may show a number of signs indicating aortic rupture, of which mediastinal widening is considered the most reliable. Some physicians recommend that aortography be performed in all patients suspected of rupture of the thoracic aorta by virtue of the mechanism of injury. Most patients should be operated on immediately by a left fourth intercostal thoracotomy. Several surgical techniques are available, but there is still no agreement on what constitutes the safest technique. Paraplegia remains the most feared complication of cross-clamping. The simple clamp repair technique appears to be just as reliable as other techniques in avoiding paraplegia.

Based on a total population of approximately 240,000 inhabitants served by Rogaland Central County Hospital, the incidence of traumatic rupture of the thoracic aorta was 1 in 53,000 inhabitants.

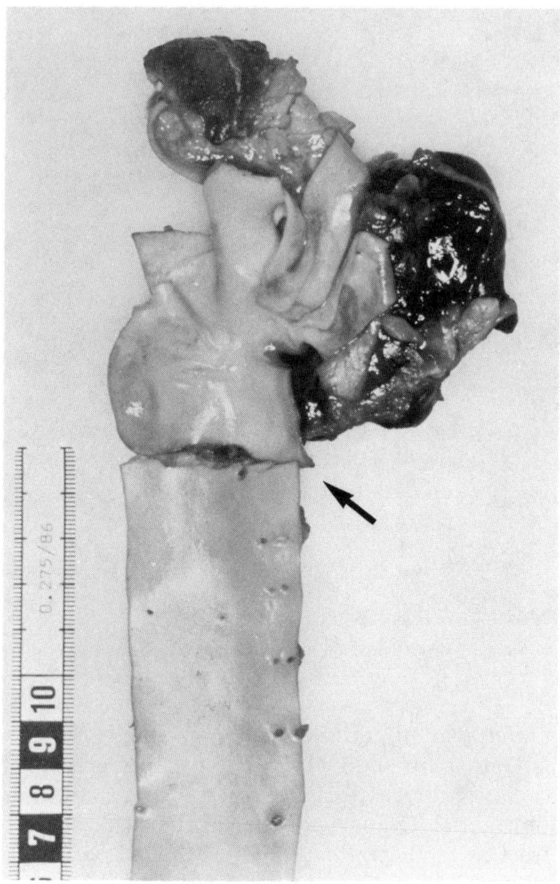

Fig 7–14.—Necropsy specimen shows complete transection of the aorta just distal to the left subclavian artery. (Courtesy of Søndenaa K, Tveit B, Kordt KF, et al: *Acta Chir Scand* 156:137–143, 1990.)

Therefore, this type of traumatic injury occurs more often than is generally thought.

▶ Rapid transport after trauma is now providing emergency physicians with more cases of traumatic rupture of the aorta. it is disappointing that bypass or simple clamp repair is still associated with a high rate of paraplegia. In effecting repair, it is important to decrease clamp time to less than 30 minutes and, if possible, maintain distal aortic perfusion above 60 mm Hg.

8 Abdominal Aortic Aneurysms

Epidemiological Aspects of Abdominal Aortic Aneurysm
Collin J (John Radcliffe Hosp, Oxford, England)
Eur J Vasc Surg 4:113–116, 1990 8–1

The incidence of abdominal aortic aneurysms (AAAs) increased by sevenfold between 1951 and 1980. The greatest increase occurred in small, asymptomatic, and uncomplicated AAAs, suggesting that improved diagnosis and the introduction of effective therapy were the most important factors.

A disease of the elderly, AAA becomes more common with advancing age. Few people younger than age 60 years die of a ruptured AAA. More men than women die of the disease, with the death rate for men peaking in the 70- to 74-year age group. In women the peak occurs a decade later. Results of studies of racial differences in the incidence of AAA are conflicting. One study that compared patients with AAA and those with aortoiliac disease found that the former were 9 times more likely to be male, were on average 11 years older, and were much less likely to have had previous arterial surgery.

The value of screening for AAA has been the subject of a number of studies. Men old enough to have a high risk for AAA but young enough to benefit from prophylactic elective surgery appear to be likely candidates for screening. Because abdominal ultrasonography has become a routine primary investigation for nonspecific abdominal symptoms, many patients are already being screened.

There may be a familial ingredient in the etiology of AAA, although studies have not been conclusive. It is clear, however, that risk increases with the diameter of the AAA. Even the smallest AAA may grow to life-threatening size within a few years of diagnosis. Thus elective surgery for AAA is advisable, especially in younger men.

▶ Common, lethal, curable, and readily found if sought, AAA seems tailor-made for widespread prospective surveillance programs. But screening works only if it is cost effective and results in clear social benefits, either in averting premature mortality or in significantly enhancing the quality of life. Collin's pioneering AAA screening models, and his evaluation of these paradigms in the community setting, provide the crucial epidemiologic substrate for any future studies of the efficacy of AAA screening programs.—Kaj Johansen, M.D., Universit of Washington, School of Medicine, Seattle, Washington.

Are Familial Abdominal Aortic Aneurysms Different?

Darling RC III, Brewster DC, Darling RC, LaMuraglia GM, Moncure AC, Cambria RP, Abbott WM (Massachusetts Gen Hosp, Boston; Harvard Med School)

J Vasc Surg 10:39–43, 1989 8–2

The incidence, clinical behavior, and anatomical characteristics of familial abdominal aortic aneurysms (AAAs) were evaluated in a 9-year prospective study involving 542 consecutive patients undergoing surgery for AAAs. A control group included 500 patients of similar age and sex without aneurysmal disease. A detailed analysis was made of the pedigree charts of patients with a positive family history of aneurysm.

A total of 82 patients (15%) with AAAs had first-degree relatives with aneurysm, compared to only 9 of 500 patients (2%) without aneurysmal disease; the difference was highly significant. Analysis of the pedigree charts showed 86 families with 209 first-degree relatives with AAAs. When compared to 460 patients operated on for AAAs with no family history of AAAs, those with familial AAAs were more likely to be women, and men with familial AAAs tended to be about 5 years younger than those in the nonfamilial AAA group. These 2 groups were comparable in terms of smoking history and presence of hypertension or diabetes. Similarly, the anatomical extent of aneurysmal disease, multiplicity of aneurysms, associated occlusive disease, and blood type did not differ significantly between the 2 groups.

The incidence of aneurysm rupture was 41% in families with familial AAAs and was significantly higher in female than in male patients (30% versus 17%). A positive female marker, i.e., identification of a family with AAAs and a female member with an aneurysm, strongly correlated with the risk of rupture. The term black widow syndrome is suggested as appropriate and analogous to the unusual but potentially fatal trait of female members of families with AAAs.

Familial AAA is a real entity. All patients should have pedigree charts when a diagnosis of AAA is made. The possibility of rupture or death from rupture of the aneurysm should be considered in male or female relatives when a positive female marker is identified.

▶ The question asked in the title of this article is answered, No. Abdominal aortic aneurysms are of multifocal origin; they occur in families and should be removed from the circulation for exactly the same indications as AAAs found outside of the family connection.

Ultrasonographic Screening of the Abdominal Aorta Among Siblings of Patients With Abdominal Aortic Aneurysms

Bengtsson H, Norrgård Ö, Ängquist KA, Ekberg O, Öberg L, Bergqvist D (Univ of Lund; Malmö Gen Hosp, Sweden; Univ of Umeå, Sweden)

Br J Surg 76:589–591, 1989 8–3

Siblings of patients with abdominal aortic aneurysms (AAAs) are potential targets for a screening program. An ultrasonographic screening study was undertaken to assess the prevalence of abdominal aortic dilatations among asymptomatic brothers and sisters of patients operated on for AAAs. Of the 102 siblings invited, 87 (35 men and 52 women) from 32 different families participated in the study. The median age was 63 years (range, 39–82).

Aortic dilatation was found in 10 brothers (29%) and 3 sisters (6%). A localized dilatation caudal to the celiac axis was noted in 10 siblings, and in the remaining 3 general dilatation of the abdominal aorta was noted with the diameter at the celiac axis being more than 29 mm. All aortic dilatations were asymptomatic and had not been recognized before the study. Blood pressure was higher and history of drug-treated hypertension was more common in siblings with aortic dilatation than in those without. Myocardial infarction was more common in men with aortic dilatations.

The prevalence of asymptomatic abdominal aortic dilatations among brothers of patients operated on for AAAs is high. This group should be considered for further screening studies.

▶ Certainly, screening of first-order relatives of patients with AAAs should be done. An extension of such screening should probably include hypertensive males, men older than age 65, and patients attending cardiac vascular clinics.

Prognosis of Abdominal Aortic Aneurysms: A Population-Based Study

Nevitt MP, Ballard DJ, Hallet JW Jr (Mayo Clinic and Mayo Found; Northeastern Ohio Univ Univs, Rootstown, Ohio)

N Engl J Med 321:1009–1014, 1989 8–4

Previous case-series studies from referral centers have indicated a mean rate of expansion for small abdominal aneurysms of approximately .4–.5 cm/year and a risk of rupture of 6% per year. These data have influenced recent recommendations for more aggressive screening and elective repair of aneurysms. Because these studies are subject to considerable bias, a population-based study was conducted among residents of Rochester, Minnesota, in whom an abdominal aortic aneurysm (AAA) was initially diagnosed between 1951 and 1984 to determine the rate of change in size and risk of rupture.

Among 370 residents with a clinically recognized AAA, 181 had at least 1 ultrasound examination that documented the presence of the aneursym. Of the 103 patients who had more than 1 ultrasound study of the initially unruptured aneurysm, no change or a reported decrease was noted in the diameter of the aneurysm was noted in 17%, 59% had an increase of less than .4 cm/yr, and 24% had an increase of at least .4 cm/yr. The overall median rate of increase in the diameter of the aneurysms was .21 cm/yr.

Among the 176 patients who had an unruptured aneurysm at time of the first ultrasound study, the cumulative incidence of rupture was 6% after 5 years and 8% after 10 years. However, the risk of rupture within 5 years was 0% for the 130 patients with an aneurym of less than 5 cm in diameter and 25% for the 46 patients with an aneurysm 5 cm or more in diameter. All ruptured aneurysms measured 5 cm or more in diameter at the time of rupture.

These population-based data challenge the validity of previous estimates of the rate of expansion and risk of rupture of aneurysms. The risk of rupture is considerably lower than previously reported in aneurysms of less than 5 cm in diameter, but larger aneurysms are associated with a clinically important risk of rupture and should be considered for elective repair.

▶ This presentation has been much criticized and for good reason. Anyone interested in this subject realizes that aneurysms do not decrease in size. It is only the technique used in measuring that suggests a decrease in size. Further, the usual anticipated expansion rate is .4 cm/yr, and it is acknowledged that some patients will have unpredictable expansion and others will remain static. The danger of this presentation is that physicians watching patients with AAAs will wait until the magic number of 5-cm diameter is reached. There is no magic number.

Collagen Types and Matrix Protein Content in Human Abdominal Aortic Aneurysms

Rizzo RJ, McCarthy WJ, Dixit SN, Lilly MP, Shively VP, Flinn WR, Yao JST (Northwestern Univ)

J Vasc Surg 10:365–373, 1989 8–5

The etiology of atherosclerotic aneurysms is not well understood. Alterations in the collagen concentration of the aortic extracellular matrix, specifically, a decrease in type III collagen, may lead to atherosclerotic aneurysm formation. An attempt was made to identify the structural and biochemical changes that occur throughout the atherosclerotic aortic wall.

Full-thickness sections of the infrarenal aorta were collected from 19 patients (mean age, 70 years) who were undergoing repair of an abdominal aortic aneurysm (AAA) and from 13 fresh cadavers with a mean age of 63 years at the time of autopsy who had no AAA. All specimens were submitted for histologic analysis and measurement of total collagen, elastin, collagen solubility, and percentage of collagen types I and III after digestion with cyanogen bromide.

Control and aneurysmal specimens had similar aortic wall thicknesses. Abdominal aortic aneurysm wall sections revealed prominent inflammatory cell infiltration and deficient, fragmented elastin. The mean collagen concentration in AAA sections was increased by 54% and the mean elastin concentration was decreased by 92% when compared with those in control specimens. There was no significant difference in the percentages of type I or type III collagen between AAA and control specimens. Atherosclerotic aneurysms are associated with an inflammatory process and may be the result of elastin degradation, but they are not associated with type III collagen deficiency.

▶ Fundamental studies such as this one will reveal errors in aortic wall proteins that possibly may be corrected by drug therapy.

Expression of Elastase Activity by Human Monocyte-Macrophages Is Modulated by Cellular Cholesterol Content, Inflammatory Mediators, and Phorbol Myristate Acetate

Rouis M, Nigon F, Lafuma C, Hornebeck W, Chapman MJ (Hôp de la Pitié, Paris; Université Paris-Val de Marne, Creteil, France)

8–6

The elastase activity of human monocyte-derived macrophages may promote atherogenesis by affecting the arterial wall. Agents that stimulate production of elastase-type enzymes and the effects of stimulation on the cholesterol content of cells were studied in vitro.

Cell-associated elastase-like activity was detected in these macrophages. Activity was increased considerably by the stimulatory agents phorbol myristate acetate (PMA) and opsonized zymosan (OZ), a model for necrotic products, but not by platelet-activating factor (PAF) or lipopolysaccharide (LPS).

Latent elastinolytic activity was present in the extracellular medium only when macrophages were activated by stimulation. Greater stimulatory effects were produced by PMA and OZ than by PAF and LPS.

Cell-associated elastolytic activity increased with cholesterol loading of cells with acetylated low-density lipoprotein but decreased with cholesterol depletion of cells by incubation with high-density lipoprotein. The effects of stimulatory agents were similar to those seen in noncholesterol-loaded cells. As for the extracellular latent elastinolytic activity of cholesterol-loaded cells, PMA and OZ had greater stimulatory effects than PAF and LPS. The effects of PMA and OZ were greater on noncholesterol-loaded cells.

Human monocyte-macrophages express both cell-associated and latent extracellular elastase-like activities. Inflammatory mediators and the cholesterol content of cells, by differing actions on these activities, may affect their role in atherogenesis.

▶ Conclusions of this study are that mononuclear elastase is present when cells are activated by stimulation, and inflammatory mediators may play a part in such activation. One is less interested in the atherogenic potential of such activity than in the effects on the strength of the arterial wall.

Genetic Variation on Chromosome 16 Is Associated With Abdominal Aortic Aneurysm

Powell JT, Bashir A, Dawson S, Vine N, Henney AM, Humphries SE, Greenhalgh RM (Charing Cross and Westminster Med School; Charing Cross Sunley Research Ctr, London)
Clin Sci 78:13–16, 1990 8–7

Deaths attributed to rupture of abdominal aortic aneurysms (AAAs) reportedly are increasing. Although emergency surgery for the disorder has a high mortality rate, elective procedures are safe. Risk factors for aortic aneurysms include smoking and hypetension. Results of recent studies suggest that a familial disposition may also play a role in the development of AAAs. Because an association between AAAs and the haptoglobin 2–1 phenotype might provide a basis for screening studies of at-risk populations, 3 groups of patients were studied.

The study groups included patients who had undergone elective repair of an AAA in the preceding 1–3 years, patients with atherosclerotic stenosing disease of the abdominal aorta who had undergone aortic grafting in the preceding 1–3 years, and healthy controls. Genotyping of the patient samples was performed blind as to the nature of the aortic disease.

Patients with aneurysms had a higher frequency of the haptoglobin α^1 allele and a higher frequency of a rare polymorphism at the cholesterol ester transfer protein locus than healthy controls. The 2 genetic markers appear to act independently. Dilatation of the abdominal aorta may be influenced by genetic variation in the haptoglobin and cholesterol ester transfer protein genes. The former might affect the degradation of elastin in the atherosclerotic aorta, whereas the latter could affect lipid metabolism and promote atherosclerosis. This study provides the first evidence of an association between AAAs and specific genes on the long arm of chromosome 16.

▶ Further evidence accumulates that certain aortic aneurysms have a familial link. Screening of family members may uncover more aneurysms.

Influence of Coronary Artery Disease on Morbidity and Mortality After Abdominal Aortic Aneurysmectomy: A Population-Based Study, 1971–1987

Roger VL, Ballard DJ, Hallet JW Jr, Osmundson PJ, Peutz PA, Gersh BJ (Hôp Tenon, Paris; Mayo Clinic and Found, Rochester, Minn)
J Am Coll Cardiol 14:1245–1252, 1989 8–8

In an aging patient population, management of multisystem cardiovascular disease becomes increasingly important. The prognostic influence of coronary artery disease after abdominal aortic aneurysmectomy was investigated in a 10-year population-based study in Olmsted County, Minnesota. Data on 131 Olmsted County residents who underwent elective surgery with aneurysmectomy as the primary indication for surgery in 1971–1987 were reviewed. Patients were followed until 1988 for death and cardiac events, including myocardial infarction, coronary bypass surgery, and angioplasty.

Patients were divided into 3 groups: 75 patients in group 1, no clinically recognized coronary disease before aneurysmectomy; 47 patients in group 2, suspected or overt uncorrected coronary artery disease defined as a history of previous myocardial infarction, angina, or positive stress test; and 9 patients in group 3, previous coronary angioplasty or coronary bypass grafting.

The 30-day operative mortality was 3% in group 1 and 9% in group 2. The estimated 8-year survival was 59% in group 1 and 34% in group 2. The expected survival rate was 68% for group 1 and 61% for group 2. The cumulative incidence rate of cardiac events at 8 years was 15% for group 1 and 61% for group 2.

Patients with uncorrected coronary artery disease had a twofold increased risk of death and a fourfold increased risk of cardiac events. These data suggest that an aggressive life-long approach to the management of coronary artery disease is appropriate in patients undergoing abdominal aortic aneurysmectomy.

► Not a bad idea.

Aortic Surgery in the Presence of Cholelithiasis: Should Simultaneous Cholecystectomy Be Performed?

Innocenti C, Defraigne JO, Limet R (Centre Hospitalier Universitaire Liège, Liège, Belgium)

J Chir (Paris) 126:159–162, 1989 8–9

Between 10% and 20% of all patients older than age 50 years have gallstones. Patients with biliary lithiasis who require aortic vascular surgery because of atherosclerotic lesions or an abdominal aortic aneurysm (AAA) present a surgical dilemma. If the gallbladder is not removed during the vascular procedure, postoperative symptoms of lithiasis may develop, with the attendant risk for increased morbidity. Removing the gallbladder simultaneously with the vascular repair increases operating time and the risk of prosthetic contamination.

Between 1984 and 1987, 17 men and 4 women aged 54–79 years underwent simultaneous cholecystectomy and vascular reconstruction procedures. Sixteen patients had an AAA and 5 had occlusive atherosclerotic disease of the abdominal aorta. Of the 11 patients who had biliary lithiasis before operation, 8 were symptomatic. In the other 10 patients the diagnosis was made during operation by systematic palpation. All 21 patients were given prophylactic antibiotics for 48 hours after operation. The vascular repair was always done first, and cholecystectomy was not performed until after the retroperitoneum was closed.

One patient died on day 9 after operation of cardiogenic shock; another patient died on day 10 of complete intestinal necrosis. In 1 patient the drainage catheter broke on day 10 after operation and reoperation was required to remove the piece left in the abdomen. One patient acquired bronchopneumonia, and another had an uncomplicated infarct. After a median follow-up of 18 months, none of the patients had symptoms of digestive disease. Combining intra-abdominal arterial grafting with cholecystectomy in patients with gallbladder disease who require vascular procedures appears to be a safe policy.

▶ A critical look at the data presented in this article would suggest that staged surgical procedures are better than the simultaneous performance of multiple operations. The advent of laparoscopic cholecystectomy has certainly changed this picture. It increasingly favors staging such surgical procedures.

Transperitoneal Versus Retroperitoneal Approach for Aortic Reconstruction: A Randomized Prospective Study

Cambria RP, Brewster DC, Abbott WM, Freehan M, Megerman J, LaMuraglia G, Wilson R, Wilson D, Teplick R, Davison JK (Massachusetts Gen Hosp, Boston; Harvard Med School)

J Vasc Surg 11:314–325, 1990 8–10

Most reports recommending use of the retroperitoneal approach for aortic reconstruction (AR) are retrospective. The merits of the retroperitoneal approach for AR were compared to those of the midline transpertioneal approach in a randomized, prospective trial of 113 patients admitted for elective, infrarenal AR between march 1987 and October 1988. The record of 56 patients who underwent a transperitoneal approach for AR performed by the same surgeons from 1984 to 1985 also were reviewed retrospectively.

Clinical and demographic features (e.g., age, male to female ratio, smoking history, incidence and severity of cardiopulmonary disease, indication for operation, and use of epidural anesthetics) did not differ between the randomized patients undergoing the transperitoneal approach and those undergoing the retroperitoneal approach. Similarly, operative details such as operative and aortic cross-clamp times, crystalloid and transfusion requirements, degree of hypothermia on arrival at the intensive care unit, and perioperative fluid and blood requirements did not differ according to approach.

The postoperative course, defined in terms of recovery of gastrointestinal function, requirements for narcotics, metabolic parameters of operative stress, incidence of major and minor complications, and duration of hostpial stay, was similar after both approaches. However, when compared with the retrospectively reviewed patients, randomized patients undergoing either transperitoneal or retroperitoneal operations had significant reductions in postoperative ventilation, transfusion requirements, resumption of oral alimentation, and duration of hospital stay. These findings do not support adoption of the retroperitoneal approach as the preferred technqiue for routine AR.

▶ A classic example of type II statistical error, although this study was elegantly structured and carefully performed.

Ibuprofen Pretreatment Inhibits Prostacyclin Release During Abdominal Exploration in Aortic Surgery

Hudson JC, Wurm WH, O'Donnell TF Jr, Kane FR, Mackey WC, Su Y-F, Watkins WD (Tufts Univ; Duke Univ; Med College of Virginia, Richmond)
Anesthesiology 72:443–449, 1990 8–11

Mesenteric traction and bowel eventration during aortic surgery produce facial flushing, lower the arterial pressure, and increase the cardiac index. Prostacyclin is the probable mediator, because increased levels of 6-keto-prostaglandin-$F_{1\alpha}$ are noted when symptoms occur. Ibuprofen, a cy-

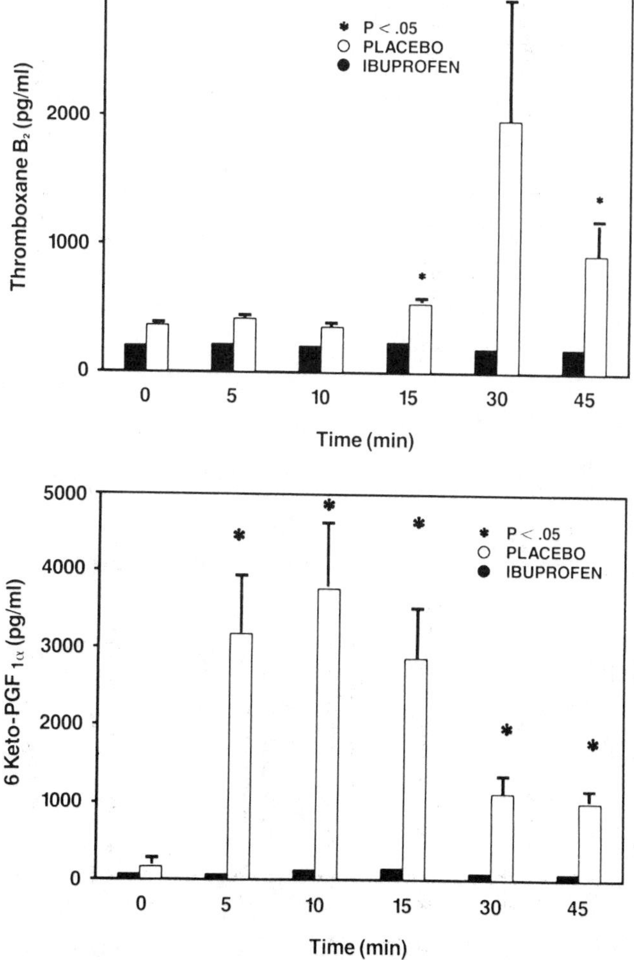

Fig 8–1.—Plasma concentrations of 6-keto-prostaglandin-$F_{1\alpha}$ (pg/mL) and thromboxane B_2 (pg/mL) in 13 patients given placebo and 14 given ibuprofen at abdominal exploration during aortic surgery. Values are means ± 1 SEM. *P* values were determined using the 2-way ANOVA and applying the Bonferroni correction. (Courtesy of Hudson JC, Wurm WH, O'Donnell TF Jr, et al: *Anesthesiology* 72:443–449, 1990.)

clooxygenase inhibitor, was administered to 14 patients scheduled for aortic reconstruction; 13 others received a placebo in a double-blind design.

Plasma levels of 6-keto-prostaglandin-$F_{1\alpha}$ increased markedly in placebo recipients, and there was a late rise in thromboxane B_2 levels. In ibuprofen-treated patients there were no significant changes in either hemodynamics or prostanoid concentrations (Fig 8–1).

The findings are consistent with the view that high levels of prostacyclin are released during manipulation of the bowel at aortic surgery. Inhibition of prostanoid synthesis by ibuprofen confirms that prostacyclin probably is the cause of symptoms in this setting.

▶ Another example of interesting information of questionable utility.

Pulmonary Edema After Aneurysm Surgery Is Modified by Mannitol

Paterson IS, Klausner JM, Goldman G, Pugatch R, Feingold H, Allen P, Mannick JA, Valeri CR, Shepro D, Hechtman HB (Brigham and Women's Hosp, Boston; Boston Univ)

Ann Surg 210:796–801, 1989 8–12

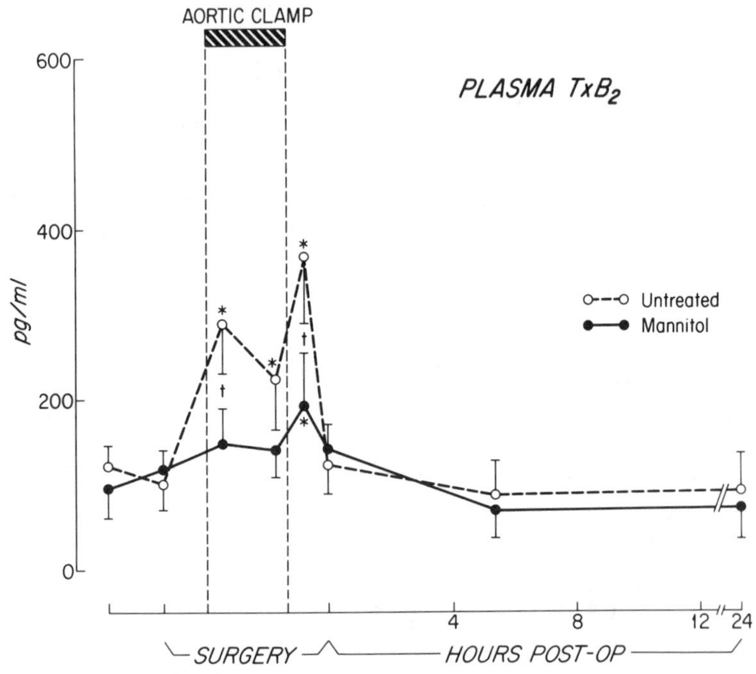

Fig 8–2.—Aortic cross-clamping and clamp removal led to transient increases in plasma thromboxane B_2 levels. Mannitol did not alter baseline plasma thromboxane B_2 levels but reduced ischemia-induced thromboxane B_2-synthesis. *Asterisks* and *daggers* refer to significance relative to baseline and between groups, respectively. (Courtesy of Paterson IS, Klausner JM, Goldman G, et al: *Ann Surg* 210:796–801, 1989.)

Reperfusion of ischemic tissue during abdominal aortic aneurysmectomy results in thromboxane A_2 generation, increased mean pulmonary artery pressure (MPAP), leukopenia, and noncardiogenic pulmonary edema. To determine whether the hydroxyl radical scavenger mannitol can modify the pulmonary injury in abdominal aortic aneurysmectomy, 26 patients undergoing elective infrarenal abdominal aortic aneurysmectomy were randomly assigned to receive mannitol, .2 g/kg, or saline intravenously before infrarenal aortic clamping. Hemodynamic, hematologic, and pulmonary function studies were obtained.

With saline, 30 minutes after aortic clamping, plasma thromboxane B_2 and MPAP increased significantly, whereas white blood cell and platelet counts were reduced significantly. With removal of the aortic cross-clamp, further increases in thromboxane B_2 and MPAP were noted. Four to 8 hours after surgery, pulmonary dysfunction occurred in all patients, as shown by significant increases in physiologic shunting and peak inspiratory pressure. Chest radiographs revealed pulmonary edema in all patients, but the pulmonary wedge pressure remained within normal limits.

Mannitol treatment before aortic cross-clamp application significantly reduced the rise in plasma thromboxane B_2 and MPAP levels relative to saline treatment (Fig 8–2), and lessened the decline in the white blood cell count and postoperative rise in physiologic shunting. No pulmonary edema was evident on chest radiography in any of the 11 patients 4–8 hours after surgery. In vitro studies showed that mannitol, $1-10^{-4}$M, prevented thromboxane B_2 synthesis by adenosine diphosphate-activated platelets in a dose-dependent manner, whereas dextrose was ineffective in preventing thromboxane synthesis. Mannitol prevents the lung injury that occurs after abdominal aortic aneurysmectomy by inhibiting ischemia-induced thromboxane synthesis.

▶ Although urine output and weight gain were the same for the study and control groups, one still suspects that it was the hyperosmolaric effect of the mannitol rather than inhibition of ischemic-induced thromboxane synthesis that was acting.

The Endoscopic Spectrum of Colonic Mucosal Injury Following Aortic Aneurysm Resection

Scherpenisse J, van Hees PAM (St Antonius Hosp, Nieuwegein, The Netherlands)

Endoscopy 21:174–176, 1989 8–13

Ischemic colitis is a serious complication of aortic aneurysm resection. To determine which patients need early exploratory laparotomy to prevent bowel perforation, the endoscopic findings and clinical course of such colonic mucosal defects in 48 patients were studied.

No complications resulted from endoscopy. The mucosal defects were nonspecific in 24 patients, 11 of whom had diffuse hyperemia with multiple submucosal hemorrhagic spots; the spots resolved within 5–10 days. Localized nonspecific injury consisted of edema and hyperemia in 11 patients and an ulcer in 2, all of which resolved within 7–31 days. Of 24 patients with ischemic colitis, ulceration without gangrene occurred in 15, which healed within 14–43 days. Of 9 patients with mucosal gangrene, the necrosis was patchy in 5; 4 others who had diffuse gangrene with a mosaic structure underwent exploratory laparotomy. One patient died after perforation, 2 had late stenosis, and 6 experienced healing.

Colonoscopy can be performed safely soon after surgery. Patients with necrosis should be monitored carefully and considered for exploratory surgery. Repeated colonoscopy 48 hours later may be sufficient for patients with ulcerating ischemic colitis but no gangrene.

▶ The original article contains beautiful photographs in color, but the conclusions of the presentation are little different from those of Ernst in 1976 (1).

Reference

1. Ernst CB, et al: *Surgery* 80:417, 1976.

Experience With PGE_1 in Patients With Postoperative Trashfoot

Gruss JD (Kurhessisches Krankenhaus, Kassel, Germany)

Vasa Suppl 28:57–60, 1989 8–14

The trash syndrome is characterized by more or less extensive diffuse peripheral embolization of atherosclerotic debris into the lower vascular system. The syndrome may occur with or without the loss of pedal pulses and always causes pain in the ischemic areas. Reportedly, intravenous prostaglandin E_1 (PGE_1) administration is efficacious in the treatment of severe foot ischemia caused by a trash syndrome. Clinical experience with intravenous PGE_1 therapy in the treatment of trash syndrome was reviewed.

During a 16-year observation period, severe trash syndrome developed in 13 patients who had undergone operation for infrarenal abdominal aortic aneurysm (AAA) and 2 patients who had had an aortobifemoral bypass in the treatment of arteriosclerotic occlusive disease. All patients had painful, cold, blue-white discoloration of the skin of both legs, the buttocks, and the lower abdomen. Arterial blood pressures were always high, and peripheral pulses were palpable only during the immediate postoperative period. Seven patients with AAA and 1 patient with arteriosclerotic occlusive disease were treated twice daily with 3 ampules of PGE_1, 60 μg, administered via a central venous catheter. Each infusion lasted for 2 hours. Patients were also given standard heparin therapy.

All 8 PGE_1-treated patients survived and only 1 required thigh amputation. The other 7 patients recovered completely without limb loss. In contrast, 2 of 7 untreated patients died within the first 3 postoperative days. A third patient who required thigh amputation also died. Another patient recovered, but lost both lower legs to amputation. The remaining 3 patients recovered completely without the need for amputation. Prostaglandin E_1 may be effective in the treatment of the trash syndrome.

▶ Prostaglandin E_1 may or may not be effective in the treatment of atheromatous embolization, but it is sad to witness the penetration of Americanisms into perfectly good continental language.

Two Year Prospective Analysis of the Oxford Experience With Surgical Treatment of Abdominal Aortic Aneurysm

Collin J, Murie J, Morris PJ (Univ of Oxford; John Radcliffe Hosp, Oxford, England)

Surg Gynecol Obstet 169:527–531, 1989 8–15

Although the operative mortality rate associated with elective surgery for abdominal aorta aneurysm (AAA) has improved considerably, the mortality rate after treatment of ruptured aneurysm has changed little. Recent experience with surgical treatment of 177 patients with AAA was reviewed.

From 1985 to 1987, 177 patients aged 53–96 years were hospitalized with the diagnosis of AAA. Of these, 103 were admitted under emergency conditions and 74 were referred for elective operation. Eighty-eight patients had a ruptured AAA, and 75 underwent surgery, with an operative mortality rate of 36%. The remaining 13 patients did not undergo surgery; 2 died before transfer to the operating room, 10 patients did not undergo surgery because of advanced age (85 years or more), and 1 had debilitating Parkinson's disease. Another 15 patients underwent emergent operations, including 11 with an acute AAA and 4 in whom symptoms were not caused by an aneurysm. Overall, 55% of all operations for AAA were for ruptured AAA or acute AAA. Seventy-four patients were referred for elective treatment. Of those, 70 underwent surgery, with an operative mortality rate of 1.4%.

There has been a recent threefold increase in the number of patients treated for AAA in Oxford, compared with earlier reports. The large proportion of patients treated emergently for ruptured or acute aneurysm contrasts markedly with the low number of referrals for elective operation. The 24-fold difference in mortality rates between procedures performed electively and those performed for ruptured aneurysm suggests that increased referral of patients with asymptomatic aortic aneurysms may have an impact on the overall mortality among patients with AAA.

▶ Collin et al. make a very solid case for community screening in detection of AAA.

Ten-Year Review of Non-Ruptured Aortic Aneurysms

Mutirangura P, Stonebridge PA, Clason AE, McClure JH, Wildsmith JAW, Nolan B, Ruckley CV, Jenkins AMcL (Royal Infirmary, Edinburgh)
Br J Surg 76:1251–1254, 1989 8–16

Whether early, elective repair of abdominal aortic aneurysms (AAAs) before rupture is justified depends on the risk of morbidity and mortality from surgery. Data were reviewed on 587 AAAs operated on in 1 hospital between 1978 and 1987.

Among the 309 patients with unruptured AAAs were 175 with no symptoms, 84 with symptoms, and 50 with acute symptoms. In 278 patients rupture had occurred. There were 91 operations for unruptured aneurysms in the first 5 years and 218 in the second 5 years.

Overall mortality for patients with unruptured aneurysms was 2.9%. Mortality for those who had elective surgery was 1.9%. For those with symptoms mortality was 3.6% and for those without, it was 1.1%. For patients who had emergency surgery mortality was 4%. In contrast, mortality associated with ruptured aneurysms during the past 5 years has averaged 28%. Recovery after surgery for unruptured aneurysms was uneventful in 106 patients, but others encountered such problems as chest infection, congestive heart failure, myocardial infarction, or renal failure.

The number of patients operated on for AAAs has risen sharply. The low mortality in this study compares favorably with that reported elsewhere and supports the view that such aneurysms should be repaired electively before they rupture.

▶ The low mortality reported for elective repair of AAAs confirms the previously observed fact that comfortable life is extended in patients subjected to this operation.

Eleven Years of Aortic Aneurysm Surgery: Changes in Techniques and Results

Berggren U, Norgren L, Pärsson H, Ribbe E, Thörne J (Lund Univ, Sweden)
Vasa 18:291–294, 1989 8–17

Elective operation for abdominal aortic aneurysms (AAAs) has become a relatively safe procedure with reported mortality rates ranging from 2% to 6%. However, the mortality associated with ruptured AAAs remains at around 50%. A few institutions have recently reported lower mortality rates of 15% to 23%. Data on all patients operated on for AAA in an 11-year period were reviewed to identify differences in complications and mortality rates as they related to changes in anesthesiologic and surgical treatment of patients.

The series included 181 men and 30 women aged 25–91 years (mean age, 70 years) were operated on from 1974 to 1984 because of AAA. Sixty-nine patients had concomitant cardiovascular disease, 32 had signs of cerebrovascular disease, and 10 had diabetes mellitus. Between 1974 and 1981 most patients were operated on with the use of general anesthesia with α- and β-blocking drugs to control hemodynamics. Between 1982 and 1984 most patients were given distal thoracic or lumbar epidural analgesia in combination with light general anesthesia. Emergency operations were still performed under general anesthesia. During the latter period the operative technique also changed in that more straight grafts were used, and graft material was changed from plain Dacron to collagen-impregnated Dacron. There were 131 patients in the early group and 80 in the late group.

The proportion of patients operated on electively increased significantly from 44% in the early period to 65% in the later period. Blood loss in the emergency group decreased from a mean of 6,000 mL to 2,900 mL, and in the elective group from a mean of 4,300 mL to 1,700 mL. There were 9 operative deaths in the early period and 1 in the late period. The hospital mortality rate among acute patients was reduced from 58% to 43% and among elective patients from 12% to 6%. By the end of the survey period in 1986, 130 of the 211 patients had died. Generalized atherosclerotic disease, mainly myocardial failure, remained the main cause of death and postoperative complications throughout both study periods.

▶ The greatest changes in technique of aortic aneurysm surgery have been in the nonoperative phases of the procedure. Tube grafts were being advocated in the early 1970s and apparently came to Sweden after 1984. Better intensive care medicine and better management of the general anesthetic phases of the operation have contributed greatly to decreased mortality. Now, the combination of epidural control of pain in the postoperative period and the occasional use of the retroperitoneal approach is making a similar contribution.

Bacteriology of Aortic Aneurysm Sac Contents

Stonebridge PA, Mutirangura P, Clason AE, Ruckley CV, Jenkins AML (Royal Infirmary, Edinburgh)

J R Coll Surg Edinb 35:42–43, 1990 8–18

Infections that develop in prosthetic grafts are the most serious complications of arterial reconstructive surgery. Factors implicated in graft infection include poor aseptic technique, emergency aneurysm repair, and bacteremia. The incidence of positive bacterial culture from an aortic aneurysm thrombus was assessed and the relationship between culture results and graft infection was determined.

Aerobic and anaerobic cultures from the intraluminal thrombus of infrarenal aortic aneurysms were obtained from 239 patients who underwent surgery at a single institution. The cases were divided into 4 groups: ruptured aneurysms (41), acute symptomatic aneurysms (30), elective

Positive Thrombus Bacterial Species

Species	Number
Staphylococcus aureus	6
Coagulase-negative staphylococci	10*
α-haemolytic streptococci	6
Streptococcus faecium	1
Escherichia coli	4*
Clostridium perfringens	3*
Bacteroides	1
Total	31*

*Two species were cultured in 4 cases.
(Courtesy of Stonebridge PA, Mutirangura P, Clason AE, et al: *J R Coll Surg Edinb* 35:42–43, 1990.)

symptomatic aneurysms (59), and asymptomatic aneurysms (101). Prophylactic cephalosporin and a single dose of intraoperative gentamicin were administered to all patients. Unless there was evidence of wound complication or a continuing pyrexia, antibiotic therapy was discontinued at 48 hours.

Patients who survived surgery were followed for a mean of 39.2 months for evidence of late graft infection. Positive cultures were obtained in 27 patients (11.3%). Gram-positive organisms predominated among the 7 species of bacteria identified (table). The incidence of positive cultures ranged from 8.3% in asymptomatic aneurysms to 20% in acute symptomatic aneurysms, but the differences were not statistically significant. No relationship was noted between thrombus bacteriology and early or late graft infection. Thus the problem of graft infection is multifactorial, and culture data from intraluminal thrombi have little clinical relevance.

▶ Interest in the bacteriology of the aortic sac contents goes back beyond 1965. Ultimately, delayed graft infection occurs both in patients with negative cultures and in those with positive cultures.

Symptomatic Abdominal Aortic Aneurysms in Long-Term Survivors of Cardiac Transplantation

Reichman W, Dyke C, Lee HM, Hanrahan J, Szentpetery S, Sobel M (HH McGuire VA Med Ctr, Richmond, Va; Virginia Commonwealth Univ)

J Vasc Surg 11:476–479, 1990 8–19

Two long-term survivors of cardiac transplantation underwent successful repair of a symptomatic abdominal aortic aneurysm (AAA). These are the only such patients to be reported since the advent of cyclosporine therapy in 1983. The number of atherosclerotic complications, including

AAA, is likely to increase as more patients survive for a significant time after cardiac transplantation.

The systemic nature of atherosclerosis helps explain why transplant recipients are disposed to aneurysm formation. In addition, older patients now receive heart transplants, and they tend to have more advanced atherosclerotic disease. Hypertension may be an important factor in aneurysm development in this population, especially with the incrased use of cyclosporine. The exact role of immunosuppression in accelerating atherosclerosis remains uncertain.

The ideal immunosuppressive regimen has not been established. Cyclosporine has significant long-term side effects warranting continued surveillance for progressive atherosclerosis and other vascular sequelae.

▶ Because atherosclerotic cardiomyopathy is a common cause of the cardiac deterioration that necessitates transplantation, it would be expected that generalized atherosclerosis elsewhere would occur in these patients. Although the patients are younger than one would expect, the severity of the atherosclerotic process remains the common denominator in causing the arteriosclerotic heart disease and the aortic atherosclerosis that results in aneurysm formation.

Sealed Rupture of Abdominal Aortic Aneurysms

Sterpetti AV, Blair EA, Schultz RD, Feldhaus RJ, Cisternino S, Chasan P (Creighton Univ, Omaha)

J Vasc Surg 11:430–435, 1990 8–20

Sealed chronic rupture of an abdominal aortic aneurysm (AAA) is not frequent. The records of 486 patients having resection of an AAA in 1974–1986 were reviewed, and 16 patients with chronic sealed rupture, defined as evidence of perforation contained by organized blood, fibrosis, or anatomical structures, were identified.

Ten of 16 patients had distal occlusive arterial disease. Only 1 was hypertensive, and this patient had acute rupture as well as signs of sealed rupture. All but 3 patients had previous symptoms referable to the aneurysm. The perforation was located posteriorly in 10 patients (Fig 8–3). Most of these patients had a small hematoma. The 3 patients with a rupture on the left lateral wall just below the renal artery origin had extremely small hematomas. One patient died after operation; the others survived resection and had regression of symptoms.

Sealed rupture of an AAA should be considered when an elderly patient has unexplained back pain or femoral neuropathy. Computed tomography is more useful than ultrasonography in making this diagnosis.

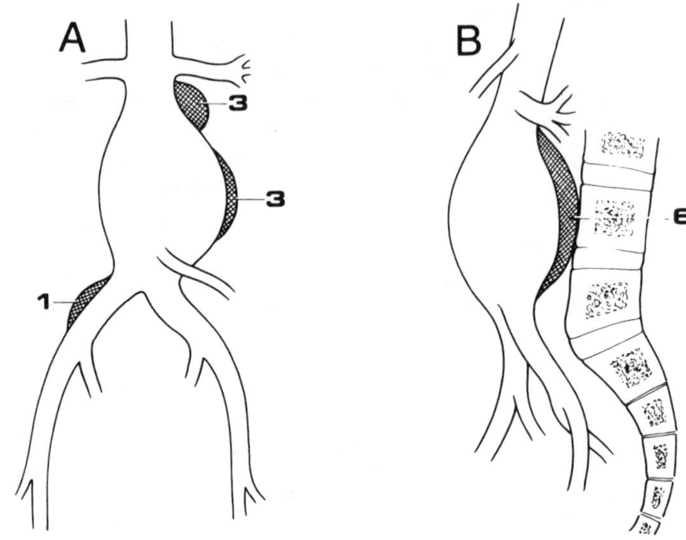

Fig 8–3.—The site of rupture was ascertained in 13 of 16 patients. Numerals indicate the number of patients with ruptures at each site. **A** and **B**, site of perforation. (Courtesy of Sterpetti AV, Blair EA, Schultz RD, et al: *J Vasc Surg* 11:430–435, 1990.)

▶ Actually, contained rupture of an AAA is relatively common, as CT has shown. As this presentation confirms, abdominal ultrasonography misses the sealed rupture.

Prognosis of Patients Over 75 Years of Age With a Ruptured Abdominal Aortic Aneurysm

Salo JA, Perhoniemi VJ, Lepäntalo MJA, Mattila PS (Helsinki Univ)
World J Surg 13:484–487, 1989 8–21

Results of emergency aneurysmectomy as well the factors influencing the outcome of emergency surgery were assessed in 47 patients (mean age, 79.7 years) who underwent emergency aneurysmectomy for a ruptured abdominal aortic aneurysm (AAA) between 1977 and 1986. In 16 patients the aneurysm had been diagnosed previously. Surgery was delayed for 6 hours or more in 17 patients and 26 were in shock preoperatively.

The mean diameter of the aneurysm was 8.9 cm (range, 5–15 cm). The mean operative time was 220 minutes, and the mean amount of operative bleeding was 8.5 L. The 1-month mortality rate was 60%, and most deaths were the result of multiorgan failure. Postoperative complications occurred in 63% of the survivors, most commonly pneumonia. The 5-year survival rate was 26%. Preoperative shock, advanced age, and a previously diagnosed but untreated AAA were associated with a significantly poor prognosis.

Mortality from a ruptured AAA in patients older than age 75 years remains high. Diagnosis of a ruptured AAA should be made quickly, preferably by clinical findings, to allow rapid initiation of therapy. Elective aneurysmectomy is recommended as soon as possible in patients with a diagnosed AAA if its diameter exceeds 4.4 cm.

▶ That the mortality from ruptured AAAs in patients older than age 75 is so high is another firm argument for community or selective screening for AAAs in patients 15 years younger.

Intra-Abdominal Compartment Syndrome as a Complication of Ruptured Abdominal Aortic Aneurysm Repair

Fietsam R Jr, Villalba M, Glover JL, Clark K (William Beaumont Hosp, Royal Oak, Mich)

Am Surg 55:396–402, 1989 8–22

Compartment syndromes are seen most commonly in the extremities, usually as a result of fractures, soft tissue injury, or arterial injury. The pathophysiology of compartment syndromes involves an increase in intracellular and extracellular fluid, which causes pressure, decreased capillary perfusion, tissue hypoxia, and ischemic necrosis that in turn lead to more swelling. A similar pathophysiology process has been observed after the emergency repair of ruptured abdominal aortic aneurysms (AAAs).

During a 10-year period, 104 patients underwent emergency operation for ruptured AAAs; in 4 an intra-abdominal compartment syndrome developed within 24 hours after operation. The syndrome was characterized by decreased urinary output, decreased ventilation, and increased central venous pressures. Each patient underwent decompressive laparotomy with placement of Marlex mesh, which rapidly reversed the symptoms.

All 4 patients had received more than 25 L of fluid resuscitation during and within 16 hours of operation, and all 4 had massive abdominal distention. Opening the abdominal incision led to dramatic improvement in central venous pressure, urinary output, ventilatory pressure, arterial carbon dioxide tension, and oxygenation. One patient who underwent removal of the Marlex mesh and closure of the abdomen on postoperative day 7 was discharged 3 days later. Two patients died of cardiac failure before closure of the abdomen on postoperative days 5 and 6. The fourth patient underwent removal of the Marlex mesh on postoperative day 13, but died on postoperative day 38 of multiple organ system failure.

In another 2 patients who had emergency aneurysm repairs, intraoperative recognition of a potential abdominal compartment syndrome led to the decision to leave the abdominal incision open after initial closure with Marlex mesh on completion of the aneurysmectomy. These patients remained hemodynamically stable and had no oliguria or ventilatory problems. Their wounds were subsequently closed with removal of Marlex mesh. One of these 2 patients died of adult respiratory distress syndrome within 30 hours of operation.

Some patients with ruptured AAAs do not tolerate closure of the abdominal wall. Opening the abdominal wound may reverse the oliguria and improve oxygenation. Delayed closure of the abdomen may be a way to prevent the development of abdominal compression syndrome.

▶ Is the condition observed here a curiosity, or does it actually happened more frequently than we have recognized?

Case Report: Ultrasonic and Comparative Angiographic Appearances of a Spontaneous Aorto-Caval Fistula

Cook AM, Dyet JF, Mann SL (Hull Royal Infirmary, Hull, England)

Clin Radiol 41:286–288, 1990 8–23

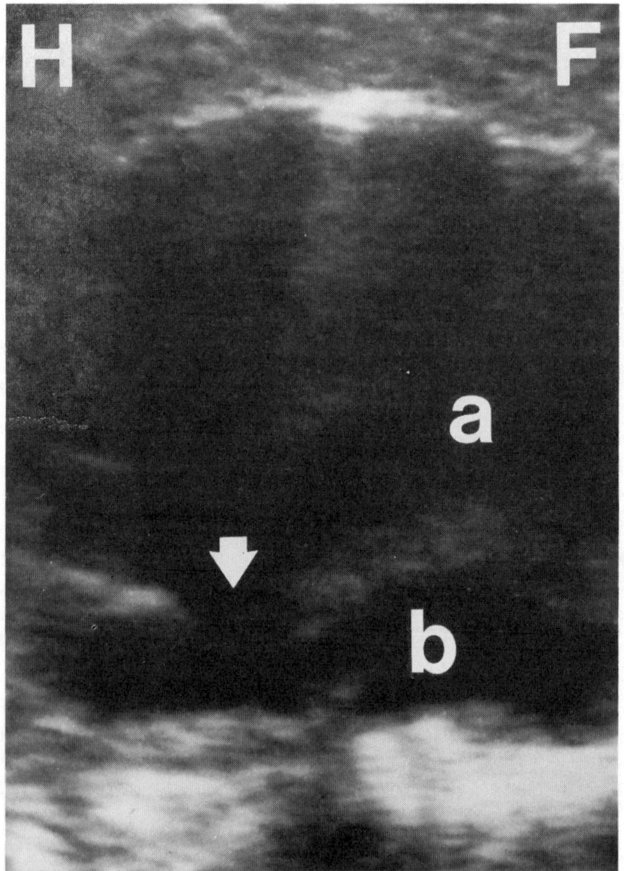

Fig 8–4.—Longitudinal midline abdominal ultrasound scan with the probe angled slightly to the right showing the aortic aneurysm, *a*, and inferior vena cava, *b*, with the fistula between them *(arrow)*. (Courtesy of Cook AM, Dyet JF, Mann SL: *Clin Radiol* 41:286–288, 1990.)

Aortocaval fistula is a rare complication of an abdominal aortic aneurysm (AAA). Its preoperative diagnosis will help to avoid complications by modifying the surgical technique. Ultrasonography can serve to localize noninvasively the site of an aortocaval fistula.

Man, 71, who had lower abdominal pain for 3 days, became jaundiced and passed little urine. Two transient episodes of back pain had occurred in the preceding 3 weeks. The patient was dyspneic and had elevated jugular venous pressure but no peripheral edema. The liver was tender and enlarged, and a pulsatile central abdominal mass was present. Renal and hepatic failure was documented. Curvilinear calcification typical of an aortic aneurysm was seen on abdominal radiographs. Ultrasonography showed a 6.9-cm aortic aneurysm and a separate lumen posteriorly that communicated directly with the aneurysm via a 2-cm channel (Fig 8–4). Aortography confirmed the presence of a fistula between the aorta

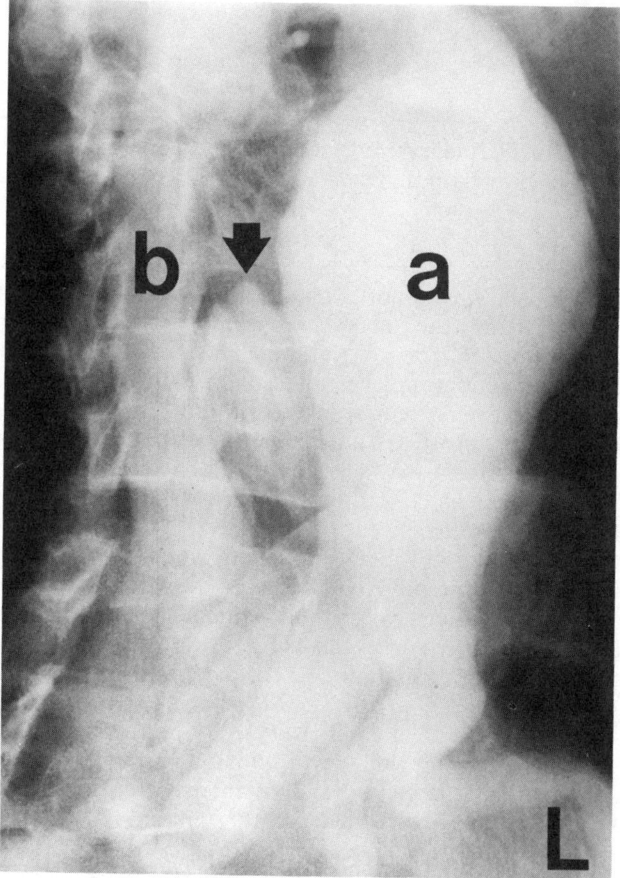

Fig 8–5.—Aortogram in right anterior oblique position that shows the aortic aneurysm, *a*, and inferior vena cava, *b*, with the fistula between them *(arrow)*. (Courtesy of Cook AM, Dyet JF, Mann SL: *Clin Radiol* 41: 286–288, 1990.)

and the inferior vena cava (Fig 8–5). The fistula was closed and the aorta was replaced with a Dacron graft, but the patient died of irreversible liver and kidney failure.

Aortocaval fistulas may be spontaneous, usually secondary to atherosclerotic aneurysms, or traumatic in origin. If not diagnosed preoperatively, clot may embolize from the aneurysm into the inferior cava, or there may be excessive venous bleeding when the aneurysm is opened. Clinical signs include abdominal or back pain, a continuous abdominal bruit, and high-output heart failure. Renal failure and venous congestion of the liver may also occur. Ultrasonography appears to be an alternative to aortography for diagnosing aortocaval fistula.

▶ Ultrasound is indeed the ain method of imaging used in the initial corroboration of the diagnosis of an AAA. However, more sophisticated and accurate methods of imaging such as CT scanning, and now magnetic resonance techniques, are much more accurate. Once a complicated situation such as aortocaval fistula is suspected, more precise imaging is in order.

Inflammatory Aortic Aneurysm: Diagnosis, Therapy, Results

Kniemeyer HW, Kolvenbach R, Rohde E, Godehardt E, Sandman W (Universität Düsseldorf, Germany)

Chirurg 61:27–31, 1990 8–24

Inflammatory abdominal aortic aneurysms (AAAs) differ from arteriosclerotic AAAs in that the aneurysmal surface has a whitish to red-yellowish appearance and the arterial wall shows fibrotic thickening. Inflammatory AAAs tend to involve adjacent structures, notably the duodenum, vena cava, left renal vein, transverse colon, and ureter. The intimate connection between the AAA and adjacent structures impedes surgical access, and the aneurysm may seem inoperable. The diagnostic and therapeutic problems associated with inflammatory AAAs were reviewed and the prognosis for this disease entity defined.

Between 1970 and 1987, of 964 patients who underwent aortic graft replacement of an infrarenal AAA, 52 were found to have an inflammatory AAA. Of 93 patients who underwent aortic graft replacement of thoracoabdominal aortic aneurysms (TAAs), only 1 had an inflammatory aneurysm. The patient population consisted of 51 men and 2 women aged 28–92 years (mean, 65 years).

Forty-two patients with inflammatory AAA were symptomatic at the time of operation and 11 were asymptomatic. Back pain was the most common complaint, followed by abdominal symptoms. All patients had more than 1 risk factor, including cigarette smoking (70%), hypertension (42%), hyperlipidemia (36%), and diabetes (4%). Except for those who needed emergency operation, all patients underwent diagnostic contrast-enhanced CT, which was not always conclusive. However, with increasing experience in the use of CT, approximately 80% of the patients received the correct diagnosis before operation (Fig 8–6). Except for the

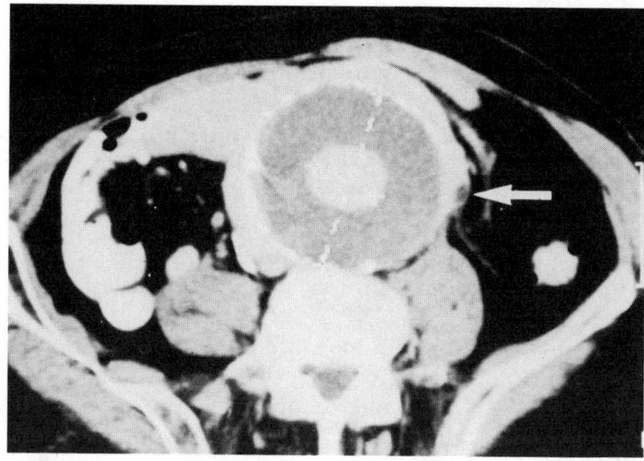

Fig 8–6.—Strong contrast-medium-enhanced widening of the ventrolateral wall of the inflammatory aneurysm. There is no widening of the dorsal and dorsolateral wall. The left ureter is involved in the inflammatory process of the aneurysmal wall *(arrow)*. (Courtesy of Kniemeyer HW, Kolvenbach R, Rohde E, et al: *Chirurg* 61:27–31, 1990.)

1 patient with a TAA, access was obtained via a median laparotomy.

The overall mortality rate was 15%. Six patients died of cardiopulmonary insufficiency, 1 of peritonitis, and 1 of coagulopathy. Rupture occurred in 8 patients, 4 of whom died. After a mean follow-up of 28 months, 35 patients were available for examination. Seven patients had died in the meantime, yielding a late mortality rate of 13.2%. Three patients could not be traced. Seven of the 35 reexamined patients had late complications, including an atrophied kidney in 3 and anastomotic aneurysms in 4. The expected 5-year survival rate was 57%, and the expected 10-year survival rate was 48%.

Inflammatory AAAs are associated with a higher morbidity and mortality than atherosclerotic AAAs. Morbidity and mortality can be lowered by a correct preoperative diagnosis and the use of modified surgical procedures.

▶ Each analysis of patients with inflammatory aneurysms comes to similar conclusions. They occur regularly and their operative treatment is associated with a higher morbidity and even mortality. Difficulties in surgery can be obviated for the most part by preoperative diagnosis, which is easily achieved by CT scanning. Whereas magnetic resonance is similarly useful, CT shows the location of the ureters much more easily and preoperative ureteral cannulation can be accomplished when difficulties are anticipated.

Histological and Clinical Markers of Inflammatory Infrarenal Abdominal Aortic Aneurysms

Hofmann W, Müller-Bühl U, Bährle S, Diehm C, Allenberg JR (Universität Heidelberg, Germany)

Pathologe 10:219–227, 1989 8–25

Inflammatory aneurysms of the abdominal aorta (IAA) differ histologically from arteriosclerotic abdominal aortic aneurysms (AAA). Inflammatory aneurysms of the abdominal aorta are characterized by plasma cell infiltration in the media, adventitia, and periadventitia, and fibrotic thickening of the aneurysmal wall. The incidence of IAA has been estimated at 2% to 23% of all AAAs, with a 10% incidence reported most often. Macroscopically, an IAA typically has dense, whitish, porcelain-like fibrotic thickening at the ventral and lateral parts of the aneurysmal wall. Adjacent organs usually adhere closely to the vessel wall, causing problems during operation. Features that distinguish IAA from AAA were identified.

During a 15-month period, 43 men and 4 women were operated on for AAA. Based on histopathologic criteria, the patients were classified into 3 categories: 33 had AAA with microscopically confirmed sclerosis of the intima; 7 had a transitional type of IAA in which the number of inflammatory cells in the media and adventitia was clearly increased, but the typical fibrotic reaction was absent; and 7 had a true IAA, in that the inflammatory process extended over the media, adventitia, and periadventitial tissues. Inflammation was especially pronounced around the vasa vasorum and around localized necrotic areas that obscured the demarcation between the vessel wall and the inflammatory reaction. The infiltrate consisted mostly of lymphocytes and plasma cells. Foreign cell particles, macrophages (including histiocytes and fibroblasts), and a few granulocytes also were seen. Because the transitory and full-blown forms of IAA differed histologically only in the extent of expression of the inflammatory process, both groups were combined for statistical analysis.

Males accounted for 97% of the 33 AAA patients and for 78.6% of the 14 IAA patients. The difference was statistically not significant. Laboratory studies indicated that IAA patients had significantly higher levels of C-reactive protein and immunoglobulins G and A than AAA patients. An IAA is a distinct disease entity characterized by inflammatory as well as degenerative processes. However, the inflammatory component does not fall into the general category of inflammatory vascular diseases; rather, it represents a secondary reactive-resorptive process resulting from arteriosclerotic changes in the vessel wall.

▶ A clue to the fundamental etiology of inflammatory aneurysms rests on the observation of plasma cell infiltration into the media. This abstract suggests that this is a reaction to the arteriosclerotic changes in the vessel wall. However, there is no proof of that. There are more attractive hypotheses.

The Response of Peri-Aneurysmal Fibrosis—the "Inflammatory" Aneurysm—to Surgery and Steroid Therapy

Stotter AT, Grigg MJ, Mansfield AO (St Mary's Hosp, London)

Eur J Vasc Surg 4:201–205, 1990 8–26

The so-called inflammatory aortic aneurysms, those associated with dense, white, periaortic fibrosis, occur in up to 15% of cases. Surgical treatment is especially difficult because of adherence of the aortic wall to adjacent structures. Steroid therapy, which reduces periaortic thickening, may facilitate surgery. However, the risk of rupture persists. Also, prosthetic repair of the aneurysm may even accelerate the inflammatory process.

Man, 59, referred for treatment of an asymptomatic aneurysm, underwent laparotomy. The wall had the typical appearance of an inflammatory aneurysm. After minimal dissection a 20-mm straight Dacron graft repair was performed. Because flow into the right common iliac artery was inadequate, an 8-mm Dacron graft was interposed between the aortic prosthesis and the right common iliac artery. On the 22nd postoperative day the patient returned to the hospital complaining of anorexia, abdominal discomfort, and episodes of sweating. Computed tomography showed increased thickening of the aneurysm wall, edema and thickening in the root of the small bowel mesentery, and obstruction of the right ureter with hydronephrosis. The patient was treated with broad-spectrum antibiotics, but his condition worsened. Treatment with steroids brought improvement, and the patient returned home. He died suddenly at 5 months after operation of varicella viremia, which suggests that he may have been immunocompromised from the outset.

The patient appeared to have an extension of the periaortic inflammation after uneventful surgical repair. Graft sepsis was suspected, but cultures proved negative. His response to steroid therapy offers circumstantial evidence for acceleration of the original process.

▶ It is unusual to see progression of the retroperitoneal fibrosis after surgical decompression. Suppression of the process by corticosteroid therapy suggests an immune mechanism that, unfortunately in this case, was suppressed sufficiently that the patient died of viremia.

Inflammatory Abdominal Aortic Aneurysms and Ureteric Obstruction
Radomski SB, Ameli FM, Jewett MAS (Wellesley Hosp; Univ of Toronto)
Can J Surg 33:49–52, 1990 8–27

Inflammatory abdominal aortic aneurysms (AAAs) are rare but can involve the ureters in the perianeurysmal fibrosis. The best treatment for ureteric involvement is debated. Ureteric obstruction associated with an inflammatory AAA was diagnosed in an elderly patient.

Woman, 73, was hospitalized for elective repair of an AAA. Computed tomography showed an infrarenal AAA with a thickened wall. She had right hydronephrosis, and her right ureter was involved in the aneurysm wall (Fig 8–7). At surgery a thick-walled, shiny AAA was seen. The level of obstruction was just above the left sacroiliac joint. Ureterolysis of the right ureter was needed. The

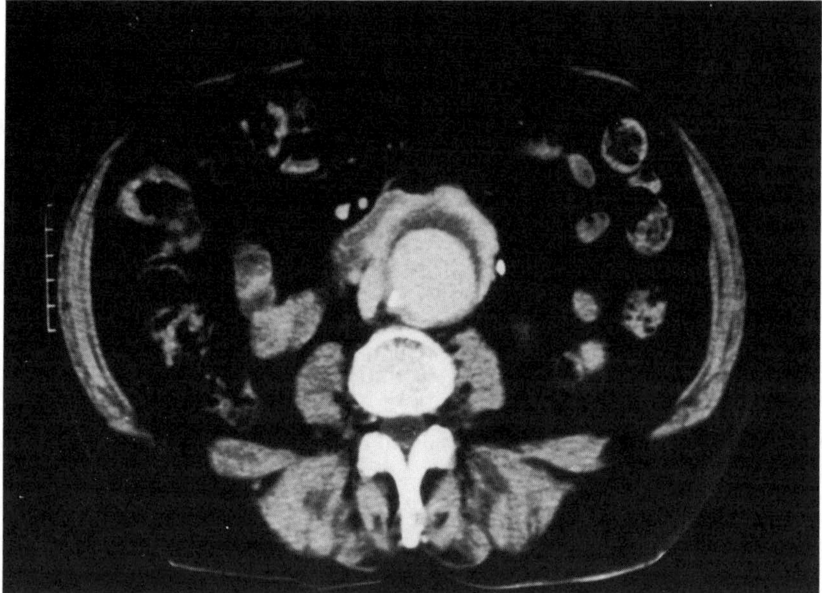

Fig 8–7.—Computed tomogram reveals infrarenal AAA measuring 5.5 cm with thickened wall. Note right ureter involved in wall of aneurysm. (Courtesy of Radomski SB, Ameli FM, Jewett MAS: *Can J Surg* 33:49–52, 1990.)

duodenum adhered to the aorta, and a severe inflammatory reaction was observed around the iliac vessels. A 16-mm Dacron graft was inserted. The aneurysm was repaired without difficulty. The ureteral stent was left in place for 7 days after surgery, during which time the patient was given antibiotics. The postoperative course was uneventful, and the patient was discharged 11 days after the operation. At her 3-month follow-up examination, she was well, and an intravenous pyelogram appeared normal.

The diagnosis of ureteric obstruction secondary to inflammatory AAAs can be made initially with CT followed by retrograde pyelography. After the diagnosis has been established, treatment consists of inserting a ureteral stent and ureterolysis. This can be done safely and effectively during repair of the inflammatory AAA. Both the vascular surgeon and urologist should suspect ureteral involvement in cases of inflammatory aortic aneurysms.

▶ After the diagnosis of an inflammatory aneurysm has been made by CT, ureteral stenting may greatly simplify surgical decompression of the retroperitoneum and removal of the aortic aneurysm from the arterial circulation. Whether or not the ureters need decompression depends on their degree of obstruction, but one would predict regularly that the retroperitoneal fibrotic process would abate after midline retroperitoneal decompression.

Inflammatory Abdominal Aortic Aneurysm: A Cause of Urinary Obstruction and Acute Renal Failure

Bartlett P, Woods D, Dobranowski J (McMaster Univ; St Joseph's Hosp, Hamilton, Ont)

J Can Assoc Radiol 40:164–166, 1989 8–28

Abdominal aortic aneurysms (AAAs) are rare causes of ureteric obstruction. Among the 122 patients with AAA operated on during a 4-year period, 3 had inflammatory AAAs presenting with urinary obstruction.

Inflammatory AAAs producing hydronephrosis, occurred in 3 elderly patients, 2 of whom had acute renal failure. Retrograde pyelography confirmed the presence of hydronephrosis secondary to extrinsic compression of the displaced ureters. Computed tomography provided an accu-

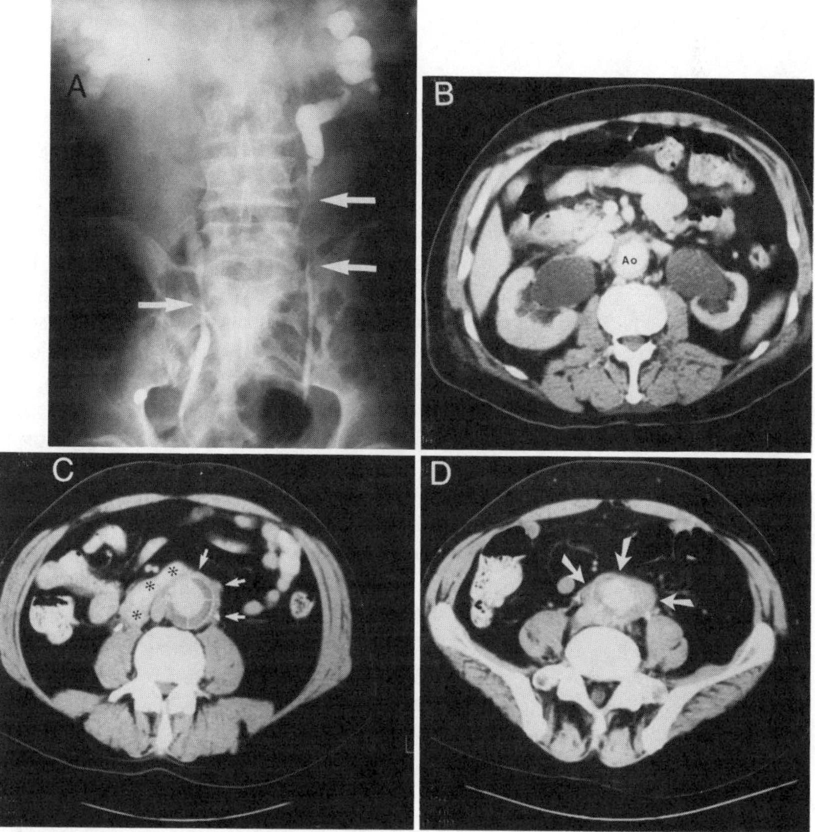

Fig 8–8.—**A,** bilateral retrograde pyelogram shows hydronephrosis and bilateral midureteric narrowing *(arrows)*. **B,** the CT scan of the upper abdomen demonstrates atherosclerotic changes in the aorta *(Ao)* and bilateral hydronephrosis with dilated extrarenal pelvises. **C,** the CT scan of the lower abdomen identifies calcification in the wall of the AAA, mural thrombus, small rim of periaortic fibrosis *(arrows)*, and adjacent small bowel loop *(asterisks)*. **D,** at the level of the aortic bifurcation, CT shows enhancing, larger periaortic fibrous mantle *(arrows)*. (Courtesy of Bartlett P, Woods D, Dobranowski J: *J Can Assoc Radiol* 40:164–166, 1989.)

rate assessment of the size and extent of the AAA. The CT findings consisted of mural thrombus, wall calcification, and an enhancing periaortic soft tissue mantle (Fig 8–8).

Inflammatory AAAs can cause urinary obstruction and acute renal failure. It is important to recognize this disease preoperatively, as it alerts the surgeon to complications, such as adherent viscera and excessive blood loss. The diagnosis can be established by CT. Treatment is directed toward ureteric decompression, either through percutaneous or retrograde catheterization, and repair of the AAA.

▶ Although retroperitoneal fibrosis has long been recognized as a cause of renal failure attributable to ureteral obstruction, the knowledge of this has come to vascular surgery lately. The process of an inflammatory aneurysm and that of retroperitoneal fibrosis is virtually indistinguishable. Only the single difference of earlier diagnosis in cases of inflammatory aneurysm separates the 2 entities.

Arteriosclerotic Abdominal Aortic Aneurysm Infected With *Yersinia enterocolitica*

Van Steen J, Vercruysse J, Wilms G, Nevelsteen A (Univ Hosps, Leuven, Belgium)

Fortschr Röntgenstr 151:625–626, 1989 8–29

Infection with *Yersinia enterocolitica* is an important cause of gastroenteritis. Bacteremia and deep tissue infections caused by *Y. enterocolitica,* however, are rare and generally are associated with underlying illness. *Yersinia enterocolitica* serotype 3 was isolated from aneurysmal blood obtained from a patient with a ruptured aneurysm of the abdominal aorta.

Man, 91, had experienced mesogastric pains, nausea, and absence of stools for 2 days. Chest roentgenography showed a generalized interstitial lung disease and an enlarged heart shadow. The only abnormal laboratory finding was a high erythrocyte sedimentation rate. The symptoms subsided and the patient was discharged from the hospital. Severe mesogastric pain returned about 2 weeks later. Computed tomography revealed an infrarenal calcified aortic aneurysm surrounded by a soft tissue mass (Fig 8–9). The patient recovered quickly after surgical resection of the aneurysm, but his condition soon deteriorated. Computed tomography showed a retroperitoneal abscess surrounding the Dacron graft. After a second operation, the patient died.

Blood from the aneurysm content and specimens from the aneurysm wall obtained at the initial operation were positive for *Y enterocolitica* serotype 3. It was suspected that the patient's infection was caused by colonization of an arteriosclerotic vessel by a cryptogenic bacteremia with a preexisting arteriosclerotic anerysm or by contiguous spread of in-

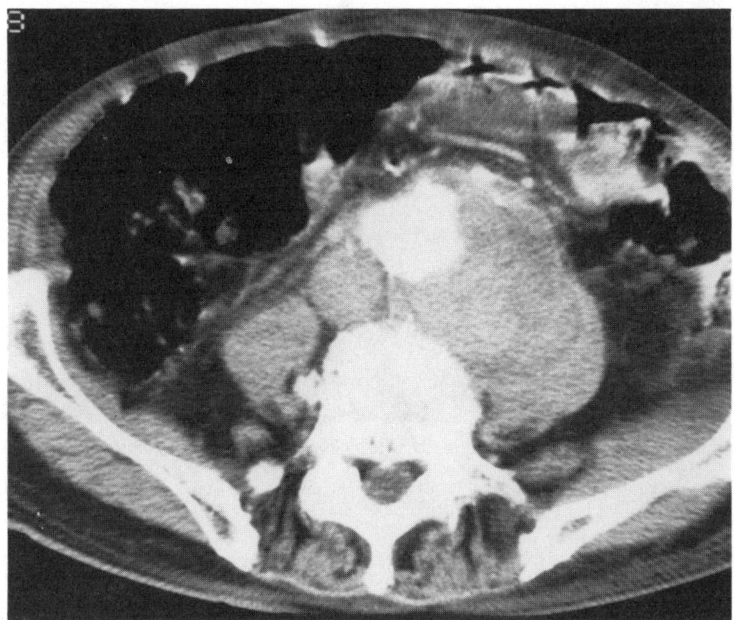

Fig 8–9.—Computed tomographic scan reveals an infrarenal calcified aortic aneurysm surrounded by a soft tissue mass. Intravenous administration of contrast material shows peripheral and slightly delayed enhancement. (Courtesy of Van Steen J, Vercruysse J, Wilms G, et al: *Fortschr Röntgenstr* 151:625–626, 1989.)

fection from an adjacent lymph node. Previous studies have found a high percentage of infected abdominal aortic aneurysms in women.

Ultrasonography and CT scanning can confirm the rapid enlargement characteristic of infected aneurysms. When bacteremia with *Y. enterocolitica* is diagnosed, especially among the elderly, long-term antibiotic treatment should be considered because of the risk of an endovascular infection, aneurysm, or endocarditis.

▶ This organism is commonly associated with gastroenteritis and mesenteric adenitis, and an erroneous diagnosis of acute appendicitis is common. It is not surprising that this organism would ultimately be found in ruptured aortic sepsis. The CT scans in this case suggest that the aneurysm was present before the septic complication occurred.

Prostatic Infarction Associated With Aortic and Iliac Aneurysm Repair

Feero P, Nickel JC, Brown P, Young I (Queen's Univ, Kingston, Ont)

J Urol 143:367–368, 1990 8–30

Acute urinary retention in male patients after abdominal aortic operation is usually caused by preexisting prostatic obstruction from benign prostatic hyperplasia. Prostatic infarction as a cause of acute urinary re-

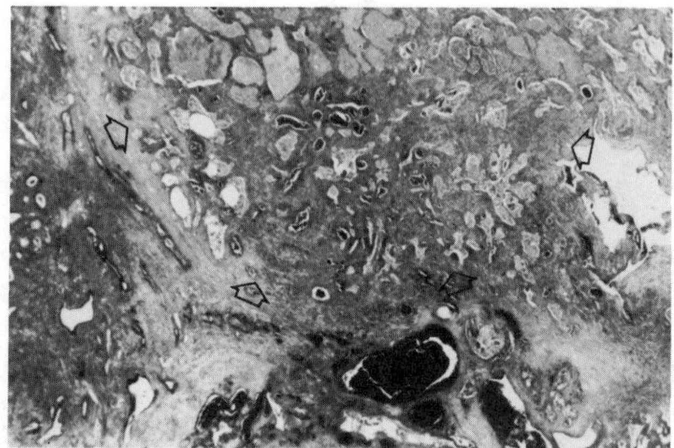

Fig 8–10.—Prostatic curette specimens obtained by transurethral resection contain extensive areas of recent infarction *(arrowheads)* that are rimmed by zones of hemorrhage and edema. Uninvolved region of prostate is shown at lower left side. Hematoxylin-phloxine-saffron stain, reduced from ×18. (Courtesy of Feero P, Nickel JC, Brown P, et al: *J Urol* 143:367–368, 1990.)

tention after aortic repair was observed in 2 men aged 66 and 80 years.

Acute bladder outlet obstruction developed after repair of both iliac artery aneurysms in 1 and a ruptured infrarenal aortic aneurysm in the other. Both men had perioperative hypotension and an indwelling urinary catheter. The right lobes of the prostate were grossly enlarged. Transurethral resection of the prostate was performed and pathologic examination revealed recent prostatic infarctions, as well as epithelial and fibromuscular hyperplasia (Fig 8–10).

Prostatic infarction should be added to the list of complications after aneurysm repair of the abdominal aorta and iliac arteries. These procedures pose a risk to the blood supply of the prostate. The infarcted prostatic tissue, as well as the secondary edema, cause acute urinary obstruction. Other factors that contribute to the pathogenesis of acute prostatic infarction include prostatitis, periods of hypotension, urethral instrumentation and catheterization, and size of the accompanying prostatic adenoma.

▶ As the blood supply to the prostate is derived from the internal iliac circulation through vesical arteries, it is important to note that in both of these cases the internal iliac arteries were excluded from the reconstruction circulation. This fact makes a stronger case for attempting to revascularize at least 1 internal iliac artery when performing reconstructive operations.

The Impact of Computed Tomography in the Diagnosis and Postoperative Follow-Up of Ureteric Obstruction in Aorto-Iliac Aneurysmal Disease

Nachbur B, Marineck B, Jakob R, Ackerman D (Univ of Berne, Switzerland)

Eur J Vasc Surg 3:475–492, 1989 8–31

The diagnosis of ureteric obstruction associated with aortoiliac aneurysmal disease has been greatly enhanced by the introduction of CT. Between 1979 and 1987, 20 patients with unilateral or bilateral ureteral stenosis secondary to aortoiliac aneurysms were examined by CT. All but 1 of these patients constituted the 8.6% of 221 patients with symptomatic nonruptured aortoiliac aneurysms treated in this period. The diagnosis was verified at surgery in 19 patients; 1 patient refused surgery.

The association between ureteric entrapment and aortoiliac aneurysm was documented clearly by CT in all 20 patients. Ureteric entrapment was caused by an inflammatory aneurysm in 8 patients. On CT, the in-

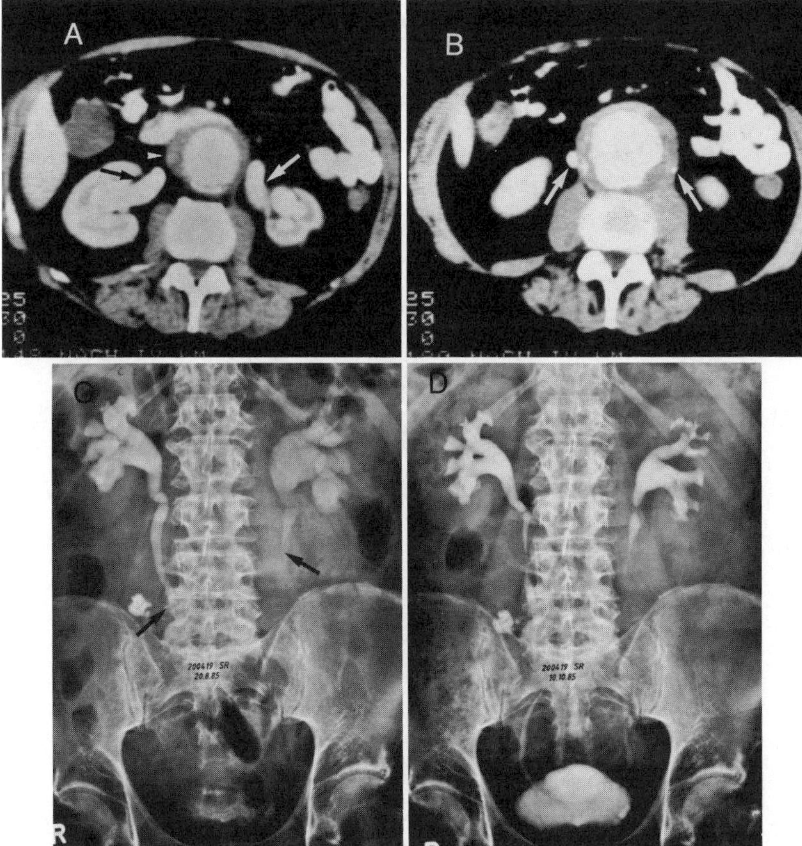

Fig 8–11.—Bilateral ureteric stenosis in a patient with inflammatory aneurysm. Preoperative CT scans after nephrostomy of the left kidney for 10 days and treatment with steroids for 6 weeks. **A,** bilateral caliceal dilatation *(arrows)*. Entrapment of the inferior vena cava (IVC) in the perianeurysmal fibrotic tissue *(arrowhead)*. **B,** 2 ureters are obstructed by fibrotic perianeurysmal tissue *(arrows)*. The lumen of the IVC with a high degree of narrowing. Broad contact of fibrotic tissue with psoas muscle on the left. **C,** intravenous pyelogram showing bilateral caliceal dilatation with blunting and ureteric obstruction alongside the inflammatory aortic aneurysm *(arrows)*. **D,** intravenous pyelogram 7 weeks after disconnection of the inflammatory aneurysm and interposition of a prosthetic bifurcation graft. (Courtesy of Nachbur B, Marincek B, Jakob R, et al: *Eur J Vasc Surg* 3:475–492, 1989.)

flammatory aneurysm was characterized by a patent vascular lumen at the center surrounded by an eccentric mass of thrombus. This layer was covered by a sheath of fibrous tissue of varying thickness (5–18 mm) arranged in a horseshoe shape around the ventral and lateral circmference of the aorta (Fig 8–11). The encased ureter was released in 3 patients,

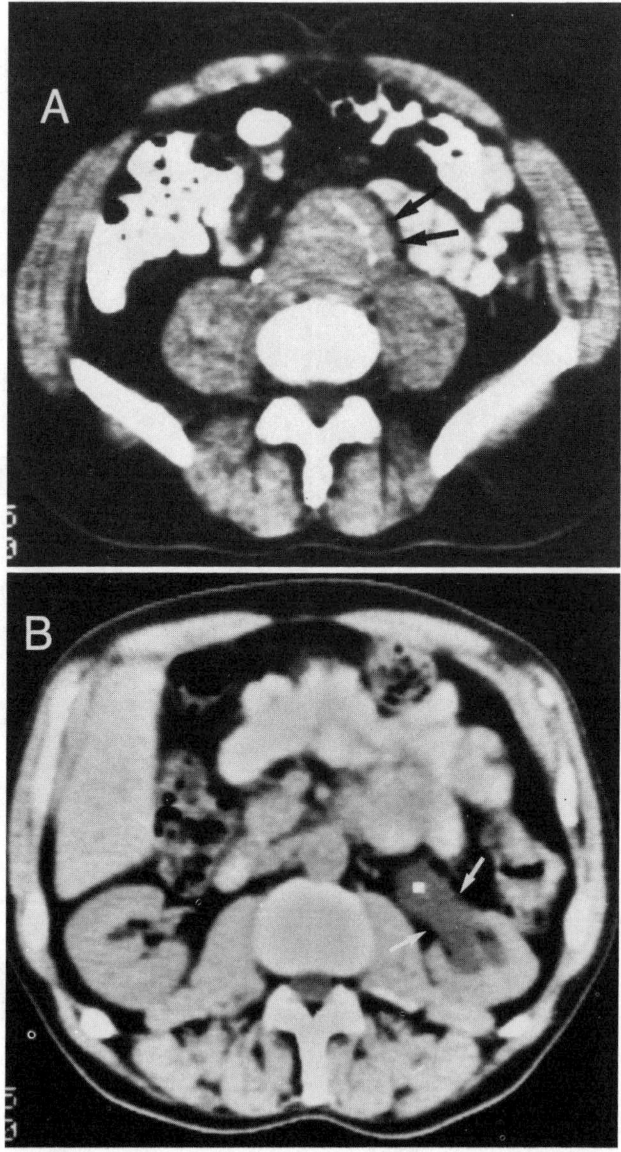

Fig 8–12.—Inflammatory aneurysm with left-sided hydronephrosis caused by ureteric entrapment. **A,** there is a thick layer of perianeurysmal fibrotic tissue on the left side *(arrow)* and anteriorly. **B,** a CT scan 9 weeks postoperatively shows no trace of regression of pyelectasis *(arrow)*.

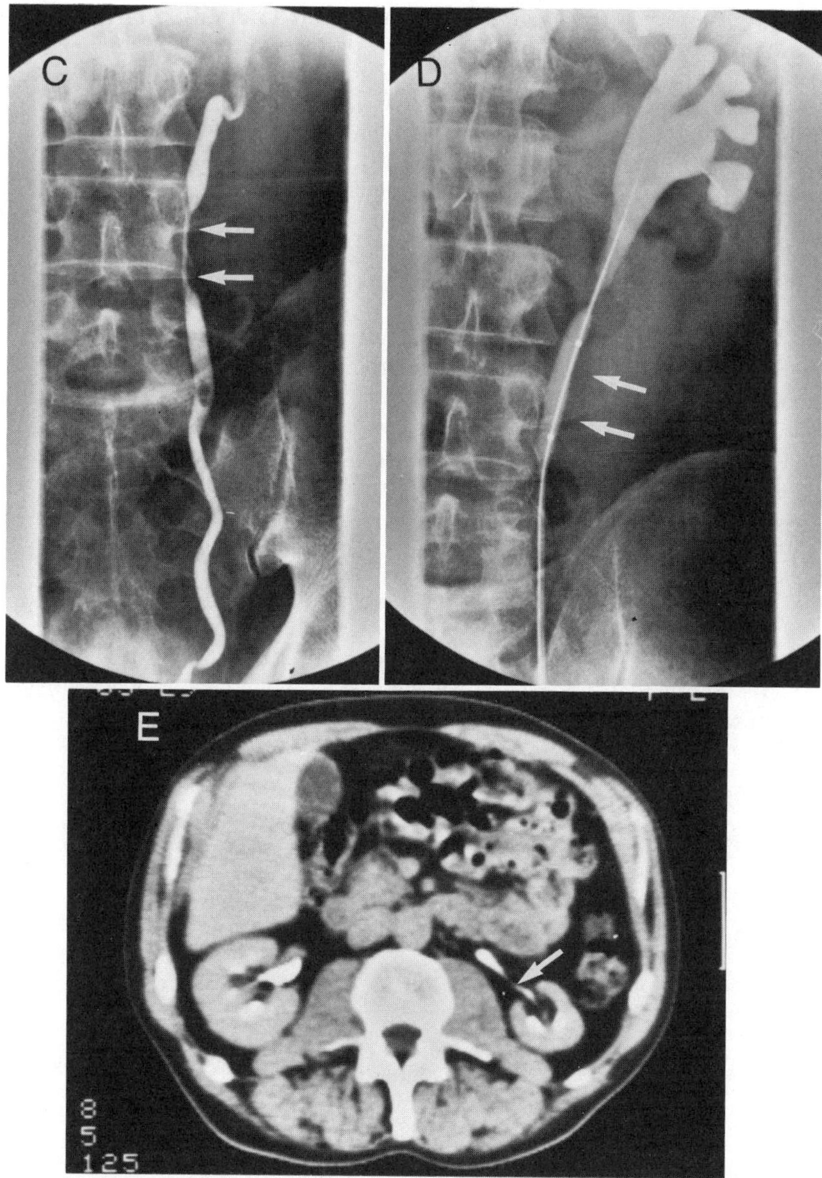

(**Fig 8–12,** *cont'd*).—**C,** the ureter had not been released during insertion of the bifurcation graft. A stenotic segment of the left ureter *(double arrows)* remains. **D,** treatment of the stenotic ureteric segment with retrograde balloon dilatation *(double arrows)*. Note caliceal dilatation with blunting. **E,** control CT 8 months later shows normalization of pyelocaliectasis. (Courtesy of Nachbur B, Marineck B, Jakob R, et al: *Eur J Vasc Surg* 3:475–492, 1989.)

whereas the other 5 had an interposition graft inserted without freeing the ureter. Follow-up CT scans in these patients revealed a time-dependent regression of perianeurysmal fibrosis, resulting in complete resolution in 4 patients at 24–52 months postoperatively. Relief of ureteral obstruction was achieved in all but 1 patient, who underwent balloon dilatation for persistent pyelectasis and caliectasis resulting from a stenotic ureteric segment (Fig 8–12). Ureteric entrapment was caused by an arteriosclerotic aneurysm in 12 patients. Ureteric entrapment generally was situated where the ureter crossed the iliac artery. The ureter was freed and an interposition graft was inserted in all patients, providing immediate relief of ureteric obstruction.

Computed tomography is the single most important imaging procedure in the diagnosis and follow-up of aortoiliac aneurysms with associated ureteric obstruction. Because of the potential difficulties associated with the surgical treatment of inflammatory aneurysms, it is important to identify the location and extent of the perivascular fibrosis preoperatively, which can be achieved only with CT. In addition, CT offers information on the occurrence and degree of pyelectasis and caliceal dilatation, identifies the location of ureteric entrapment, defines the extent of aneurysmal disease of the iliac arteries, and has the most to offer if contrast medium enhancement is contraindicated because of renal failure.

▶ Once again, CT scanning has shown the regression of retroperitoneal fibrosis after resection of abdominal aortic aneurysms. When the iliac aneurysm has entrapped the ureter, removing the aneurysm from the circulation is similarly effective. In the postoperative period the CT scan once again is extremely valuable in following the progress of ureteric obstruction.

9 Aortoiliac Occlusions

Variations in Geometry and Shear Rate Distribution in Casts of Human Aortic Bifurcations

Mark FF, Bargeron CB, Deters OJ, Friedman MH (Johns Hopkins Univ Applied Physics Lab, Laurel, Md)

J Biomechanics 22:577–582, 1989 9–1

The finding that atherosclerotic lesions are not uniformly distributed throughout the vascular system provides indirect evidence that local hemodynamic phenomena may be involved in the atherogenetic process. Many hypotheses regarding the role of hemodynamics in atherogenesis are based on the distribution of atheromatous lesions in the vasculature. Atherosclerotic lesions often develop near bifurcations, ostia, and vessel curvatures, suggesting that the complex flow patterns occurring at such locations may have a role in these hemodynamic phenomena. Previous studies have used flow-through casts of arterial segments to reproduce arterial flow fields in man. Shear rates were measured at sites along the walls of casts made of 10 human aortic bifurcations obtained at autopsy.

Casts were made after injection of a silicone rubber compound into the arteries. Fluid velocity measurements were made in the casts using a laser Doppler velocimeter. Eugenol was used as the working fluid. Pulsatile flow velocities were measured at sites immediately distal to the flow divider tip and along the lateral walls of the aorta and both iliac arteries.

Generally, the more geometrically symmetric casts showed a more symmetric distribution of shear rate values along their lateral wall. However, the variability in shear distribution among individuals was so great that generalizations regarding the shear environment of the vessel wall should be made with caution.

▶ Ever since the observation of Leriche, there has been interest in the hemodynamic cause of aortoiliac occlusive disease. Patients observed by Leriche had a shorter aorta, longer iliac arteries, and a completely patent distal circulation. As similar patients are seen in the modern era, they represent the ideal candidates for direct arterial reconstruction because their hemodynamic status can be normalized by successful operation. Further, they do not have the stigmata of arteriosclerotic heart disease or cerebrovascular disease. Further investigations such as the one reported in this abstract should be fruitful and will emphasize the fact that there are different populations of patients with aortoiliac occlusive disease and each should be managed in an individual fashion.

LDL Accumulation in the Grossly Normal Human Iliac Bifurcation and Common Iliac Arteries

Spring PM, Hoff HF (Cleveland Clinic Found)

Exp Mol Pathol 51:179–185, 1989 9–2

An earlier study described the topographic distribution of low-density-lipoprotein (LDL) accumulation in the aortic intima of normolipemic swine using an electrophoretic transfer procedure. With a similar procedure, the topographic distribution of LDL accumulation in grossly normal human iliac bifurcation and common iliac arteries was studied to assess the relationship between LDL accumulation and intimal thickening. Aortic samples were obtained from 6 recently dead persons aged 16–36 years. The technique used was the transfer by electrophoresis of LDL from the tissues into an agarose gel containing anti-LDL, and then staining the immunofixed LDL in the gel for lipid. On the basis of control studies, the level of lipid staining at the 37 ng apoB/mm^2 intimal surface area was used as the cut-off value between LDL-rich and LDL-poor sites.

The LDL-rich sites were found in all but 2 of the 6 cases. Intimal thickening was threefold greater in LDL-rich than in LDL-poor zones. Previous immunohistochemical studies suggesting a preferential accumulation of LDL at areas of diffuse and focal intimal thickening in human arteries were supported. The immunotransfer approach provides valuable information on the association of LDL with altered hemodynamics and formation of atherosclerotic lesions.

▶ The LDL accumulates at sites of intimal thickening. Correlation of such areas with demonstrated altered shear stress would be most valuable.

Percutaneous Transluminal Angioplasty of the Distal Abdominal Aorta

Belli A-M, Hemingway AP, Cumberland DC, Welsh CL (Northern Gen Hosp, Sheffield, England)

Eur J Vasc Surg 3:449–453, 1989 9–3

Percutaneous transluminal angioplasty (PTA) was used in the treatment of isolated, short-segment abdominal aortic stenoses in 13 patients with a mean age of 53 years. The mean follow-up was 27 months (range, 7–70 months). The femoral artery route was used, and the method of dilatation was by single- or double-balloon technique. Primary success was defined as a loss of systolic pressure gradient across the lesion or a residual gradient of less than 50% of the initial predilatation value.

All 13 stenotic aortas were dilated successfully with no complications (Fig 9–1). All patients reported symptomatic improvement, including 11 (85%) who became completely asymptomatic. Percutaneous transluminal angioplasty is a safe and effective procedure in selected patients with seg-

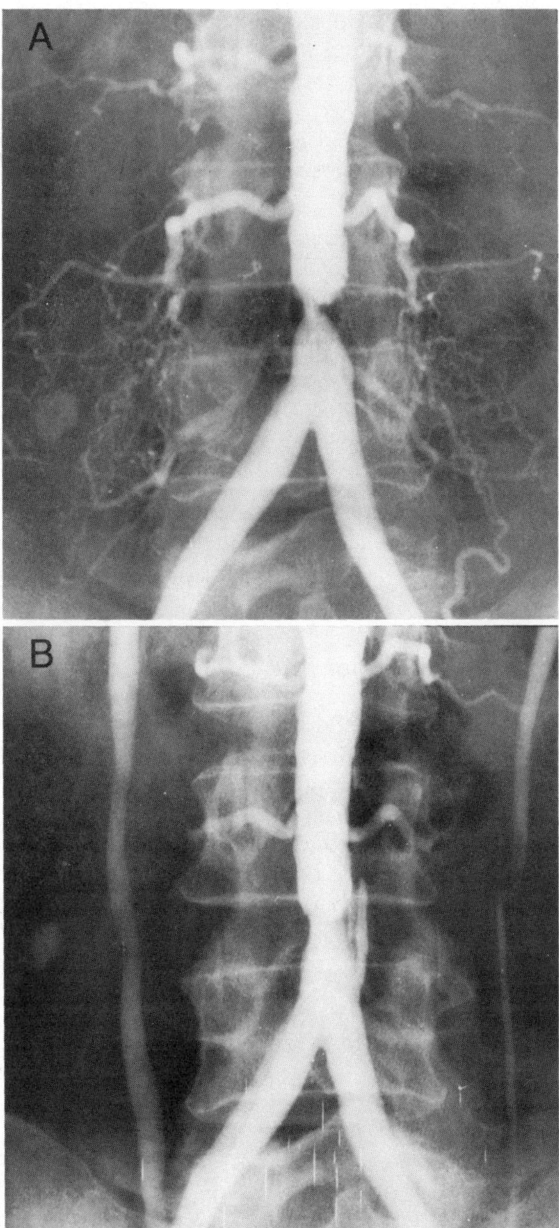

Fig 9–1.—A, stenosis of distal abdominal aorta. **B,** postangioplasty, "dissection" or subintimal cleft is visible, but the diameter of aortic lumen is wider and the pressure gradient was abolished. (Courtesy of Belli A-M, Hemingway AP, Cumberland DC, et al: *Eur J Vasc Surg* 3:449–453, 1989.)

mental distal aortic stenoses. Surgical intervention may not be necessary, at least in the short and medium term.

▶ The availability of nonsurgical relief of aortoiliac occlusive disease stimulates investigation of patients with claudication and diminished femoral pulsation. It is perfectly justified to treat patients with such claudication by PTA or surgical bypass techniques.

Aortoiliac Endarterectomy: An 11-Year Review

Naylor AR, Ah-See AK, Engeset J (Aberdeen Royal Infirmary, Scotland)

Br J Surg 77:190–193, 1990 9–4

Aortoiliac endarterectomy, once the most common form of reconstructive surgery for the severely diseased aortoiliac segment, has been replaced primarily by aortofemoral bypass (Fig 9–2). To determine whether this switch in procedure is justified, an 11-year review of 57 patients who underwent aortoiliac endarterectomy was initiated.

Although none of these patients died in the immediate postoperative period, 9 had significant complications. The cumulative survival rate was 98% at 1 year, 94% at 5 years, and 78% at 10 years. The cumulative segment patency rate was 92% at 5 years and 68% at 10 years. Smokers had significantly poorer rates for patency, limb failure, and symptom status than nonsmokers had. During the follow-up period, symptoms worsened in 27 patients, and 24 of these required secondary vascular intervention. In 14 cases this involved aortofemoral bypass. Recurrent disease in the external iliac artery was the most common cause of treatment failure.

Aortoiliac endarterectomy should be considered in young patients with localized disease not involving the external iliac artery. Patients who do not fit this description should be considered for primary aortofemoral bypass. The likelihood of success with either operation is decreased if the patient continues to smoke.

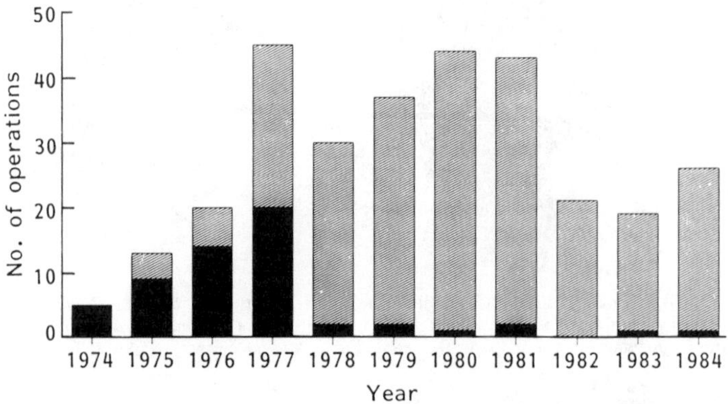

Fig 9–2.—Frequency of 2 forms of aortoiliac reconstruction, 1974–1984: *solid column,* aortoiliac endarterectomy; *shaded column,* aortofemoral bypass. (Courtesy of Naylor AR, Ah-See AK, Engeset J: *Br J Surg* 77:190–193, 1990.)

▶ The authors examined the results of a modest number of aortoiliac endarterectomies (52) in an 11-year period. The reader must wonder, with an average of 5 per year, how many surgeons with varied technical skill were responsible for the experience? It is a fact that technical excellence is responsible for superior results with the operation under study.

The pattern of aortoiliac atherosclerosis was not uniform. Only 17% of lesions terminated at the common iliac bifurcation, the level we use for performing either endarterectomy, or aortofemoral bypass if the disease exceeds the external iliac artery. This diffuse disease is responsible for the high early occlusion rate (4%) and the later failures, which were presumably the result of progression of untreated external iliac disease.

The conduct of the operation is critical for success. The authors, for reasons unknown, switched the arteriotomy orientation. They used transverse aorta, not longitudinal, and longitudinal in iliac arteries, not transverse. A few were closed with vein patches, but longitudinal primary closure of most segments produces narrowing and later occlusion. End points were tacked, but if the operation is tailored to the extent of iliac disease, no end point tacking is required because a clean transition occurs at the proper termination using the correct plane. The 2 patients who had a primary reconstruction failure and the 5 who needed another procedure underline the probability of technical imperfection that may exist.

This paper reviews the results of aortoiliac endarterectomy, and even considering the critique of this reviewer, the outcome was comparable to that achieved with prosthetic bypass, *without* introducing a foreign body, in their relatively young patients.— Ronald J. Stoney, M.D., Professor of Surgery, University of California Medical Center, San Francisco

---

Simultaneous Aortic and Renal Artery Reconstruction

Cooper GG, Atkinson AB, Barros D'Sa AAB (Royal Victoria Hosp, Belfast)

Br J Surg 77:194–198, 1990 9–5

Atheromatous renal artery stenosis is common in patients with peripheral vascular disease. When surgery is indicated for infrarenal aortic disease, simultaneous aortic and renal artery reconstruction can be considered in patients with difficult-to-treat hypertension or impaired renal functioning.

Nine patients were treated with simultaneous aortic reconstruction and renal artery revascularization. Seven had aneurysmal and 2 had occlusive aortic disease. In 4 patients this was associated with unilateral atheromatous renal artery stenosis, whereas it was bilateral in the other 5. The indications for renal revascularization were hypertension refractory to medical treatment (8 patients) and chronic renal failure (1). Postoperative complications developed in 5 patients, and 1 fatality occurred.

The remaining 8 patients were followed for 7 months to 4 years. Blood pressure control improved in 6 of the 7 hypertensive patients in this group. Serum creatinine levels stabilized or fell in 5 patients. Although simultaneous aortic and renal artery reconstruction has a high postoperative morbidity rate, it can improve hypertension control and stabilize renal function in selected patients.

▶ Increasingly, it has become recognized that when patients actually need simultaneous renal artery reconstruction with aortic reconstruction, this can be performed without the morbidity and mortality reported many years ago. However, the increased morbidity to be expected in combined procedures should be countered by meticulous intensive care management of such patients, both before and after the surgical procedure.

Retroperitoneal Lymphocele After Abdominal Aortic Surgery

Garrett HE Jr, Richardson JW, Howard HS, Garrett HE (Univ of Tennessee, Memphis)

J Vasc Surg 10:245–253, 1989 9–6

Lymphoceles resulting from traumatic injury to retroperitoneal lymphatics during abdominal aortic reconstruction are rare, only 5 symptomatic and 3 incidentally discovered asymptomatic lymphoceles having been reported. A record review of 4,000 patients who underwent abdominal aortic operations between 1974 and 1987 identified 4 (.1%) who were treated for persistent retroperitoneal lymph collections eventually diagnosed as groin lymphoceles.

The 3 men and 1 woman, who ranged in age from 46 to 85 years, had undergone aortofemoral bypass operations in the treatment of occlusive or aneurysmal arterial disease. The lymphoceles in the groin were not discovered until 2 to 8 years after operation. Three patients had bilateral lymphatic fluid collections and 1 had an unilateral lymphocele. Because the problem was not recognized initially, 3 patients were treated erroneously with repeated aspirations of lymphatic fluid, which failed to control the drainage. The repeated use of an irrigation-suction system ultimately introduced infection that required removal of the aortobifemoral graft and replacement with an axillofemoral graft. Reexploration of the retroperitoneum in these patients confirmed lymphatic injury, which was then treated by ligation of the lymphatics and suture. One patient in whom the initial diagnosis was correct underwent surgical drainage of the lymphocele; the graft was covered with sartorius and rectus muscle flaps.

Diagnosing lymphoceles is difficult as symptoms may mimic graft infection or pseudoaneurysm. Knowledge of the lymphatic anatomy (Fig 9–3) and recognition of the potential for infection with inappropriate drainage will help to prevent such complications. Direct surgical repair or suture ligation of lymphatic structures is recommended in a patient with postoperative chylous lymphocele as a complication of abdominal aortic reconstruction.

▶ Lymphocele development presents a recurring problem after aortofemoral reconstruction. Fortunately, intra-abdominal and pelvic lymphatics are decom-

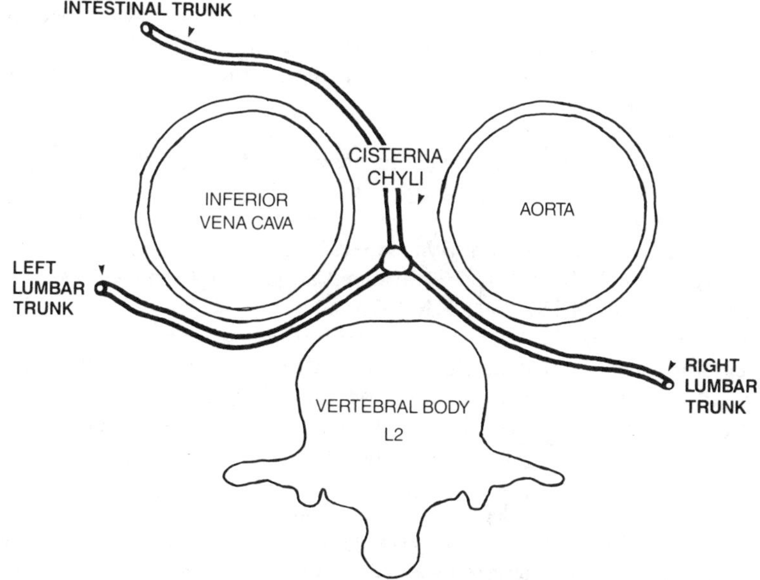

Fig 9–3.—Cross-sectional relationship of the cisterna chyli to surrounding structures. (Courtesy of Garrett HE Jr, Richardson JW, Howard HS, et al: *J Vasc Surg* 10:245–253, 1989.)

pressed by the retroperitoneal incision. In the groin, no absorptive surface such as the peritoneum or undersurface of the diaphragm is available. Furthermore, electrocoagulation used extensively in the reconstruction does not seal lymphatics. The lessons learned are that lymphatics should be occluded by ligature or clip and not cautery, and that repeated aspirations of lymphatic fluid can introduce the infection that one wishes to avoid.

Vacuum Drainage of Groin Wounds After Vascular Surgery: A Controlled Trial

Dunlop MG, Fox JN, Stonebridge PA, Clason AE, Ruckley CV (Western Gen Hosp; Royal Infirmary, Edinburgh; Royal Infirmary, Hull, England)
Br J Surg 77:562–563, 1990 9–7

The main lymphatic trunks of the legs, which converge in the inguinal region, are inevitably disrupted during femoral artery exploration, which may result in clinically important lymph leakage. The extent of lymph leakage and other complications in patients with groin wounds was investigated. The effect of suction drainage on lymph leakage and wound infection in 100 consecutive patients with groin wounds after vascular surgery was evaluated in a randomized, blind, controlled study. Lymph leakage occurred in 12% of patients and was significantly related to wound infection and prolongation of hospital stay. Subsequently, 127 wounds were randomly assigned to drainage or no drainage. The wounds were evaluated blindly by independent observers. There was no difference in the incidence of lymph leakage or wound infection between the 2 groups. The routine use of vacuum drainage was ineffective in controlling this complication.

▶ Sometimes controlled trials provide an answer, sometimes they don't.

Pregnancy After Aortofemoral Bypass Grafting in a Diabetic Patient

Bradley-Watson PJ (West Wales Gen Hosp, Carmarthen, Dyfed, Wales)

Am J Obstet Gynecol 161:200–201, 1989 9–8

Pregnancy after aortofemoral bypass grafting has been reported previously. However, there are no cases on record of pregnancy after aortofemoral bypass complicated by insulin-dependent diabetes. Both conditions were present in a patient who had an uncomplicated pregnancy.

Woman, 32, had insulin-dependent diabetes since age 9 years. At age 20, she delivered a healthy infant after 35 weeks' gestation. At age 30 years she underwent left renal aortoendarterectomy and end-to-end aortobifemoral bypass grafting with a knitted Dacron graft because of complete block of the aorta just below the level of the renal arteries. At age 32 years she was seen in the tenth week of her second pregnancy, which she was adamant about continuing. The patient was monitored at home with a glucometer, and a capillary blood glucose series was done twice a week. Retinas were examined throughout the pregnancy, and there were no adverse changes. Fetal well-being was monitored clinically and by serial ultrasonography. There was no evidence of intrauterine growth retardation or diabetic macrosomia. The patient was admitted at 38 weeks' gestation for planned induction of labor because of diabetes. She had a normal delivery of a healthy infant weighing 3.4 kg. Postpartum recovery was uneventful. The infant was observed in the special care baby unit for 48 hours and needed only early feeding to maintain adequate blood glucose levels.

Despite an earlier bypass operation, the blood supply to the pelvic organs in this patient did not appear to have been compromised enough to cause intrauterine growth retardation. Because of the added complication of diabetes, no prophylactic anticoagulant therapy was used.

▶ An interesting and informative case.

10 Femorodistal Occlusions

The Incidence of Congenitally Absent Foot Pulses

Robertson GSM, Bullen BR, Ristic CD (George Eliot Hosp, Nuneaton; Walsgrave Hosp, Coventry, England)

Ann R Coll Surg Engl 72:99–100, 1990 10–1

To determine the frequency of absent pedal pulses in healthy young persons, studies were made in 323 school children aged 9–10 years and 224 randomly chosen persons aged 15–30 years. The dorsalis pedis pulse was absent on both sides in 1.8% of the study population, and on 1 side in 6 others. The posterior tibial pulse was absent in only 1 person (.2%). In some children the posterior tibial pulses were impalpable but were detected using the Doppler probe.

The infrequent finding of congenitally absent foot pulses makes the absence of a pedal pulse in later life a more meaningful marker of peripheral vascular disease than previously recognized. If there is no pulse on Doppler probe study, the finding is especially significant.

▶ Because physical findings are so definitive in all forms of vascular disease, the findings of this simple study become extremely important.

Fluorescence-Guided Laser-Assisted Balloon Angioplasty in Patients With Femoropopliteal Occlusions

Leon MB, Almagor Y, Bartorelli AL, Prevosti LG, Teirstein PS, Chang R, Miller DL, Smith PD, Bonner RF (Natl Insts of Health, Bethesda, Md)

Circulation 81:143–155, 1990 10–2

The frequency of vessel wall perforations and limited recanalization efficacy have decreased the success rate of laser angioplasty in patients with peripheral vascular disease. The solutions to these problems focus largely on the use of more sophisticated pulsed laser systems. The clinical application of an integrated dual laser system that makes use of laser-excited fluorescence guidance to control pulsed laser ablation of plaque was evaluated.

In 12 patients with femoropopliteal occlusions that could not be recanalized by standard guidewire-balloon angioplasty techniques, percutaneous laser-assisted balloon angioplasty was performed using a new fluorescence-guided dual-laser system. Plaque detection by 325-nm laser-excited fluorescence spectroscopy gave real-time feedback control to a

480-nm pulsed dye laser for atheroma ablation. After diagnostic fluorescence sensing, using a common 200-μm optical fiber, computer algorithms directed a fire or no-fire signal to the treatment laser to selectively remove plaque.

Laser recanalization was successful in 10 patients. The procedure was followed by definitive balloon angioplasty in 7 patients with increased ankle/arm indexes. All femoropopliteal occlusions in the treatment failures were heavily calcified. There were 2 mechanical guidewire perforations without clinical sequelae. Ablation of calcified lesions required higher pulse energies and greater total energy per centimeter of recanalized tissue. Fluorescence spectroscopy was useful in flush occlusions, and correctly identified plaque, underlying media, and thrombus by changes in fluorescence intensity, shape, and peak position.

In this subgroup of patients refractory to standard angioplasty procedures, primary recanalization of femoropopliteal occlusions was successful in 83% of patients, and subsequent balloon angioplasty was successful in 58%. Heavily calcified lesions accounted for all of the failures. These lesions will require modified delivery systems to create larger primary channels and increase catheter-tip control.

▶ Engineers involved in adapting new technology to medical applications have done a marvelous job. The equipment described in this abstract and in the original article is enormously complex but does offer a tantalizing technique for restoring circulation through blocked arteries. Sadly, it is not the avoidance of perforation that is important in laser techniques. Rather, it is modification of the arterial wall response to injury.

A Confidence Profile Analysis of the Results of Femoropopliteal Percutaneous Transluminal Angioplasty in the Treatment of Lower-Extremity Ischemia

Adar R, Critchfield GC, Eddy DM (Duke Univ)
J Vasc Surg 10:57–67, 1989 10–3

Despite numerous reports there remains some uncertainty on the role of percutaneous transluminal angioplasty (PTA) in the treatment of lower extremity ischemia, possibly because of the lack of standardized reporting. The Confidence Profile Method consists of bayesian formulas and a computer system that incorporates subjective judgments and assumptions and gives quantitative and visual representations of the effect of the technology on the specific health outcome being measured and the range of uncertainty associated with it. Data from 12 selected clinical reports were used to ascertain the outcomes of femoropopliteal PTA in patients with intermittent claudication (IC) and with more severe extremity-threatening ischemia ("salvage").

The early success rate was estimated at 89% after PTA for IC, compared with 77% after PTA for salvage. Most failures occurred during the first 6–12 months. The patency rate at 3 years was 62% for IC and 43% for salvage, with little further loss at 5 years. The risk of procedure-related mortality was .5%, and the rate of PTA-related extremity loss was 1%. The risk of serious procedure-related complications that required surgical repair was 2.4%.

The Confidence Profile Method combines data from several reports into single best estimates of the outcomes that are considered important for decision making. The estimates derived in this study can be used for any decision concerning the use of PTA in the femoropopliteal segment.

▶ As the authors say, "Application of the confidence profile method is not easy."

Transluminal Iliac Angioplasty With Distal Bypass Surgery in Patients With Critical Limb Ischaemia

Griffith CDM, Harrison JD, Gregson RHS, Makin GS, Hopkinson BR (Queen's Med Ctr, Nottingham, England)

J R Coll Surg Edinb 34:253–255, 1989 10–4

Transluminal balloon angioplasty of the iliac artery has been used in combination with distal bypass procedures in high-risk patients who require treatment of critical ischemia in a lower limb. This approach improves arterial inflow to distal grafts while eliminating the need for major aortic reconstructive or extra-anatomical bypass procedures. Data on 25 patients with critical limb ischemia who underwent transluminal iliac angioplasty combined with distal arterial bypass grafts were reviewed.

The 17 men and 8 women aged 48–79 years had critical lower-limb ischemia with rest pain, ischemic ulceration, or digital gangrene. Of the patients, 16 were smokers, 7 had ischemic heart disease, and 5 had chronic airway disease at the time of operation. Iliac angioplasty was performed during bypass surgery with direct exposure of the femoral artery in 11 patients. The other 14 had percutaneous iliac angioplasty under radiologic guidance 2–7 days before undergoing bypass operation. All patients received intravenous antibiotic prophylaxis with amoxycillin and clavulanic acid at anesthesia induction and after operation. Femoropopliteal grafts were performed in 20 patients, and femorofemoral grafts in 5.

Iliac angioplasty was effective in all 25 patients; 2 patients died in the immediate postoperative period and 2 others died after 4 months and 26 months of follow-up. Postoperative complications, occurred in 5 patients, including myocardial infarction, pulmonary embolism, prosthetic graft infection, and minor superficial wound infections. Limb salvage rates were 75% at 12 months and 24 months, with graft patency rates of 63% at 12 months and 50% at 24 months. Transluminal balloon angioplasty combined with distal bypass grafting procedures in high-risk patients who require treatment for limb-threatening ischemia gives acceptable long-term limb salvage and graft patency rates.

▶ There is no doubt that proximal disobliteration and distal bypass is an effective technique. Removal of 2 hemodynamically significant blockages in sequence goes far to restoring near-normal circulation in a limb that has been severely compromised. However, basing a distal bypass on a tenuous percutaneous transluminal angioplasty in the iliac system can be dangerous. Inevitably, restenosis at the iliac level will once again severely compromise the distal limb and, of course, the distal bypass.

Femoropopliteal Arterial Fibrodysplasia

van den Dungen JJAM, Boontje AH, Oosterhuis JW (Univ Hosp, Gronigen, The Netherlands)

Br J Surg 77:396–399, 1990 10–5

Atherosclerotic occlusive disease causes most obstructions in the femoral and popliteal vessels. A rare cause, fibrodysplasia, was identified in 3 young patients with different types of dysplastic disease.

Case 1.—Girl, 15 years, had experienced claudication in her right leg for more than a year. Normal pulsations were found over the femoral arteries and over the left pedal arteries, but none over the right pedal arteries. Angiography revealed an occlusion of the entire length of the right superficial femoral artery. The patient underwent a femoropopliteal bypass to the proximal popliteal artery with autologous saphenous vein. At 12-year follow-up she continued to function well with no recurrence of symptoms. Histologic examination classified this patient's lesion as perimedial fibroplasia.

Case 2.—Man, 21, had medial dissection with secondary intimal fibroplasia—the first such case to be described. He recovered temporarily after undergoing lumbar sympathectomy, but claudication developed again. Four years later total occlusion of the entire superficial femoral, popliteal, and anterior tibial arteries occurred. Histologic examination of the artery showed an abnormal configuration (Fig 10–1). Occlusion of the bypass developed, and thrombectomy was unsuccessful. Two years later an iliac obstruction led to amputation of the patient's left lower leg because of severe rest pain.

The third patient, a 36-year-old man, was treated successfully for histologically verified intimal fibroplasia (Fig 10–2), only the second known case.

Fibrodysplasia, first described in 1938, remains an enigma. Because most of the patients described in the literature have been female, the condition may be influenced by hormones. Some cases may be related to an autoimmune process. Neither etiologic factor, however, seems to apply in these 3 patients.

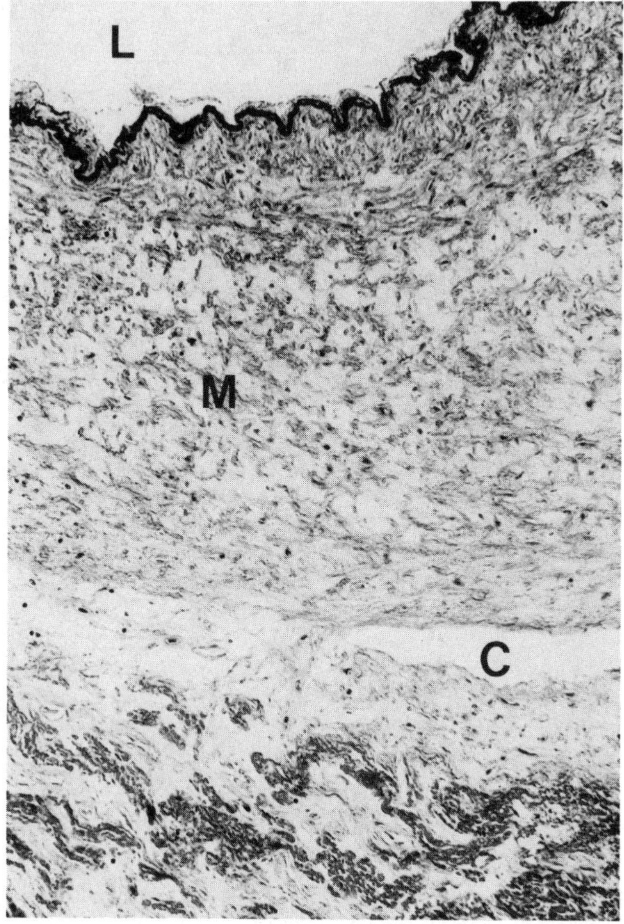

Fig 10–1.—Histologic section of medial dissection in case 2. The media is broad with irregular elastic fibers. In the outer zone of the media a channel is formed on the basis of mucoid degeneration. *L*, lumen; *M*, media; *C*, channel. Verhoeff stain; original magnification, ×140. (Courtesy of van den Dungen JJAM, Boontje AH, Oosterhuis JW: *Br J Surg* 77:396–399, 1990.)

▶ Several unusual conditions affecting the femoral popliteal segment appear at irregular intervals. Among the rarest is arterial dysplasia.

Cystic Adventitial Disease of the Popliteal Artery: A Case of Spontaneous Resolution

Owen ERTC, Speechly-Dick EM, Kour NW, Wilkins RA, Lewis JD (Northwick Park Hosp and MRC Clinical Research Ctr, Harrow, England)

Eur J Vasc Surg 4:319–321, 1990 10–6

Cystic adventitial disease (CAD) is a rare cause of intermittent claudication. The mucin-containing adventitial cysts occur most often in the

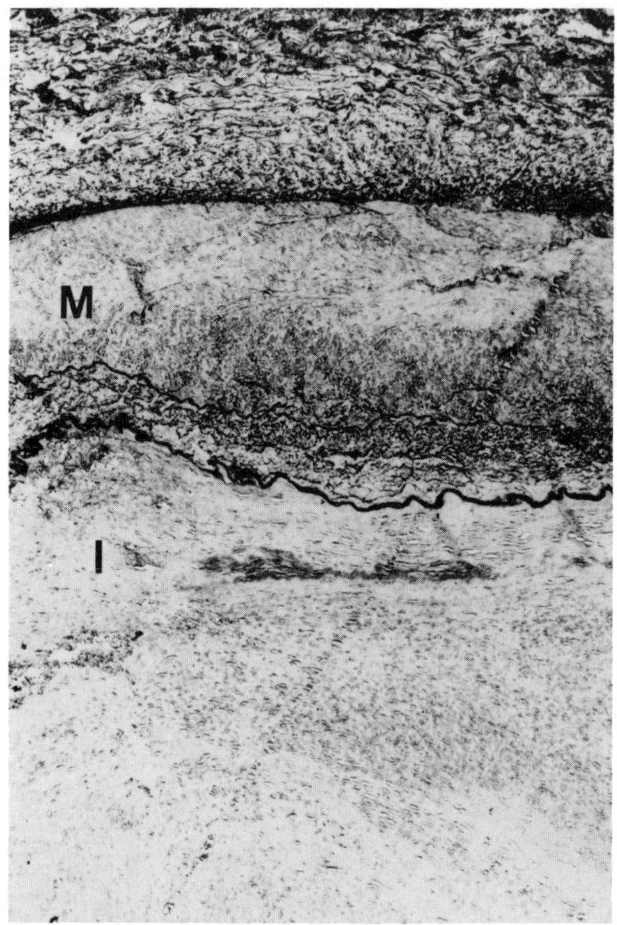

Fig 10–2.—Histologic section of intimal fibroplasia in patient aged 36. Intimal proliferation *(I)*, reduplication of the internal elastic lamina, and irregularity of elastic fibers in the media *(M)* are present. Verhoeff stain; original magnification, ×35. (Courtesy of van den Dungen JJAM, Boontje AH, Oosterhuis JW: *Br J Surg* 77:396–399, 1990.)

popliteal artery; they narrow the lumen but do not usually occlude the vessel. Spontaneously resolving CAD of the popliteal artery, the first such case reported occurred in previously healthy man.

Man, 35, nonsmoker, experienced intermittent claudication in the right calf for 6 weeks. No pulse was felt below the femoral artery, and the brachial pressure index at the ankle was .75. Angiography showed 80% stenosis of the right popliteal artery. A CT scan showed compression caused by a cystic lesion within the wall of the popliteal artery. After 15 months the patient's symptoms were much improved and distal pulses were present in the extremity. The pressure index was normal. Angiography showed significant luminal improvement. Symptoms were absent 6 months later.

It appears that spontaneous resolution of the lesion resulted from extravasation of the cyst contents. if adequate imaging facilities are available, conservative management or cyst aspiration may be considered before invasive surgery in cases of CAD.

▶ Cystic adventitial disease of the popliteal artery is rare. Its spontaneous resolution is equivalent to the spontaneous rupture of ganglia at the wrist. Similarly, one might predict recurrence of the lesion.

The Popliteal Artery Entrapment Syndrome: Presentation, Morphology, and Surgical Treatment of 13 Cases

Schurmann G, Mattfeldt T, Hofmann W, Hohenberger P, Allenberg JR (Heidelberg Univ, Germany)

Eur J Vasc Surg 4:223–231, 1990 10–7

About 140 patients with popliteal artery entrapment syndrome have been reported to date. This segmental vascular compression syndrome is based on an anomaly of the popliteal region. The syndrome has been seen mostly in young active persons with well-developed muscles. Typically, intermittent claudication progresses over a period of years, but symptoms also may develop abruptly.

The diagnosis is made by clinical examination, Doppler study, and angiography. Doppler pulse waves that appear normal in resting conditions may change during active plantar flexion (Fig 10–3). The popliteal artery

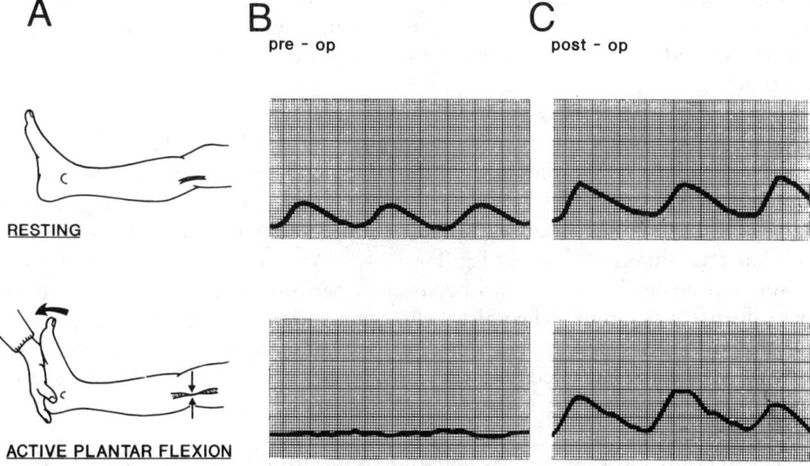

Fig 10–3.—A, during active plantar flexion (against resistance) the contracted gastrocnemius muscle causes an additional compression of the entrapped popliteal artery; **B,** Doppler pulse waves may be normal under resting conditions but disappear during active plantar flexion; **C,** evident improvement after surgical release of the entrapped vessel. (Adapted from Ferrero R, Barile L, Buzzachino A, et al: *Minerva Cardioangiol* 26:389–410, 1978, and Weiner SN, Hoffman J, Bernstein RS, et al: *Angiology* 6:418–428, 1983. (Courtesy of Schurmann G, Mattfeldt T, Hofmann W, et al: *Eur J Vasc Surg* 4:223–231, 1990.)

may be compressed between the medial gastrocnemius and the semimembranosus, or by atypically inserting muscle fibers, usually parts of the medial gastrocnemius. Intermediate types also are found.

Measures used to treat these patients have included thromboendarterectomy, vein patch placement, vein graft interposition, resection of aberrant tendon or muscle tissue, and removal of a poststenotic aneurysm. Freeing the artery may suffice in some cases but, usually, popliteal artery decompression and autologous vein graft placement are the best approach.

▶ Of the 3 rare manifestations of femoral popliteal arterial occlusive disease described in this edition of the YEAR BOOK, the most common is the entrapment phenomenon. This presentation is timely, authoritative, and emphasizes physical findings, but fails to stress the importance of CT. In fact, CT can be definitive, especially in assessing the status of the asymptomatic limb. This, of course, would dictate therapy in the asymptomatic extremity.

The Embolic Type of Popliteal Entrapment Syndrome

Haddad M, Barral X, Boissier C, Youvarlakis P, Bouilloc X, Beraud AM (Beilinson Med Ctr, Petah-Tikva, Israel; CHU Nord, Saint-Etienne, France)

VASA 19:63–67, 1990 10–8

Popliteal entrapment syndrome is ascribed to developmental anomalies. Patients usually have an acute or chronic ischemic syndrome, intermittent claudication or signs of distal ischemia, or intermittent arterial-compression-attributal symptomatology. One man had a Buerger-like syndrome and another had an acute ischemic syndrome. Both cases were characterized by embolic phenomena, which originated at the site of entrapment.

Man, 35, a heavy smoker with a history of superficial thrombophlebitis in the right leg, had a chronic ulceration of the right big toe for 9 months after surgery for an ingrown toenail. Two years earlier Buerger's disease at a mild stage II Fontaine classification had been diagnosed. Angiography revealed total occlusion of the 3 arterial trunks of the right leg (Fig 10–4). At surgery, a popliteotibialis posterior (retromalleolar) saphenous bypass was performed. The diagnosis of Buerger's disease was refuted when histologic examination of a fragment of the tibialis posterior artery showed no inflammatory reaction. A similar problem was treated in the patient's left leg 4 months later. The patient's big toe wound healed, and he was able to resume normal activities.

The second patient, an 18-year-old male athlete, was seen with acute ischemia. Popliteal artery entrapment appears to result from constantly recurring microtrauma to the deviated popliteal arterial wall by muscular contractions. This can lead to local arteriosclerosis and stenosis and ultimately to thrombosis, formation of aneurysm, occlusion, or mural microthrombi. The syndrome appears to be predominant in young men

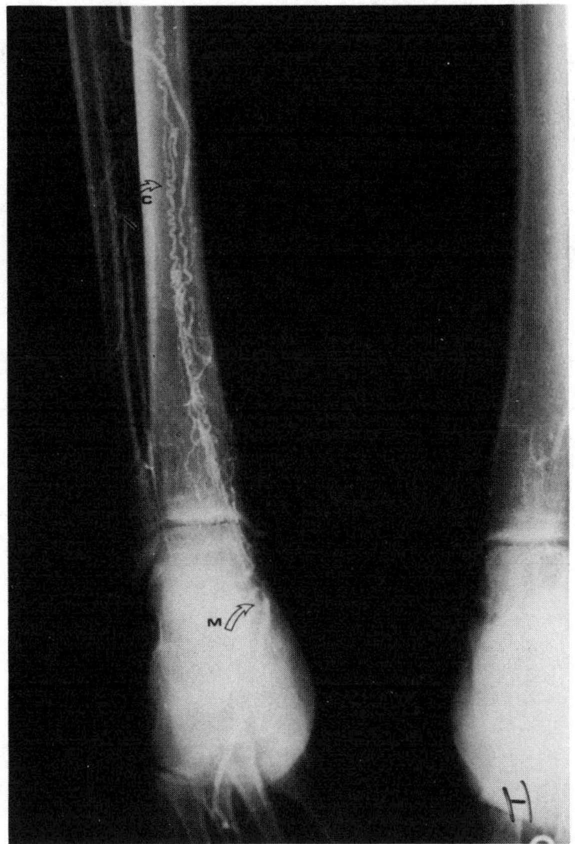

Fig 10–4.—Angiography demonstrating total occlusion of 3 arterial trunks of right leg. *C*, coiled collaterals and *M*, reappearance of healthy distal tibialis posterior at level of ankle. Peroneal artery lacks its middle third. Both have cutoff terminations characteristics of postembolic phenomenon. (Courtesy of Haddad M, Barral X, Boissier C, et al: *VASA*, 19:63–67, 1990.)

who engage in strenuous physical activity. Arterial biopsy can distinguish the condition from Buerger's disease.

▶ Distal microembolic disease in the lower extremities is chiefly a manifestation of ulcerative proximal atheroma. However, in younger individuals the congenital problems of entrapment or persistent sciatic artery can be suspected.

Isolated Popliteal Vein Entrapment
Nelson MC, Teitelbaum GP, Matsumoto AH, Stull MA (Georgetown Univ Hosp)
Cardiovasc Intervent Radiol 12:301–303, 1990 10–9

Congenital or rarely acquired abnormalities of insertion of the gastrocnemius muscle heads can cause entrapment of the popliteal artery. The

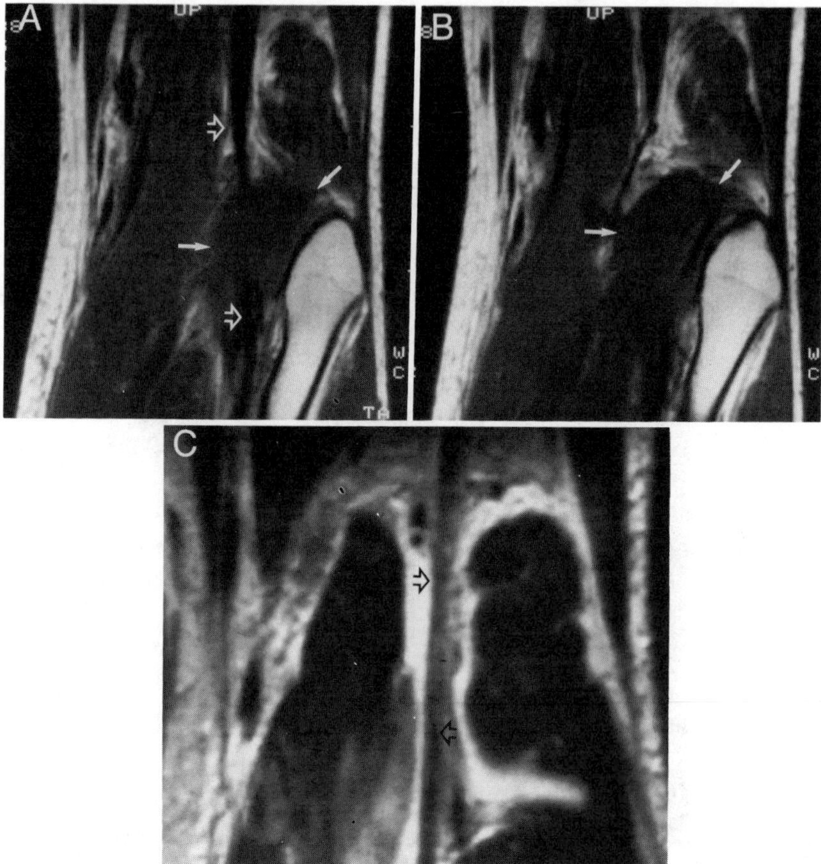

Fig 10–5.—T_1-weighted coronal spin-echo images of the popliteal fossa (**A, B**); TR, 600 ms; TE, 25 ms. **A,** compression of the popliteal vein *(open arrows)* is caused by the lateral head of the gastrocnemius muscle *(arrows)*. **B,** an image slice 3 mm more anterior to **A** shows the aberrant course of the gastrocnemius muscle *(arrows)*. **C,** a T_2-weighted coronal spin-echo image (TR, 2,000 ms; TE, 70 ms) slightly anterior to those in **A** and **B** demonstrates a normal caliber popliteal artery *(open arrows)*. (Courtesy of Nelson MC, Teitelbaum GP, Matsumoto AH, et al: *Cardiovasc Intervent Radiol* 12:301–303, 1990.)

popliteal vein may also be involved. Isolated entrapment of the popliteal vein was shown in 2 patients by venography and MRI.

Case 1.—Man, 47, had left calf tenderness and swelling exacerbated by exertion. He was treated with Naprosyn orally for nonspecific left knee arthritic changes; his symptoms persisted for about 1 month, however, at which time an MR study was done. Magnetic resonance imaging showed no mensical or ligamentous abnormalities or evidence of a Baker's cyst or mass. Assessment of the popliteal fossa, however, showed entrapment and compression of the popliteal vein secondary to the lateral head of the gastrocnemius muscle (Fig 10–5). A left leg venogram showed extrinsic compression of the popliteal vein. The patient's symptoms improved markedly with intermittent leg elevation.

Case 2.—Woman, 64, had a 1-week history of painless left calf swelling. Left lower extremity venography showed no sign of deep venous thrombosis, but there was marked extrinsic compression of the popliteal vein exacerbated by plantar flexion. Magnetic resonance imaging also revealed compression of the popliteal vein of a dynamic nature. The patient was managed with support hose and elevation of the leg.

These 2 patients had isolated popliteal vein entrapment caused by the lateral head of the gastrocnemius muscle. Their condition was confirmed by both venography and MRI of the knee.

▶ As other clinical studies have shown, any structure in the popliteal fossa can be entrapped by an abnormal gastrocnemius muscle head. The rarest form is entrapment of the nerve.

Present Status of Reversed Vein Bypass Grafting: Five-Year Results of a Modern Series

Taylor LM Jr, Edwards JM, Porter JM (Oregon Health Sciences Univ, Portland)
J Vasc Surg 11:193–206, 1990 10–10

Autogenous greater saphenous vein is thought to be the best conduit for infrainguinal bypass, but there is no consensus on the best technique to be employed. Of 564 limbs in 434 patients with infrainguinal arterial ischemia treated from January 1, 1980, through mid-December 1988, 516 limbs in 387 patients were subjected to autogenous reversed vein bypass grafting. In 285 grafts the ipsilateral greater saphenous vein was adequate; the remaining 231 operations used distal graft origins (151 grafts), alternate venous sources, or phlebophlebostomy. The distal anastomosis was to the below-knee popliteal artery in 199, the infrapopliteal artery in 241, and the above-knee popliteal artery in 76.

At 5 years the primary patency rate for all grafts was 75% and the secondary patency rate, 81%. The primary patency rate for grafts to infrapopliteal arteries was 69%, significantly worse than those for grafts to the popliteal artery, which were 77% for grafts above the knee and 80% for those below. The primary patency rate was 80% for grafts of adequate ipsilateral greater saphenous vein and 68% for all other grafts. The secondary patency rates, whatever the source of conduit or site of graft origin or distal anastomosis, ranged from 76% to 85%.

Reversed vein bypass grafting is recommended for infrainguinal revascularization. It yields excellent patency rates and is applicable to the many patients without intact ipsilateral greater saphenous vein.

▶ One is not surprised that autogenous tissue is preferred by all vascular surgeons, or, in fact, that a reversed vein bypass produces similar results to an in situ bypass. What is surprising is the fact that diabetics in this series had a better record of patency of their grafts than nondiabetics, as has been reported by LoGerfo. Clearly, there is need for nonvascular surgeons and internists to understand that there is no end-artery disease in the diabetic foot that impedes runoff from a reconstruction.

Great Saphenous Vein Protection in Arterial Reconstructive Surgery

Deriu GP, Ballotta E, Bonavina L, Alvino S, Franceschi L, Grego F, Thiene G (Univ of Padua, Italy)

Eur J Vasc Surg 3:253–260, 1989 10–11

Lower limb bypasses may be kinked or trapped at the popliteal level. Femorodistal bypasses with a distal anastomosis in the lower part of the limb may be compressed by tendinous or muscular structures. A reinforced prosthetic support, ringed polytetrafluoroethylene (PTFE) 8 mm, was used to protect the saphenous vein in 30 patients. In an additional patient with a thrombosed carotid patch graft, a new saphenous vein patch graft was covered with an onlay patch graft of PTFE.

Two patients required reoperation, but not for reasons related to the vein protection procedure. All of the protected femorodistal bypasses remained patent for 1 month to 7 years after surgery. In a patient with severe infection caused by a preexisting trophic ulcer, the distal part of the prosthesis was removed along with the thrombosed vein bypass.

This vein protection technique can improve the long-term results of long saphenous grafts in selected patients. In addition to the use of a ringed PTFE graft of adequate caliber, long-term anticoagulation is important. Vein protection may prevent aneurysm formation in vein graft bypasses.

▶ Deriu et al. describe an ingenious technique that might be utilized in particular situations.

Preoperative Correlates of Impaired Wound Healing After Saphenous Vein Excision

Utley JR, Thomason ME, Wallace DJ, Mutch DW, Staton L, Brown V, Wilde CM, Bell MS (Spartanburg Regional Med Ctr, Spartanburg, SC; Univ of South Carolina, Columbia; Med Univ of South Carolina, Charleston)

J Thorac Cardiovasc Surg 98:147–149, 1989 10–12

Major complications in leg wounds after vein graft excision are rare, whereas delayed healing associated with cellulitis, lymphangitis, edema, inflammation, and fat necrosis are more common. A study was conducted to identify preoperative clinical factors that significantly correlate with impaired healing in leg wounds after coronary artery bypass grafting. Wound healing impairment was defined as inflammation, separation, cellulitis, lymphangitis, drainage, necrosis, or abscess requiring wound dressing, antibiotics, or débridement before wound healing with complete epithelialization without eschar.

During a 5.5-year study period, 790 men and 257 women underwent coronary artery bypass grafting. Wound healing was impaired in 254 patients, including 170 men and 83 women. Statistically significant correlations were found between impaired wound healing and female sex, a body mass index indicating obesity, diabetes mellitus, left ventricular end-diastolic pressure greater than 15 mm Hg, arterial occlusive disease of the legs, and a preoperative hematocrit value of less than 35%.

Multiple regression analysis of the predictors of impaired leg wound healing showed that body mass index, female sex, and arterial occlusive disease accounted for the greatest amount of variability in the prediction of impaired leg wound healing. The other factors that correlated with impaired leg wound healing did not add significantly to the prediction.

▶ Vascular surgeons are regularly confronted with the need for revascularization after removal of a saphenous vein for coronary artery bypass grafting. Careful precardiac surgery evaluation of the lower extremities by objective techniques such as the Doppler and the ankle brachial index might prevent a number of these problems.

Femoro-Popliteal Versus Femoro-Distal Bypass Grafting for Limb Salvage in Patients With an "Isolated" Popliteal Segment

Darke S, Lamont P, Chant A, Barros D'Sa AAB, Clyne C, Harris P, Ruckley CV, Bell P (Royal Victoria Hosp, Bournemouth, England; Joint Vascular Research Group, England)

Eur J Vasc Surg 3:203–207, 1989 10–13

It is not clear what the best site is for distal anastomosis when a patent popliteal artery is "isolated" from healthy calf vessels by an occluded or stenosed segment. Fifty-nine such patients were randomized to undergo infrainguinal bypass grafting to either the popliteal segment or a reconstituted distal vessel in the calf. Fourteen femoropopliteal bypasses were above and 20 were below the knee. Eighteen femorodistal grafts were joined to the posterior tibial artery, 5 to the anterior tibial artery, and 2 to the peroneal arteries.

Limb salvage was achieved in 88% of patients who had femoropopliteal grafting and in 80% of those given femorodistal grafts. The 1-year graft patency rates were 79% in the femoropopliteal group and 70% in the femorodistal group, not a significant difference. Increases in the ankle/brachial pressure index were comparable in the 2 groups (table). Technical problems were considerably more prevalent in femorodistal bypass procedures.

If there is a choice between femoropopliteal bypass grafting and femorodistal grafting in a patient with severe limb ischemia, technical considerations alone suggest that popliteal anastomosis is preferable. A good outcome can be expected even if severe stenosis or occlusion is present between the site of anastomosis and the ischemic changes.

Mean Ankle/Brachial Pressure Indices (±SD)	Popliteal	Distal
Pre-operative	0.24±0.25	0.26±0.22
Postoperative	0.69±0.27	0.62±0.39
Change in pressure index:		
(a) Immediate post-op	+0.45±0.29	+0.37±0.27
(b) One year post-op	+0.58±0.32	+0.47±0.29

(Courtesy of Darke S, Lamont P, Chant A, et al: *Eur J Vasc Surg* 3:203–207, 1989.)

▶ Once again we find that graded runoff does not correlate with graft patency, even though logic would hold that the reverse would be true.

Routine Intraoperative Angioscopy in Lower Extremity Revascularization

Miller A, Campbell DR, Gibbons GW, Pomposelli FB Jr, Freeman DV, Jepsen SJ, Lees RS, Isaacsohn JL, Purcell D, Bolduc M, LoGerfo FW (New England Deaconess Hosp, Boston)

Arch Surg 124:604–608, 1989 10–14

The inability to see through blood and the need for complete removal of blood from the visual field are the primary obstacles to the widespread use of angioscopy during lower extremity revascularization. Whether applying the principles of irrigation and using a dedicated irrigation pump would make routine intraoperative angioscopy possible in such cases was investigated in a series of 136 intraoperative angioscopies performed during 112 peripheral bypass procedures, 15 thrombectomies, 2 embolectomies, and 7 other revascularization operations.

The total volume of irrigation fluid used in the peripheral bypasses ranged from none to 1,400 mL (average, 398 mL). The visual quality was good in more than 80% of the angioscopies. The failure rate was only 1.8%. Seventy-eight clinical or surgical decisions were made on the basis of the findings in 71 angioscopies. No complications could be attributed directly to insertion of the angioscope or use of the pump.

Routine intraoperative angioscopy can yield consistent high-quality results during surgical revascularization of the lower extremities when the basic principles of irrigation and the angioscopic pump are used. In this series, routine angioscopy was both clinically useful and safe.

▶ The era of angioscopy has arrived. The scope can be considered to be a useful addition to the armamentarium, especially during distal bypass grafting.

New Angioscopic Findings in Graft Failure After Infrainguinal Bypass
Miller A, Jepsen SJ, Stonebridge PA, Tsoukas A, Gibbons GW, Pomposelli FB Jr, Freeman DV, Campbell DR, Schoen FJ, LoGerfo FW (New England Deaconess Hosp; Brigham and Women's Hosp, Boston)
Arch Surg 125:749–755, 1990 10–15

Intraoperative angioscopy permits a direct, in vivo, 3-dimensional assessment of the interior of native vessels and grafts, and is a safe and informative means of monitoring infrainguinal bypass grafts. Videotaped recordings of intraoperative angioscopy in 25 patients having infrainguinal bypass grafts inserted unsuccessfully were reviewed to identify findings that related to graft failure. In addition, 3 failing grafts were evaluated angioscopically during graft salvage surgery. The failed grafts represented 11.5% of all infrainguinal bypasses done in the review period.

Most failures occurred within a month of surgery. Study of the early graft failures showed severe atherosclerosis with stenosis of the distal artery, poor vein graft quality (Fig 10–6), vein stenosis, improper graft tunneling, and graft torsion. Examination of the later graft failures showed severe distal outflow disease, uncut valve leaflets, and valvulotomy-induced injury.

Intraoperative angioscopy is a useful means of directly monitoring infrainguinal bypass grafting, and it provides information not otherwise obtainable. The procedure itself does not appear to heighten the risk of graft failure.

▶ It appears that the angioscopy revealed that technical factors, including improper tunneling, graft torsion, and poor vein quality, were the cause of a large number of failures. These, for the most part, can be avoided.

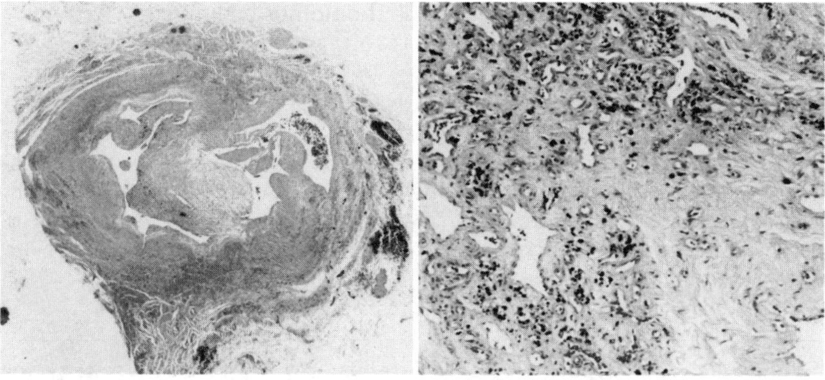

Fig 10–6.—Partially occluded saphenous vein resulting from recanalized organized thrombus. **Left,** low-power photomicrograph of vein cross-section demonstrates residual webs from recanalization of vessel; **right,** high-power photomicrograph demonstrates neovascularization with both large and small blood channels, chronic inflammation, and hemosiderin pigment indicative of organized thrombus. Hematoxylin-eosin; original magnification, ×20 *(left)* and ×150 *(right)*. (Courtesy of Miller A, Jepsen SJ, Stonebridge PA, et al: *Arch Surg* 125:749–755, 1990.)

Below-the-Knee Angioplasty: Tibioperoneal Vessels, the Acute Outcome

Dorros G, Lewin RF, Jamnadas P, Mathiak LM (St Luke's Med Ctr, Milwaukee; William Dorros-Isadore Feuer Found for Interventional Cardiovascular Diseases, Milwaukee)

Cathet Cardiovasc Diagn 19:170–178, 1990 10–16

Conventional balloon angioplasty, or peripheral angioplasty (PTA), has been applied reticently to the distal popliteal and tibioperoneal vessels because of potential complications. Peripheral angioplasty was attempted in 111 patients (mean age, 67 years) who had lesions in 168 below-the-knee tibioperoneal vessels (TPVs). The most common presenting symptoms were claudication, nonhealing ulcer or gangrene, and pain at rest. In 56% of patients an above-the-knee vessel was dilated before TPV angioplasty.

Successful PTA was achieved in 90% of the TPVs, in 99% of stenoses, and 65% of occlusions. Complications included contrast-induced renal failure in 4% of cases, distal embolization in 4%, entry site arterial repair or embolectomy in 2%, dissection or occlusion in 2%, and groin hematoma in 2%. Significant complications occurred in 3%: 1 patient died, 1 needed emergency bypass surgery, and 1 had distal embolization. Ninety percent of the patients had no complication. At discharge 95% of the patients were clinically improved.

Forty percent had a restenosis or a second PTA, or both, at a mean of 9 months after the initial procedure. Only 36% had lesion recurrence with or without new disease, and 64% had evidence of disease progression with symptoms. In 96% of the patients who had a second PTA the procedure was successful angiographically and clinically.

Balloon angioplasty can be used successfully in patients with symptomatic obliterative disease of the TPVs. In this series the results were excellent. There was good clinical improvement and a low risk of complications. Thus PTA of below-knee vessels should not be limited to extremity salvage situations.

▶ Vascular surgeons looking at the results of this large experience would come to exactly the opposite conclusions. Nearly half of the patients were treated for claudication. Even though technical success was achieved in 90%, actual success was achieved in only 65% of the occlusions. A significant complication, including death, occurred in 3% of the patients and a major complication in 14%. With all of this as background, 40% of patients needed a redo procedure within 9 months.

Saphenous Vein Bypass to Pedal Arteries: An Aggressive Strategy for Foot Salvage

Harris HW, Rapp JH, Reilly LM, Orlando PA, Krupski WC, Goldstone J (Univ of California, San Francisco)

Arch Surg 124:1232–1236, 1989 10–17

Forefoot ischemia caused by advanced tibial artery disease presents a challenge to revascularization. Success with saphenous vein bypass to more proximal vessels led to a trial of this approach in 24 men with critical lower limb ischemia involving the foot. Two thirds were diabetics, half were hypertensive, and most were currently smoking. Multiple tibial artery occlusions were present in all cases.

The authors' preference has been to originate the in situ saphenous vein graft from the common femoral artery. When vein length is inadequate the superficial femoral artery is used for graft inflow. A single vein sufficed in 23 cases. A modified Mills valvulotome was introduced through side branches of the vein to cut the valve leaflets. Heparin was given before the arteries were occluded, and low-molecular-weight dextran was infused.

Foot salvage was achieved in 83% of cases during a mean follow-up of 14 months. The mean flow velocity in the bypass graft at the ankle was 60 cm/sec at discharge. Two grafts were treated successfully by percutaneous balloon angioplasty. Only 5 grafts failed, 3 of them within 2 months of surgery. Six major wound complications occurred.

Saphenous vein bypass to the pedal arteries provides limb salvage in patients with severe infrapopliteal arteriosclerosis and critical foot ischemia. Careful technique can reduce wound complications to an acceptable level.

▶ A definition of the distal limits of revascularization is being achieved by this experience and that of other workers.

Is Arterial Reconstruction to the Ankle Worthwhile in the Absence of Autologous Vein?

Tyrell MR, Grigg MJ, Wolfe JHN (St Mary's Hosp, London)

Eur J Vasc Surg 3:429–434, 1989 10–18

Autologous vein from the arm or leg is the preferred conduit for femorodistal bypass procedures. In the absence of suitable veins, some surgeons suggest that primary amputation should be considered because of poor extremity salvage rates with prosthetic grafts. A technique that created a compliant, wide-diameter vein collar at the distal anastomosis was used in 30 patients with critical ischemia, which was defined as rest pain with distal tissue loss or Doppler ankle pressure of 40 mm Hg or less, or both. A 6-mm externally supported polytetrafluoroethylene (PTFE) graft with interposed vein collars to a distal calf or pedal vessel (Fig 10–7) was used in the reconstructive procedures. The mean age of the 21 male and 9 female patients was 70 years.

Ten femorodistal PTFE grafts (33%) occluded in the perioperative period, in 5 cases leading to amputation. Another 12 grafts occluded within 12 months of operation, and 4 of these cases resulted in amputation. During a mean follow-up of 14 months (range, 1–49 months) 14 grafts

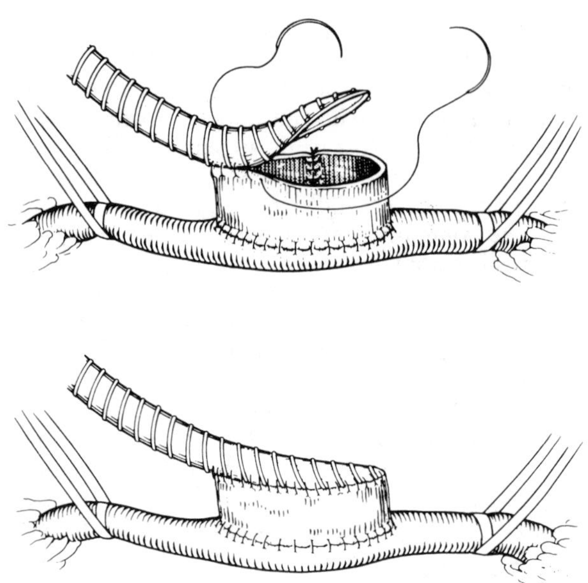

Fig 10–7.—Polytetrafluroethylene graft is anastomosed to collar by using continuous 6/0 prolene sutures. (Courtesy of Tyrell MR, Grigg MJ, Wolfe JHN: *Eur J Vasc Surg* 3:429–434, 1989.)

(47%) remained patent, with a mean duration of patency of 10 months. Six patients died.

The aim of salvage surgery was to maintain independence until death occurred, and the maximum possible number of "amputation-free months" in these 30 patients was 417; 300 months (72%) were actually achieved. In addition, 21 legs (70%) were spared amputation. If no suitable vein is available, femorocrural grafting by using PTFE with a vein collar is preferable to primary amputation in the elderly patient.

▶ Distal prosthetic grafting seems to be enhanced by the use of the Miller collar as described in this presentation.

Lateral Plantar Artery Bypass Grafting: Defining the Limits of Foot Revascularization

Andros G, Harris RW, Salles-Cunha SX, Dulawa LB, Oblath RW (St Joseph Med Ctr, Burbank, Calif)

J Vasc Surg 10:511–521, 1989 10–19

Bypass grafting to paramalleolar arteries has facilitated revascularization of ischemic lower extremities at risk for amputation. Researchers analyzed distal bypass grafting to the lateral plantar artery (Fig 10–8) to further define the limits of this procedure.

Surgeons placed 20 bypass grafts to the lateral plantar artery in 18 extremities with wet or dry gangrene. Seventy-five percent of grafts were implanted in men. Patients had a median age of 65 years. Fifteen patients

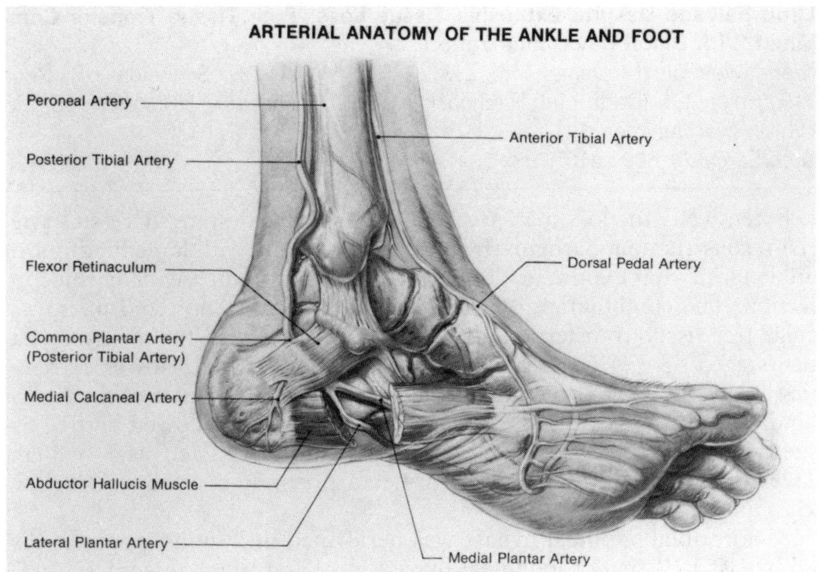

Fig 10–8.—Salient anatomical landmarks in dissection of the lateral plantar artery. (Courtesy of Andros G, Harris RW, Salles-Cunha SX, et al: *J Vasc Surg* 10:511–521, 1989.)

had diabetes, 8 of whom were insulin dependent. One patient had vasculitis with chronic lymphocytic leukemia; the remaining patient had Buerger's disease. Seventy-one percent of the patients had heart disease; 65%, a history of smoking; 53%, hypertension; and 35%, osteomyelitis in the foot. Eleven of 15 gangrenous feet in which cultures were positive had gram-negative bacilli.

Four grafts were long femoroplantar bypasses. Ten short grafts were placed from the popliteal artery; 6 jump grafts were placed distal to a femoropopliteal or tibial bypass. The median hospital stay was 16 days. There were 2 in-hospital deaths. Nine feet required transmetatarsal or button toe amputations. Of 2 patients who underwent below-knee amputations, 1 had a patent graft. At 2 months the foot salvage rate was 89%. All but 4 wounds healed within 6 months; 4 gangrenous ulcers were unhealed at 6 months. The primary and secondary patency rates were 85% at 1 month and 73% at 3 months and subsequently. Four of 5 graft failures occurred in 2 legs that had had repeat bypass grafting. All patients who achieved successful revascularization can walk, and 7 are able to work full time.

An aggressive approach to limb salvage appears to be justified. Procedures include selection of the lateral plantar artery as a distal anastomotic site.

▶ Another technique, which emphasizes use of the lateral plantar artery below the medial malleolus and is helpful in far distal bypass, is described in this presentation.

Limb Salvage Despite Extensive Tissue Loss: Free Tissue Transfer Combined With Distal Revascularization

Cronenwett JL, McDaniel MD, Zwolak RM, Walsh DB, Schneider JR, Reus WF, Colen LB (Dartmouth-Hitchcock Med Ctr, Hanover, NH; VA Med Ctr, White River Junction, Vt)

Arch Surg 124:609–615, 1989 10–20

Extensive tissue loss may preclude limb salvage despite successful arterial reconstruction, particularly in diabetic patients with large hindfoot or ankle ulcers that expose tendon and bone with accompanying chronic infection. The combination of distal arterial reconstruction and microvascular free tissue transfer avoids limb loss in these patients. Fourteen patients aged 33–74 years with extensive tissue loss in 15 lower extremities, exposing bone or tendon on the heel, ankle, lower part of the leg, or hindfoot, underwent distal arterial revascularization followed by free tissue transfer to achieve limb salvage. The mean ulcer size was 5 × 8 cm. Twelve patients were diabetic and 4 had previous contralateral below-knee amputations.

Femorotibial/popliteal bypass was performed in 7 limbs, popliteal-distal bypass in 3, femoropopliteal bypass in 4, and tibial angioplasty in 1. Muscular or fascial free flaps combined with split-thickness skin grafts or fasciocutaneous free flaps were used to obtain soft tissue coverage. Serratus anterior, scapular, latissimus dorsi, rectus abdominis, gracilis, ulnar, or temporalis free flaps were used. Both free flap and arterial reconstructive procedures were performed during the same operation in 2 patients. The mean interval between arterial reconstruction and free flap coverage was 13 days.

Limb salvage was achieved in 14 (93%) limbs during a mean follow-up of 24 months (range, 4–38 months). The single amputation occurred as a result of severe foot ischemia in a patient whose femorodistal bypass remained patent only to the viable free flap. Of the 13 patients with patent bypass grafts, 1 required subsequent vein patch angioplasty of the popliteal anastomosis to prevent thrombosis. Of the 17 free flaps, 12 healed primarily and 3 healed after minor surgical revision of the wound edges, for an 88% success rate. Of the 16 ulcers treated, 15 healed completely. Weight-bearing ambulation was achieved in 13 of 14 patients.

Lower extremity revascularization combined with free tissue transfer may allow limb salvage in a subgroup of patients with severe lower extremity ischemic tissue loss. These patients are usually diabetic, with large, deep ulcers on the hindfoot or ankle that have developed in association with peripheral neuropathy.

▶ This technique is another that aids in defining just how far vascular surgery can go to prevent amputation.

Influence of Smoking and Plasma Factors on Patency of Femoropopliteal Vein Grafts

Wiseman S, Kenchington G, Dain R, Marshall CE, McCollum CN, Greenhalgh

RM, Powell JT (Charing Cross Hosp, London; Queen Elizabeth Hosp, Birmingham, England)
Br Med J 299:643–646, 1989 10–21

To determine the effects of smoking, lipid factors, and clotting factors on the patency of saphenous vein femoropopliteal bypass grafts at 1 year, 157 patients with such grafts were studied prospectively. Forty-four had occluded grafts 1 year after surgery. The blood concentration of carboxyhemoglobin, plasma concentration of thiocyanate, and plasma levels of fibrinogen and apolipoproteins AI and (a) were all significantly higher in the patients with occluded grafts. Serum levels of cholesterol, in contrast, were higher in patients with patent grafts.

One fourth of all patients untruthfully claimed to have stopped smoking. Based on the smoking markers, graft patency at 1 year was significantly less in smokers than in nonsmokers. Patency rates were significantly higher in patients with lower plasma levels of fibrinogen. An increased level of plasma low-density lipoprotein cholesterol unexpectedly correlated with improved graft patency at 1 year. Discriminant function analysis indicated that the most powerful predictors of graft status were the plasma concentrations of fibrinogen and thiocyanate.

Thrombosis probably is more important than atherosclerosis in early failures of femoropopliteal vein bypass grafts. Patients require stronger measures to persuade them to stop smoking. Interventions to lower the plasma level of fibrinogen may be a worthwhile goal in patients with femoropopliteal grafts.

▶ Repeatedly, smoking appears to be a proven source of trouble in distal bypass grafting.

Serial Noninvasive Studies Do Not Herald Postoperative Failure of Femoropopliteal or Femorotibial Bypass Grafts

Barnes RW, Thompson BW, MacDonald CM, Nix ML, Lambeth A, Nix AD, Johnson DW, Wallace BH (Univ of Arkansas; Little Rock VA Med Ctr)
Ann Surg 210:486–494, 1989 10–22

Because the likelihood of prolonged patency after secondary intervention for graft or host-artery stenosis is greater than for correction of a thrombosed reconstruction, serial noninvasive postoperative surveillance of bypass grafts has been recommended to identify hemodynamically significant lesions that may jeopardize graft patency. To determine whether serial postoperative noninvasive studies are useful in predicting patients at risk for impending graft failure, 188 patients who underwent femoropopliteal and 44 patients who underwent femorotibial bypass were evaluated in a retrospective case-control study. Serial ankle/arm pressure indices (API) were correlated with graft patency. An interval decrease in API of .20 or greater was considered hemodynamically significant, but interventional therapy was performed only for clinically symptomatic graft failure and an API less than .20 greater than the preoperative value.

The cumulative 5-year patient survival was 63% and the cumulative 5-year limb salvage rate was 82%. A significant interval decrease in API did not correlate with subsequent graft failure. The cumulative 5-year primary graft patency rates were 60% for patients with stable and 62% for those with interval decreases in API. The lack of correlation between a decrease in interval API and adverse graft outcome was true not only for autogenous vein grafts, but also with polytetrafluoroethylene and human umbilical vein or composite grafts. These findings suggest that serial postoperative surveillance by noninvasive measurement of resting API in patients undergoing infrainguinal bypass has a limited role in predicting patients at risk of impending graft failure.

▶ In accepting the results of this study, which is at variance with surveillance techniques using duplex scanning, one should note that of the grafts being followed 22% were polytetrafluoroethylene and an additional 13% were umbilical vein or composite. Others have noted that the ankle brachial index is not as sensitive an indicator of graft failure as the velocity profile. Therefore, this report should not be taken to mean that postoperative graft surveillance is a bad idea.

Atheromatous Embolism: Varied Clinical Presentation and Prognosis

Jennings WC, Corder CN, Jarolim DR, Blackwell J, Cherian J, Chen D (Univ of Oklahoma, Tulsa; Univ of Utah)

South Med J 82:849–852, 1989 10–23

Microemboli consisting of atheromatous debris can cause sudden atheromatous embolization (AE), which may result in systemic AE syndrome (SAES) with multiple organ system failure, including involvement of the lower extremities, or in lower extremity AE syndrome (LEAES) with injuries limited to the soft tissues of the legs and feet. The records of 10 patients treated for AE were reviewed retrospectively.

During a 3-year period, 7 men and 3 women aged 49–72 years were treated for AE. Presenting symptoms and signs included acute onset of bilateral pain in the feet, lower legs, thighs, and hips, abdominal pain, mottling and discolorization of the skin, hypertension, digital ischemia with normal pulses, visual defects, hematuria, and tissue confirmation of AE (Fig 10–9). Preexisting disorders included hypertension, arteriosclerotic heart disease, and chronic pulmonary disease. In 3 patients AE was directly attributable to recent aortic surgery; 5 patients had embolic events within 48 hours after undergoing arteriography, and 2 patients had spontaneous embolic events. Four patients

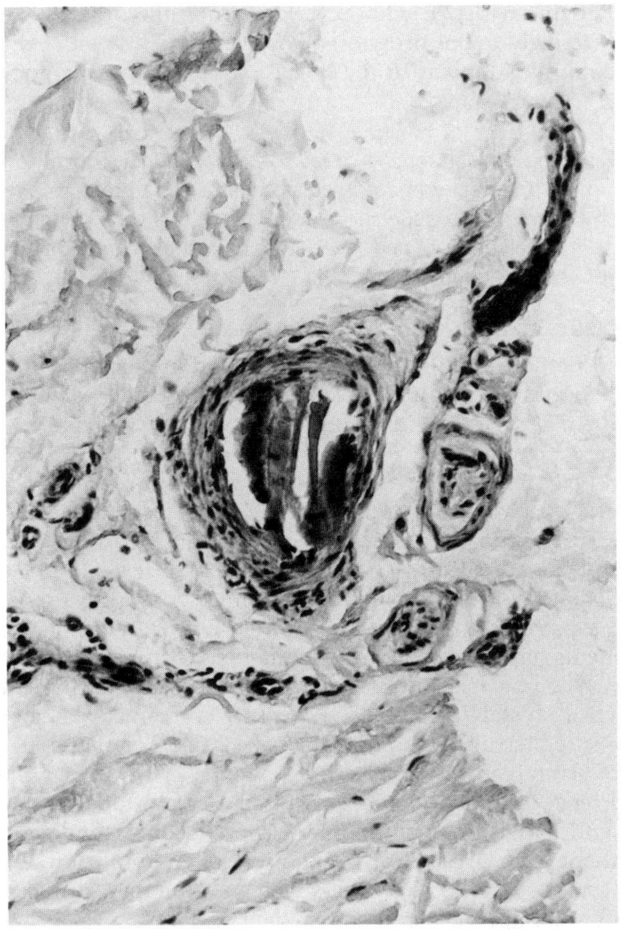

Fig 10–9.—Histologic section of soft tissue shows arteriolar occlusion by cholesterol crystal emboli (hematoxylin-eosin; original magnification, ×400). (Courtesy of Jennings WC, Corder CN, Jarolim DR, et al: *South Med J* 82:849–852, 1989.)

had SAES with multiple organ system failure and 6 patients had LEAES only.

The treatment of SAES consisted of supportive care with specific treatment of each organ system that had failed. Anticoagulation or lytic therapy appeared to be of no benefit. Calcium channel blocking agents gave immediate pain relief and improved the appearance of the ischemic feet in 4 patients with LEAES. Lumbar sympathectomy was performed on 3 patients with persistent ischemic ulceration with uniformly good results. Two patients eventually required amputation of a single digit, but both were able to walk normally. Of the 4 patients with SAES, 1 eventually died, 1 recovered, 1 was undergoing long-term dialysis, and 1 was severely debilitated at last follow-up. All 6 patients with LEAES recovered. Patients with AE who experience multiple organ system failure have an extremely grave prognosis, whereas patients with AE in whom soft tissue injury is limited to the lower extremities have a good prognosis.

▶ The devastating consequences of iatrogenically induced atheroembolization are stressed. Arteriography is a particular cause of the problem, and coronary arteriography seems to be especially dangerous in this regard. It is the multiple organ system involvement, and even the paraplegias and paraparesis produced, that become acutely dangerous.

Cholesterol Embolization: Clinical Findings and Implications

Rosman HS, Davis TP, Reddy D, Goldstein S (Henry Ford Hosp, Detroit)

J Am Coll Cardiol 15:1296–1299, 1990 10–24

This group of 13 patients with cholesterol embolization is the largest clinical series yet reported. The patients were seen between 1975 and 1988, were predominantly male, and had a mean age of 65 years. All had preexisting evidence of atherosclerotic vascular disease. In 11 cases vascular catheterization or surgery was presumed to be the cause of embolization. Six patients had definite or borderline hypertension.

Ten patients had new symptoms of angina, abdominal pain, foot pain, or blurred vision at the presumed time of embolization. Physical evidence of cholesterol crystals was noted 3 weeks to 5 months later. The mean blood pressure increased by an average of 24 mm Hg. Three patients had cholesterol crystals in retinal arterioles (Fig 10–10). All but 1 of the patients had renal dysfunction and 5 required dialysis. Elevated levels of eosinophils and a high sedimentation rate were frequent findings.

One patient died, presumably of cholesterol embolization, 2 days after coronary artery surgery. Two others died of acute myocardial infarction; 10 patients were alive 8 months after the episode.

Cholesterol embolization is most frequent in patients with atherosclerotic disease who have vascular procedures. It is not rare, but it is infrequently recognized. A prospective study is needed to determine the true frequency of subtle cholesterol embolization. Recognition is important because interventions such as hydration, blood pressure control, and dialysis may prevent major organ dysfunction.

▶ It is dangerous to say that a group of patients is the largest ever to be reported. Maybe it is even erroneous.

Cholesterol Embolism: Experience With 22 Histologically Proven Cases

Dahlberg PJ, Frecentese DF, Cogbill TH (Gundersen Clinic, Ltd, La Crosse, Wis)

Surgery 105:737–746, 1989 10–25

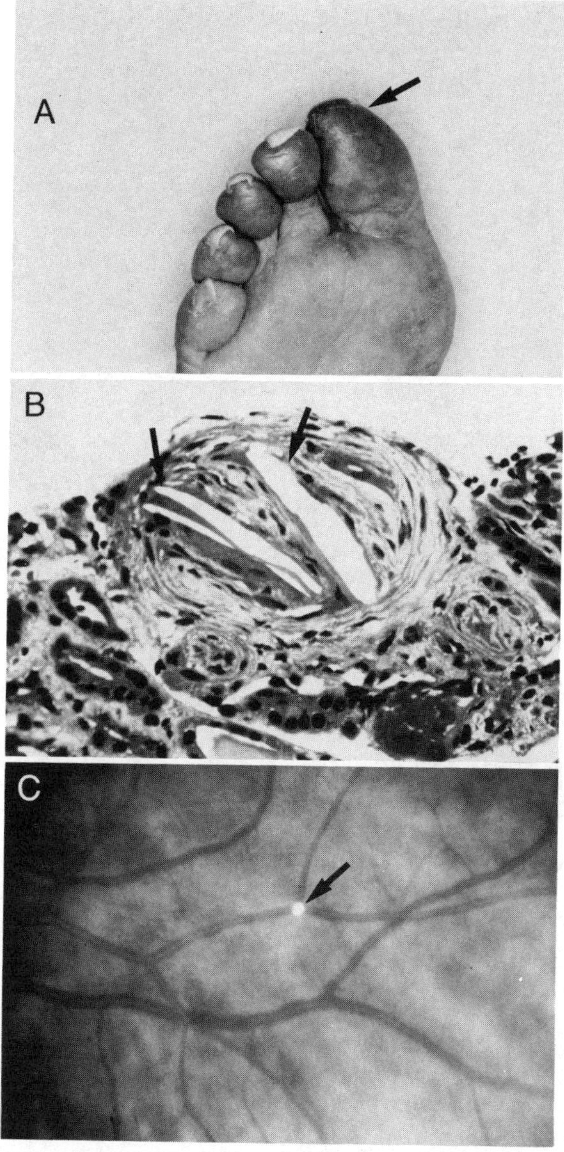

Fig 10–10.—**A,** foot of patient with severe pattern of cholesterol embolization. Great toe shows demarcated area *(arrow)* of cyanosis resulting from ischemia. **B,** renal biopsy showing multiple cholesterol clefts *(arrows)* in glomerulus. **C,** cholesterol crystal lodged inside retinal arteriole *(arrows)*. (Courtesy of Rosman HW, Davis TP, Reddy D, et al: *J Am Coll Cardiol* 15:1296–1299, 1990.)

The aortas of patients with cholesterol embolism (CE) syndrome are ulcerated, crystal laden, or lined by friable atheromatous debris (Fig 10–11). Cholesterol embolism syndrome causes disease ranging from asymp-

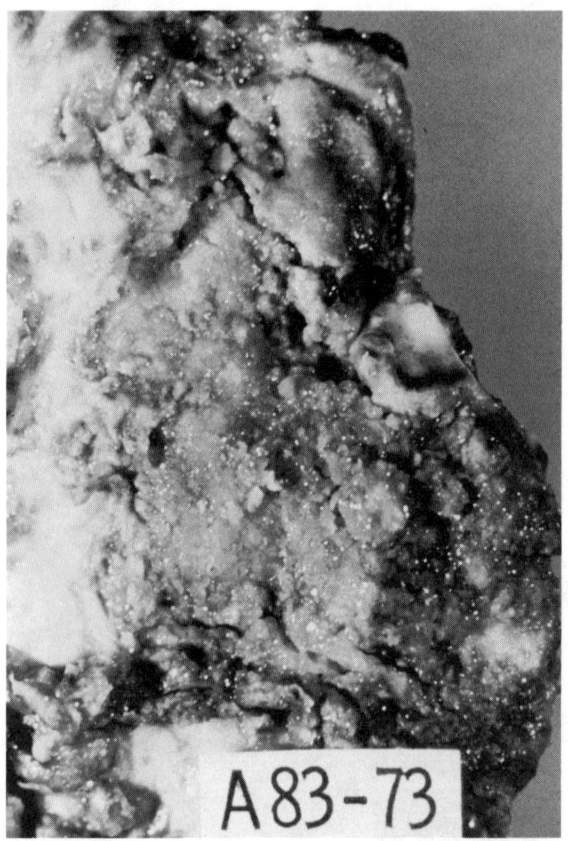

Fig 10–11.—Photograph of aorta taken at autopsy shows glistening cholesterol crystals loosely attached to the intimal surface after the overlying thrombus was removed. (Courtesy of Dahlberg PJ, Frecentese DF, Cogbill TH: *Surgery* 105:737–746, 1989.)

tomatic to rapidly progressive multiple system failure. The records of 22 patients with histologically proved CE seen in an 11-year period were reviewed (Fig 10–12). Preexisting symptomatic or known atherosclerotic illness was noted in 21 patients; 20 had 1 or more precipitating factors, such as warfarin administration, angiography, angioplasty, intra-aortic balloon pump placement, vascular surgery, aortitis, and cardiopulmonary resuscitation. These occurrences usually preceded the onset of symptoms by less than 3 weeks. Peripheral CE occurred in 8 patients, and 14 visceral CE occurred in 14, all of whom had renal CE characterized by abrupt deterioration of renal function after a precipitating event, evidence of concurrent CE to the lower extremities or other organs, accelerated hypertension, gross hematuria, or flank and back pain. Patients with visceral CE who survived initial hospitalization often needed dialysis and later hospitalizations because of complications. In 18 patients, premortem diagnoses were made from surgical or biopsy specimens. Definitive vascular surgery was possible in only 2 patients and successful in 1.

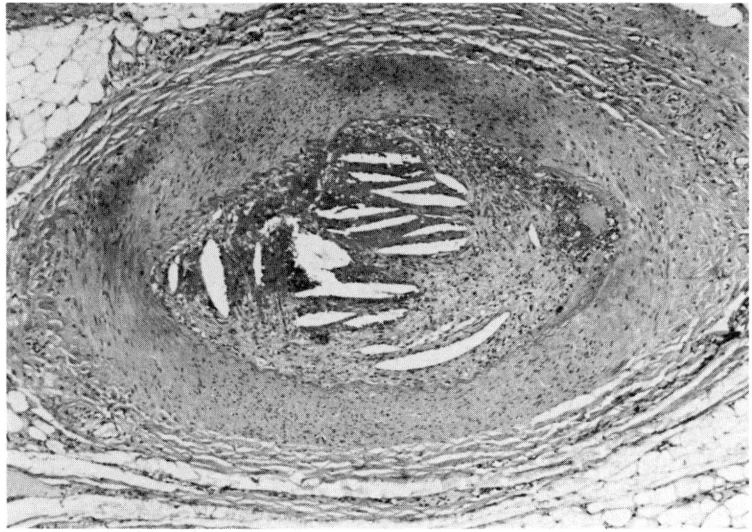

Fig 10–12.—Cross-section of a digital arteriole shows occlusion of the vessel by cholesterol emboli surrounded by birin and platelet thrombi. Cholesterol crystals are washed out during histologic processing and are represented by biconvex clefts in the specimen (hematoxylin-eosin; original magnification, ×40). (Courtesy of Dahlberg PJ, Frecentese DF, Cogbill TH: *Surgery* 105:737–746, 1989.)

Patients at risk for CE have multiple risk factors. They almost always have symptomatic atherosclerosis. In this series, efforts to diagnose and treat atherosclerotic disease were the main precipitating events resulting in CE. Intra-aortic balloon pump placement and aortitis were added to the list of previously reported interventions (anticoagulants, angiography, angioplasty, vascular surgery, and trauma) that can precipitate CE.

▶ This report stresses the devastating nature of cholesterol and other atheromatous embolization. The visceral and somatic consequences of disseminated particulate embolization are indeed extremely serious.

11 Cerebrovascular Occlusions

Early and Late Follow-Up Results After Subclavian-Carotid Transposition

Brandl R, Jauch K-W, Bae JS (Ludwig-Maximilians-Univ, München, Germany)

Chirurg 61:171–177, 1990 11–1

Subclavian steal phenomenon caused by occlusion or high-grade stenosis of the subclavian artery is characterized by a reversed blood flow in the ipsilateral vertebral artery from the basilar artery to the subclavian artery beyond the point of occlusion. Subclavian transposition is a fairly unknown extrathoracic procedure in which a direct end-to-side anastomosis is created between a point beyond the obstruction in the subclavian artery and the ipsilateral common carotid artery. In a 10-year period, 49 men and 36 women (mean age, 59 years) underwent subclavian-carotid transposition.

Of the patients, 52 had obstruction and 33 had stenosis of the subclavian artery. Most patients had cerebral symptoms suggestive of subclavian steal syndrome, and 65 had symptoms of vertebrobasilar insufficiency; 57 patients had intermittent claudication. Follow-up evaluation included clinical examination, Doppler ultrasonography, and digital subtraction angiography (Fig 11–1). Results of radiographic studies were available for 35 patients.

In contrast with the recommended supraclavicular access to obtain exposure of the proximal subclavian artery, a cervical incision was made at the anterior margin of the sternocleidomastoid (Fig 11–2). This approach allows simultaneous treatment of an ipsilateral stenosis of the internal carotid artery without having to make a second incision. Of the 85 patients, 14 required simultaneous treatment of a high-grade stenosis of the ICA; 1 patient underwent simultaneous thoracic sympathectomy. The mean clamping time was 17 minutes (range, 5–51 minutes). No shunts were used in any of the patients.

There were no perioperative deaths. Low-dose heparin therapy prevented early reocclusion. Transient ischemic attacks occurred in 2 patients; none had neurologic sequelae. Reoperation was necessary in 3 patients, 2 because of postoperative hemorrhage and 1 for a lymphatic fistula. During follow-up of 6–100 months (mean, 47.8 months), 12 patients died. At last follow-up, the reconstructed vessel had remained patent in the other 73 patients. There was evidence of restenosis in 2 patients, but both were asymptomatic. At last follow-up, 59 patients were symptom free, 13 had some subjective complaints,

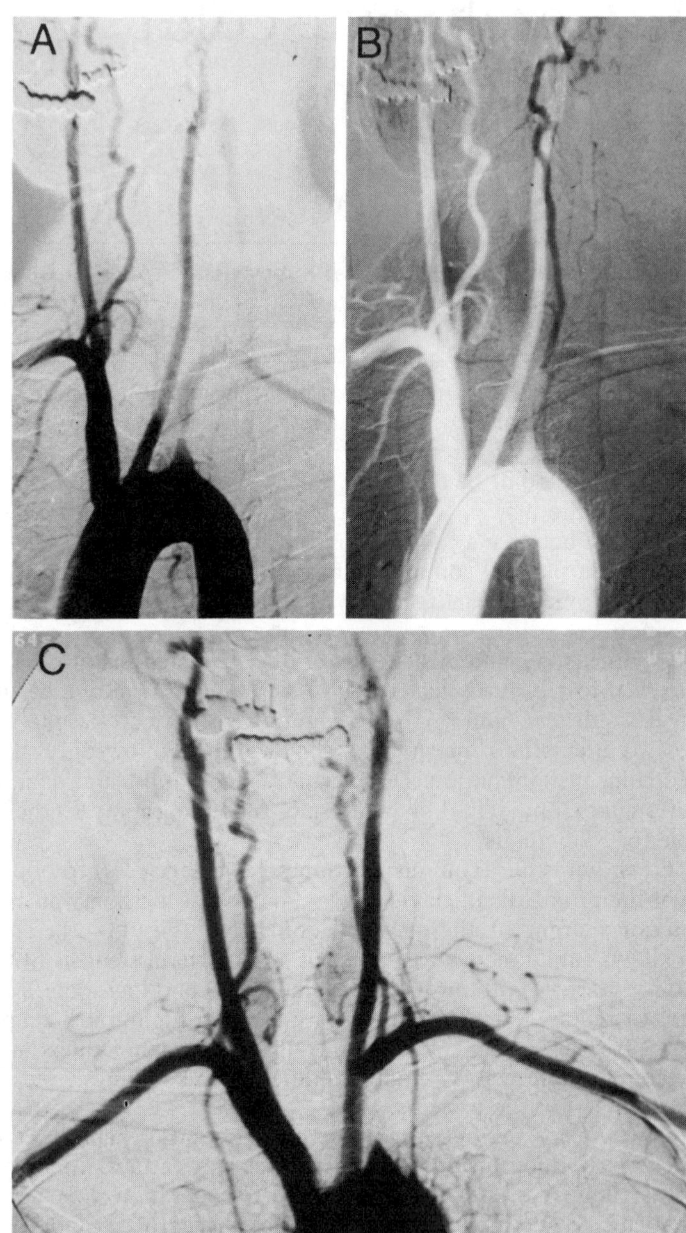

Fig 11–1.—**A,** preoperative digital subtraction angiography (DSA) with high-grade subclavian stenosis and absence of filling in the vertebral artery in the early phase. **B,** radiographic evidence of steal phenomenon with retrograde subclavian filling over the vertebral artery in the late phase. **C,** postoperative follow-up DSA with orthograde filling of the vertebral artery and hemodynamically appropriate anastomosis between the common carotid artery and the subclavian artery. (Courtesy of Brandl R, Jauch K-W, Bae JS: *Chirurg* 61:171–177, 1990.)

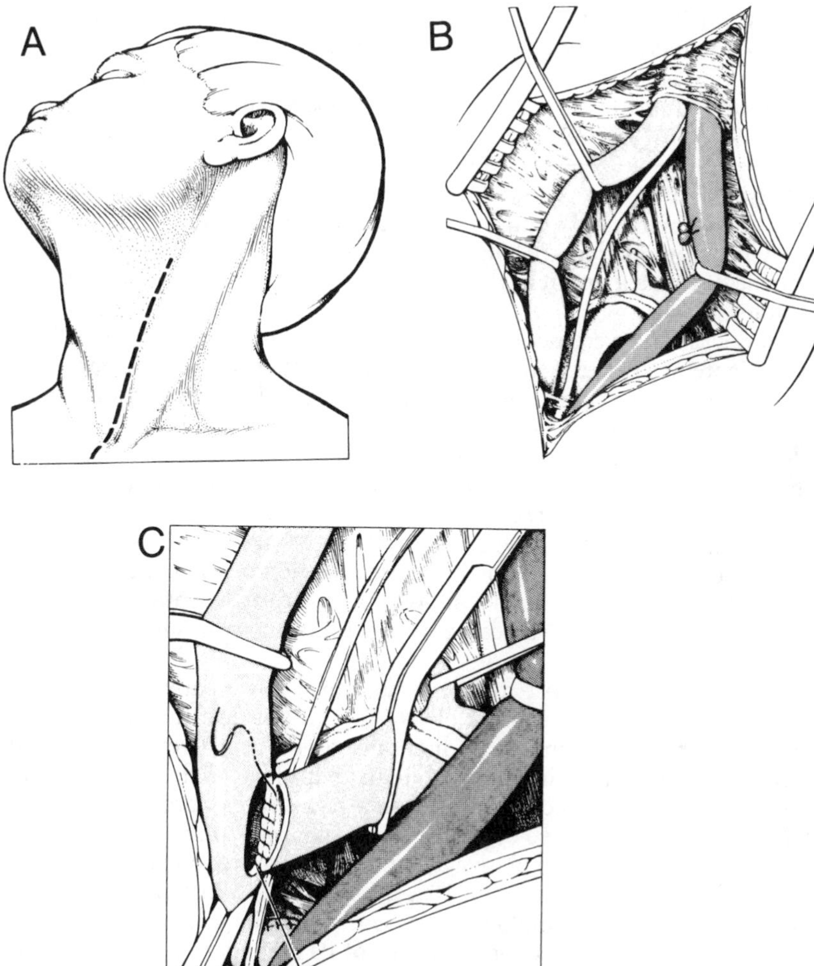

Fig 11–2.—A, incision at the margin of the sternocle; domastoid muscle. **B,** freeing the subclavian artery after exposure of the common carotid artery and the internal jugular vein. **C,** oblique anastomosis after ligation of the subclavian artery. (Courtesy of Brandl R, Jauch K-W, Bae JS: *Chirurg* 61:171–177, 1990.)

and 1 was not improved; in retrospect, the latter patient did not have steal syndrome. Subclavian-carotid transposition is safer than traditional bypass because the use of synthetic prosthesis materials is avoided, and an important source of embolism is eliminated.

▶ There is much wisdom in this article and abstract. Notice the unusual incision, the fact that shunts were not used, and that patency was quite satisfactory and the restenosis rate quite small.

Long-Term Results of Aortoinnominate and Aortocarotid Polytetrafluoroethylene Bypass Grafting for Atherosclerotic Lesions

Cormier F, Ward A, Cormier J-M, Laurian C (St Joseph's Hosp, Paris; Basingstoke and North Hampshire Health Authority, Basingstoke, England)

J Vasc Surg 10:135–142, 1989 11–2

Between 1978 and 1986, 53 patients with atherosclerotic occlusive disease of the innominate and left common carotid arteries underwent 69 polytetrafluoroethylene (PTFE) bypass grafting procedures from the ascending aorta. The mean age was 52 years, and the mean follow-up, 50.5 months.

All operations were performed via median sternotomy. About 50% of innominate artery reconstructions were associated with revascularization of at least 1 other supra-aortic trunk, including the left common carotid artery (in 16 cases) and left subclavian artery in 14. Indications for surgery included symptoms of amaurosis fugax, vertebrobasilar ischemia, and upper extremity ischemia in 36 patients and severe hemodynamically significant occlusive disease in 17.

One patient died of a myocardial infarction on the fifth postoperative day. One patient had a mnor postoperative neurologic deficit that partially regressed on subsequent follow-up. Two early asymptomatic occlusions were detected; 1 was caused by a technical error and the other by low systemic perfusion.

Two patients were lost to follow-up and 6 more patients died, for a cumulative 5-year survival rate of 84.9%. All but 2 of the evaluable patients were free of symptoms: 1 had only partial improvement of preoperative symptoms and another had a late neurologic deficit caused by internal carotid artery occlusion distal to a patent aortocarotid bypass.

There were no infective complications. There was only 1 late asymptomatic occlusion. The cumulative 5-year primary graft patency was 94.6% and secondary patency was 96.1%. There were no instances of anastomotic stenosis or morphological or hemodynamic graft changes at follow-up. Direct reconstruction by means of PTFE bypass grafting from the ascending aorta appears to be the treatment of choice for innominate or left common carotid artery occlusive disease, or both, particularly in young patients without serious risk factors.

▶ The sternotomy-ascending aorta approach to innominate and common carotid origin occlusions has proven itself to be superior. This large experience confirms the satisfactory long-term follow-up of such reconstructions using PTFE.

Risk Factors for Site Specific Extracranial Carotid Artery Plaque Distribution as Measured by B-Mode Ultrasound

Tell GS, Howard G, McKinney WM (Bowman Gray School of Medicine, Winston-Salem, NC)

J Clin Epidemiol 42:551–559, 1989 11–3

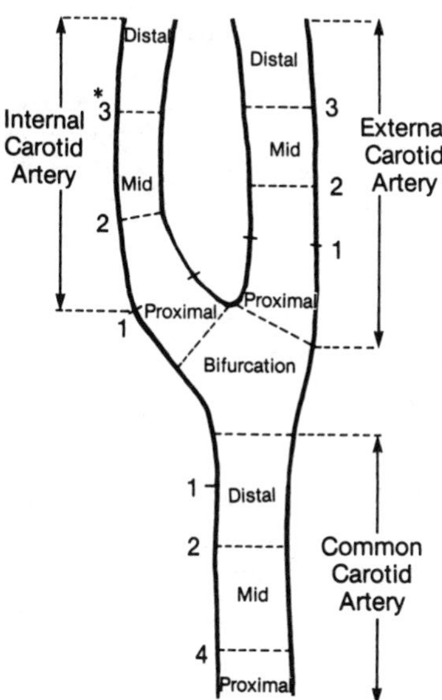

Fig 11–3.—Extracranial carotid artery sites examined by B-mode ultrasound. (Courtesy of Tell GS, Howard G, McKinney WM: *J Clin Epidemiol* 42:551–559, 1989.)

Autopsy studies have shown that the distribution of arterial plaque within arteries is not uniform, and that certain anatomical sites have a predilection for severe atherosclerotic lesions. The availability of noninvasive high-resolution B-mode scanning allows the study of even mild vascular lesions and wall irregularities of extracranial neck arteries.

The distribution of atherosclerotic lesions was examined in different regions of the extracranial carotid arteries and related to age, sex, pulse rate, diabetes, hypertension, and smoking history in 698 white men, 730 white women, 77 black men, and 76 black women, aged 24–98 years. All had been referred for diagnostic carotid ultrasound evaluation. Indications for referral included stroke (10%), transient ischemic attacks (19%), carotid bruits (29%), cerebrovascular symptoms (19%), and coronary artery disease without cerebrovascular symptoms (23%). The 8 carotid arterial locations examined bilaterally included the proximal, mid and distal common carotid, the bifurcation, and the proximal and mid internal and external carotids (Fig 11–3).

Multivariate analysis with plaque thickness at each site as the outcome variable revealed that cigarette smoking and age were the most consistent risk factors affecting plaque thickness at all investigated sites. Hypertension affected more sites than diabetes, men had more plaques than women, and white persons had more plaques than black persons. Although the data from this study may not be applicable to the general population, the findings suggest that risk factors are not uniformly associated with atherosclerosis at all sites of the extracranial carotid arterial distribution.

▶ Although this is a study of a large patient population, it should be noted that the population was, in fact, a hospital-based or sick population. Unfortunately, all this study does is confirm the obvious.

Progression of Carotid Atherosclerosis and Its Determinants: A Population-Based Ultrasonography Study
Salonen R, Salonen JT (Univ of Kuopio, Finland)
Atherosclerosis 81:33–40, 1990 11–4

The incidence of atherosclerotic lesions increases with increasing age. The progression of carotid atherosclerosis and its determinants were studied in a population-based ultrasonography study of 100 Eastern Finnish men aged 42, 48, 54, or 60 years. Each subject underwent a repeat high-resolution B-mode ultrasonographic examination after 24 months of follow-up.

The mean intimal-medial thickness in the common carotid artery increased by .12 mm, with a range of −.06 mm to .9 mm. The strongest predictors of atherosclerosis progression were age, serum low-density lipoprotein (LDL) cholesterol concentration, pack-years of smoking, blood leukocyte count, and platelet aggregability measured at baseline. Hypertension, current blood pressure level, serum high-density lipoprotein (HDL) cholesterol, and serum HLD_2 cholesterol levels at baseline were not associated with intimal medial thickness changes in 2 years.

These results confirm previous findings on the role of serum LDL cholesterol and smoking in atherosclerosis. However, there was no association between hypertension and serum HDL cholesterol and atherosclerosis progression. This needs to be reexamined in larger longitudinal population studies. These observations can be used as a basis of power calculations for studies of interventions aimed at preventing carotid atherosclerosis progression.

▶ Progression of the carotid atherosclerotic plaque is not related to the usual risk factors of atherogenesis. This suggests that the configuration of the carotid bifurcation is of greater importance.

Angiogenic Activity of the Atherosclerotic Carotid Artery Plaque
Alpern-Elran H, Morog N, Robert F, Hoover G, Kalant N, Brem S (Sir Mortimer B Davis–Jewish Gen Hosp, Montreal; McGill Univ; Univ of Montreal)
J Neurosurg 70:942–945, 1989 11–5

A prominent feature of atherogenesis is the local growth of new capillaries from the vasa vasorum into the enlarging plaque, which may provide the pathologic substrate for intraplaque hemorrhage. To determine the stimulus for angiogenesis, fragments of atherosclerotic plaque were obtained at carotid endarterectomy from 12 patients with cerebral ischemia. Angiogenesis was induced in the rabbit cornea by implanting fragments of the fibrous cap of the atherosclerotic plaque from 11 of these patients. Nonatherosclerotic human uterine arteries and normal carotid artery of rabbits were also studied.

Of 278 fragments of atherosclerotic plaques, 125 stimulated a neovascular response. In contrast, angiogenesis was induced in only 2 of the 80 control tissues, in none of the 22 samples of boiled atherosclerotic plaques, in 2 of 26 samples of normal rabbit carotid artery, and in none of the 32 samples of nonatherosclerotic human uterine artery. Histologic analysis showed that 127 of the atherosclerotic fragments were cellular, composed mainly of smooth muscle cells, and 132 were acellular, consisting of amorphic, necrotic, calcific, lipid-laden material. Cellular fragments were significantly more angiogenic than acellular fragments.

Angiogenesis in vivo is a function of the cellular component of the advanced atherosclerotic plaque, but not in the normal, stable arterial wall. These fragile new vessels may promote the growth of the plaque or be a source of hemorrhages, microinfarcts, and plaque fissures that convert a stable, silent lesion into an expanding, ulcerated, thrombotic, symptomatic plaque.

▶ As plaque accidents are an important cause of symptoms in carotid bifurcation disease, the findings in this study are of great interest to vascular surgeons.

The Origin and Distribution of Vasa Vasorum at the Bifurcation of the Common Carotid Artery With Atherosclerosis

Bo WJ, McKinney WM, Bowden RL (Wake Forest Univ, Winston-Salem, NC)

Stroke 20:1484–1487, 1989 11–6

The carotid bifurcation is predisposed to the development of atherosclerotic lesions. The plaques may exhibit intramural hemorrhage, and thromboemboli can result, leading to transient ischemia or stroke. The relation of vasa vasorum to plaque at this site was examined by preparing luminal casts from the arteries of unembalmed adult cadavers aged 40–96 years. In other specimens the arteries were cleared.

Seven of 12 cadavers exhibited extensive gross atherosclerotic plaques. The 7 specimens had a network of vasa vasorum in the area of plaque. The vasa vasorum arose from the superior thyroid and ascending pharyngeal arteries. Luminal casts from 3 of the cadavers also showed vasa vasorum arising from the internal carotid artery distal to the plaque. No extensive network of vasa vasorum was found in the cadavers without gross atherosclerosis.

Vasa vasorum are prominent in areas of marked atherosclerosis at the common carotid artery bifurcation. The findings suggest neovascularization and indicate that angiogenic factors may be operative. Compromised function of arterial branches that give rise to the vasa vasorum may be important in the ischemic and hemorrhagic changes that occur in plaques at this site.

▶ This study confirms the findings reported in Abstract 11–5.

Carotid Thrombosis Following Neck Irradiation
Call GK, Bray PF, Smoker WRK, Buys SS, Hayes JK (Univ of Utah)
Int J Radiat Oncol Biol Phys 18:635–640, 1990 11–7

Neck irradiation may have delayed cerebrovascular consequences, including the acceleration of atherosclerosis and an increased risk of carotid artery stenosis or occlusion. These changes may occur from just a few months to many years after therapeutic radiation. Histologic changes

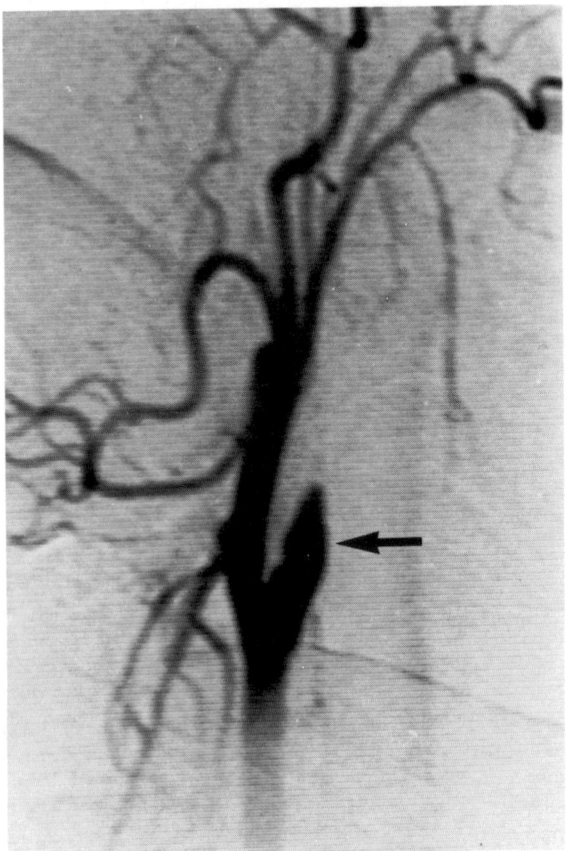

Fig 11–4.—Stump of the occluded right internal carotid artery *(arrow)*. (Courtesy of Call GK, Bray PF, Smoker WRK, et al: *Int J Radiat Oncol Biol Phys* 18:635–640, 1990.)

are those of arteriosclerosis with a modest round cell infiltrate that most closely resembles atherosclerosis. In 3 young patients aged 26–42, carotid artery occlusion occurred within 3 years of their receiving moderate-dose irradiation.

All 3 patients had carotid artery occlusion within the radiation port less than 3 years after undergoing radiation therapy of the neck in the treatment of cancer. Angiographic evaluation showed that occlusion occurred in the absence of atherosclerotic stenosis (Fig 11–4). Two patients had received radiation therapy in the treatment of Hodgkin's disease; the third patient was treated for a rhabdomyosarcoma. One patient was left with a profound aphasia, hemiplegia, and hemihypesthesia. The second patient became completely mute and was unable to follow even simple commands. The third patient had a persistent right Horner's syndrome with ptosis and miosis.

The findings that none of these 3 patients had any evidence of atherosclerosis or other angiopathy elsewhere, and that the carotid occlusion occurred within the radiation port, suggest an association between radiation therapy and carotid artery occlusion. Patients who undergo radiation therapy of the neck are at risk not only for the delayed development of diffuse atherosclerosis, but also for thrombotic occlusion within months to several years. Patients who have neurologic symptoms or signs after neck irradiation for malignant disease should be evaluated for carotid or vertebral artery disease.

▶ Patients with neck irradiation should be followed serially with duplex scans so that the complications observed in the 3 patients described here can be avoided. The technical performance of carotid endarterectomy in such cases is only flawed by achieving satisfactory vascular coverage, and this can be accomplished in virtually every case.

Alcohol Consumption and Carotid Atherosclerosis in the Lausanne Stroke Registry

Bogousslavsky J, Van Melle G, Despland PA, Regli F (Universitaire Vaudois, Lausanne, Switzerland)

Stroke 21:715–720, 1990 11–8

There is some evidence that alcohol consumption—at moderate levels—is an independent factor protecting against ischemic heart disease. At the same time, higher levels may promote coronary atherosclerotic disease. This association was examined in 261 patients older than 50 years who were admitted with a first ischemic stroke. Carotid disease was assessed by duplex scanning with spectral analysis and by real-time B-mode imaging of the bifurcation.

Light to moderate intake, with 4 or fewer standard drinks a day, was inversely related to the severity of internal carotid stenosis (Fig 11–5). The potential benefits of alcohol consumption were strongly countered by the effects of hypertension, smoking, and age in men, and by diabetes

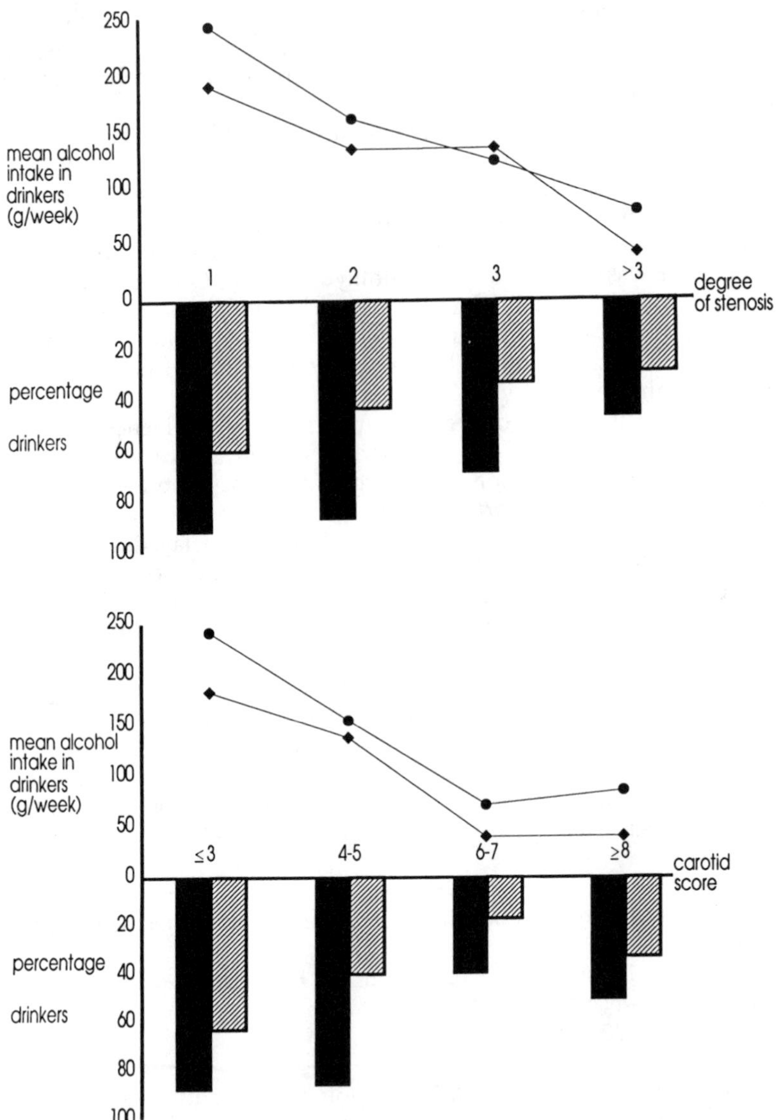

Fig 11–5.—Graphs of correlations between drinking habits and *(top)* degree of internal carotid artery stenosis (1, no visible lesion; 2, 0% to 25% stenosis; 3, 26% to 50% stenosis; >3, 51% to 100% stenosis) ipsilateral to first ischemic stroke and *(bottom)* carotid score (sum of scores [as above] for ipsilateral and contralateral internal carotid arteries). *Upper part* of each graph: mean alcohol intake among male *(circles)* and female *(diamonds)* drinkers. *Lower part* of each graph: proportion of male *(filled bars)* and female *(shaded bars)* drinkers among patients with given degree of stenosis or carotid score. (Courtesy of Bogousslavsky J, Van Melle G, Despland PA, et al: *Stroke* 21:715–720, 1990.)

and smoking in women. The protective effect of alcohol consumption was most evident in younger men who did not smoke and who were normotensive. In nondiabetic, nonsmoking women, alcohol had an effect only in the absence of hypertension.

The lack of follow-up of carotid artery morphology precludes interpreting the findings as indicating a protective effect of drinking alcohol. Future studies should evaluate a potential protective role for alcohol consumption in persons with a known intake who undergo sequential carotid ultrasonography on a prospective basis.

▶ Moderate alcohol consumption without smoking is good. Smoking and hypertension are bad.

Cigarette Smoking: A Risk Factor for Hemorrhagic and Nonhemorrhagic Stroke

Gill JS, Shipley MJ, Tsementzis SA, Hornby R, Gill SK, Hitchcock ER, Beevers DG (Dudley Road Hosp, Birmingham; Dept of Neurosurgery, Smethwick, West Midlands; London School of Hygiene and Tropical Medicine, England)

Arch Intern Med 149:2053–2057, 1989 11–9

The role of cigarette smoking in the pathogenesis of stroke remains debatable. Using case-control methods, 621 stroke patients and 573 controls were studied to determine the relationship between cigarette smoking and specific subtypes of stroke, such as subarachnoid hemorrhage (SAH), intracerebral hemorrhage (ICH), and thromboembolic cerebral infarction.

An excess of stroke patients were smokers. The risk of stroke for cigarette smokers vs. nonsmokers was significant in both men (3.22) and women (2.24). After adjusting for confounding variables, the risks of stroke in cigarette smokers were 1.8 for ICH, 3.2 for cerebral infarction, and 4.5 for SAH among men, and 1.3, 2.3, and 2.5, respectively, in women. The risk of stroke increased in daily smokers, being highest in the heaviest smokers and rising about 1.5 times for each 10 cigarettes smoked per day in both men and women.

Cigarette smoking is associated with an increased risk of hemorrhagic and nonhemorrhagic stroke. Cigarette smoking may be an important preventable risk factor for premature stroke in men and women.

▶ This study, which focuses on ICH, SAH, and cerebral infarction, merely confirms the others that link smoking to carotid bifurcation plaque and accidents within that plaque.

Duration of Cigarette Smoking Is the Strongest Predictor of Severe Extracranial Carotid Artery Atherosclerosis

Whisnant JP, Homer D, Ingall TJ, Baker HL Jr, O'Fallon WM, Wiebers DO (Mayo Clinic and Found, Rochester, Minn)

Stroke 21:707–714, 1990 11–10

The interaction of cigarette smoking with extracranial carotid atherosclerotic disease was examined in 752 patients having at least 1 carotid artery visualized. The patients, aged 40–69 years, underwent angiogra-

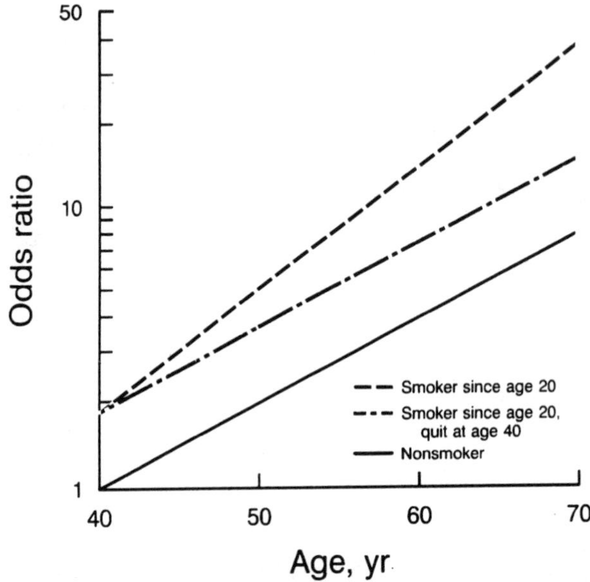

Fig 11–6.—Calculated adjusted odds ratio for likelihood of having severe carotid atherosclerosis as function of age and years of cigarette smoking. Odds ratio of 1 was assigned arbitrarily to 40-year-old person who had never smoked. (Courtesy of Whisnant JP, Homer D, Ingall TJ, et al: *Stroke* 21:707–714, 1990.)

phy between 1983 and 1986. Men constituted 61% of the group and the median age was 61 years. In 70% of cases the indication for angiography was atherosclerotic cerebrovascular disease.

Total years of smoking was the only independent predictor of whether severe carotid atherosclerosis was present. The next most influential factors were age, hypertension, diabetes, male gender, and the current systolic blood pressure. By age 60, a person who had smoked for 40 years was 3.5 times more likely to have severe carotid atherosclerotic disease than one who had never smoked. The rate at which the odds ratio rose with age was less for former smokers than for current smokers (Fig 11–6).

The duration of cigarette smoking is strongly associated with accelerated atherosclerosis of the extracranial carotid arteries. Stopping smoking is beneficial chiefly through limiting the number of years of smoking.

▶ It is not surprising that the duration of smoking has a stronger effect on atherosclerosis at the carotid bifurcation than any other factor.

Carotid Arteriosclerosis in Identical Twins Discordant for Cigarette Smoking

Haapanen A, Koskenvuo M, Kaprio J, Kesäniemi YA, Heikkilä K (Univ of Turku; Univ of Helsinki; Seinäjoki Central Hosp; Univ of Oulu, Finland)

Circulation 80:10–16, 1989 11–11

A study on smoking-discordant twin pairs has suggested an increased risk of ischemic heart disease in the smoking co-twin. To determine if this increased risk is associated with arteriosclerosis among the smoking co-twins, 49 identical twin pairs (mean age, 52) with highest discordance in cigarette smoking were studied. The smoking history was obtained in 1975, 1981, and 1986. The mean life-long smoking dose was 19.7 package-years. Duplex sonography of the carotid arteries was performed. Except for a higher use of alcohol in smoking co-twins, nonsmoking and smoking twins had similar systolic and diastolic blood pressures, total plasma cholesterol levels, body mass indexes, and certain psychosocial factors.

Carotid artery stenoses, defined as narrowing of area of the lumen by 15% or more, was found in 9 pairs (in 9 smoking co-twins and in 2 of their nonsmoking co-twins). Smoking co-twins had significantly larger mean area of carotid plaques and more marked thickness of the inner layer of carotid arteries than did nonsmoking co-twins. The size of the plaques and the degree of inner layer thickening correlated with the smoking dose, but these trends were not significant. The association of smoking with carotid arteriosclerosis remained highly significant even after controlling for confounding factors as age, total plasma cholesterol level, diastolic blood pressure, and body mass index. These findings strongly support a causal role of smoking in the development of atherosclerosis.

▶ This elegantly conceived and well-performed study provides the final and most positive link between carotid plaque severity and smoking history.

Bruit and Stenosis of the Internal Carotid Artery

Lepojärvi M, Kallanranta T, Siniluoto T, Tolonen U (Oulu Univ, Finland)

Surg Res Comm 7:173–181, 1990 11–12

Although carotid auscultation is less sensitive than duplex scanning or angiography, it remains an important measure for detecting significant carotid stenosis. The relationship between bruits and the degree of stenosis and postendarterectomy symptoms was examined in 82 patients after 100 consecutive internal carotid endarterectomies. The patients were followed for 2 years postoperatively. One third of the patients had stroke, and two thirds experienced transient ischemic attacks.

An ipsilateral bruit was detected preoperatively in 81 of 100 patients and a contralateral bruit in 41 patients. The presence of a bruit was closely related to the grade of carotid stenosis (Fig 11–7). All but 10% of arteries that were 60% stenosed had a bruit. A bruit was 59% accurate in detecting significant carotid stenosis. An ipsilateral bruit disappeared after operation in all but 4 patients. A contralateral bruit disappeared after operation in 25 of 41 patients. None of 10 patients who had an ipsilateral bruit 6 months postoperatively deteriorated clinically.

Carotid bruits most accurately reflect internal carotid stenosis of about

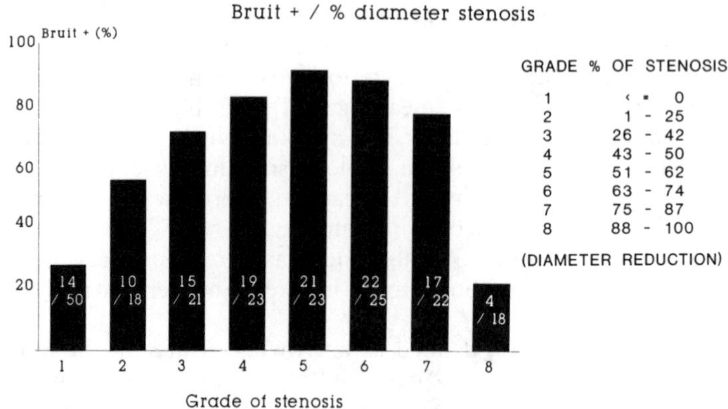

Fig 11–7.—Internal carotid artery bruit occurrence according to diameter stenosis. *Numbers inside the bars,* numbers of observations. (Courtesy of Lepojärvi M, Kallanranta T, Siniluoto T, et al: *Surg Res Comm* 7:173–181, 1990.)

50% to 70%. Disappearance of a contralateral bruit postoperatively may reflect normalized contralateral carotid flow when stenosis, which leads to compensation on the opposite site, is relieved. Most patients with critical carotid stenosis have no ipsilateral bruit.

▶ A bruit merely detects turbulent flow, nothing more.

Anatomical Variations of the Carotid Bifurcation: Implications for Digital Subtraction Angiography and Ultrasonography

Trigaux JP, Delchambre F, Van Beers B (Cliniques Univ UCL de Mont-Godinne, Yvoir; Facultés Univ Notre-Dame de la Paix, Namur, Belgium)
Br J Radiol 63:181–185, 1990 11–13

Knowledge of the anatomical variants of carotid bifurcation will aid in the accurate interpretation of digital subtraction angiographs and ultrasound studies. The findings in 100 adults undergoing intravenous digital subtraction angiography because of suspected atherosclerotic disease were reviewed.

In 48.5% of patients the external carotid artery was anteromedial to the internal carotid. The vessel was anterolateral to the internal carotid artery in 13% of bifurcations, more frequently on the right side than on the left. In the remaining patients the external carotid artery was located anterior to the internal carotid artery. The internal carotid ostium was evaluable on at least 2 projections in 74% of patients with anterior or anteromedial variants, but in only 19% of those with the anterolateral variant, a highly significant difference.

The left anterior oblique view is potentially best suited for evaluating both carotid bifurcations by digital subtraction angiography. For ultrasonography, the posterolateral approach is recommended because it utilizes the sternocleidomastoid muscle as an acoustic window.

▶ As MR angiography appears and infinite views of the carotid bifurcation become available, anatomical variance may be of less importance than at the present time.

Role of Duplex Scanning in the Selection of Patients for Carotid Endarterectomy

Farmilo RW, Scott DJA, Cole SEA, Jeans WD, Horrocks M (Bristol Royal Infirmary, England)

Br J Surg 77:388–390, 1990 11–14

Three techniques are currently used for the preoperative assessment of carotid artery disease: conventional arteriography, intra-arterial digital subtraction arteriography, and intravenous digital subtraction angiography. Duplex scanning has proved to have certain definite advantages over angiography. A retrospective review of 63 patients examined the role of duplex scanning in the preoperative assessment of carotid artery disease and the need for routine angiography before carotid endarterectomy.

The patients underwent both duplex scanning and arteriography. A consultant vascular surgeon with no knowledge of the results of the arteriograms selected patients for surgery without angiography, angiography, or conservative treatment on the basis of clinical details and the scan report. Twenty-four patients were selected for surgery. The diagnosis was correct for 41 vessels (91%). Surgery would have been inappropriate for 2 vessels diagnosed as critically stenosed by duplex scanning, because the vessels were totally occluded. Eighteen patients were referred for angiography and conventional management. In the 21 patients selected for conservative treatment, the status of 94% of carotid arteries was diagnosed accurately.

Overall, duplex scans had a sensitivity of 96% and a specificity of 95% in detecting stenosis of more than 50%. In cases of total occlusion, however, the sensitivity was 50% and specificity, 95%. Ulceration was not reliably detected with the scans. In selected cases, duplex scanning is a noninvasive, cost-effective means of selecting patients for safe carotid endarterectomy without angiography. Patients should have clear hemispheric symptoms, a satisfactory scan, a surgically accessible lesion located in the appropriate internal carotid artery, and stenosis greater than 50%. Suspected occlusions should be confirmed by angiography.

▶ Repeatedly, duplex scanning has been verified as providing sufficient information in selected patients to allow surgery to proceed. Others have found that this approach avoids the risks of arteriography (1).

Reference

1. Gelabert HA, Moore WS: *Surg Clin North Am* 70:213, 1990.

Comparison of Color Flow and 3D Image by Computer Graphics for the Evaluation of Carotid Disease

Houi K, Mochio S, Isogai Y, Miyamoto Y, Suzuki N (Jikei Univ School of Medicine, Tokyo)

Angiology 41:305–312, 1990 11–15

Doppler color-flow analysis was performed in 20 patients who had sustained cerebral infarction or experienced transient ischemic attacks. Seven patients also had 3-dimensional (3-D) imaging of the carotid bifurcation by transverse B-mode imaging.

Color-flow images of the bifurcation demonstrated transient flow reversal at peak systole in 16 of the 20 patients, always in the outer posterior wall of the carotid sinus. In 5 cases plaque formation was seen in the area of flow separation and reattachment. Three-dimensional analysis of computer graphics showed small plaques in the outer posterior wall of the carotid sinus, opposite the origin of the external carotid artery, in 5 cases. In 2 cases without flow reversal, 3-D images showed the internal carotid running straight from the common carotid artery, with plaque formation in both the anterior and posterior walls of the carotid sinus.

Comparison of color-flow and 3D images is very helpful in relating the vessel wall configuration to flow phenomena such as flow separation and stagnation. Further studies of this type might help to elucidate the pathogenesis of carotid atherosclerosis secondary to abnormal blood flow.

▶ At this point, 3-D imaging adds very little to duplex scanning. However, future developments along this line are predictable and may be promising.

Transcranial Doppler Ultrasound Findings in Middle Cerebral Artery Occlusion

Kaps M, Damian MS, Teschendorf U, Dorndorf W (Justus-Liebig Univ, Giessen, Germany)

Stroke 21:532–537, 1990 11–16

Transcranial Doppler ultrasonography (TCD) is a way of noninvasively evaluating patients in the acute phase of stroke who are unfit for angiography and of following them at brief intervals. Twenty-three patients with acute middle cerebral occluson were examined and 20 had follow-up studies. Sonography was done daily for the first week, every 3 days in the second week, and then weekly until discharge if abnormal flow velocity persisted. Eleven patients were studied angiographically.

Occlusion was most reliably diagnosed when all of the basal arteries except that affected were identified. Corroboration was provided by enhanced flow velocity in the anterior cerebral artery, reflecting leptomeningeal collateralization. Recanalization occurred gradually. Turbulent signal irregularities were the most persistent abnormality. Recanalization was seen up to 17 days after onset of stroke. It could be difficult to distinguish postischemic hyperemia from residual middle cerebral stenosis during recanalization.

Transcranial Doppler ultrasonography can accurately exclude middle cerebral artery occlusion, but its sensitivity in making this diagnosis is uncertain. Transcranial Doppler ultrasonography is much more convenient than angiography in the actue phase of stroke, and it is helpful in following patients and documenting recanalization.

▶ Transcranial Doppler technology is interesting, but is it useful in patients being considered for carotid endarterectomy?

Asymptomatic High-Grade Internal Carotid Artery Stenosis: Is Stratification According to Risk Factors or Duplex Spectral Analysis Possible?

Moneta GL, Taylor DC, Zierler RE, Kazmers A, Beach K, Strandness DE Jr (Univ of Washington; Seattle VA Med Ctr)

J Vasc Surg 10:475–483, 1989 11–17

Overall, patients with asymptomatic carotid stenosis have a low risk of stroke, but some patients with a high-grade stenosis are at significantly increased risk of having ischemic neurologic events. It would be useful to identify predictive risk factors that could differentiate high-risk patients from those with more stable lesions.

Seventy-three patients with unoperated-on high-grade asymptomatic internal carotid artery stenoses were selected by duplex scanning. Patients were followed at 3- to 6-month intervals by clinical evaluation and duplex scanning and were grouped according to whether they reached a neurologic end point. Group A included 31 patients who remained asymptomatic for at least 12 months. Group B included 25 patients who were initially asymptomatic but subsequently experienced a neurologic event. The mean time to an event was 7.4 months.

There was no significant difference between the groups in average age, sex, use of aspirin, smoking history, or prevalence of hypertension, cardiac disease, or diabetes. Whether the index lesion affected the contralateral internal carotid artery or the ipsilateral external carotid artery did not affect the risk. However, on duplex scanning, high-grade stenoses with >6.5 kHz end-diastolic frequencies were more frequently associated with an event than those with lower end-diastolic frequencies. Thirty percent of lesions with end-diastolic frequencies >6 kHz were associated with subsequent internal carotid artery occlusion compared with only 3.5% of lesions with end-diastolic frequencies ≤6 kHz.

The end-diastolic frequency of internal carotid artery lesions may help to identify a subgroup of patients with asymptomatic high-grade lesions who are at greatest risk for subsequent neurologic events. Further research is needed to confirm the hypothesis that end-diastolic frequency is a valid predictor of the behavior of asymptomatic high-grade internal carotid artery stenosis.

▶ Strandness and his group have been enormously productive in defining the high-risk patient with carotid stenosis. This addition to the facts that they have given us in the past may be extremely valuable.

Stroke Risk and Critical Carotid Stenosis

Norris JW, Zhu CZ (Univ of Toronto)

J Neurol Neurosurg Psychiatry 53:235–237, 1990 11–18

Apparently, a critical degree of carotid stenosis is associated with a maximal risk of stroke, because the risk declines when the artery becomes occluded. Degree of carotid stenosis was measured by continuous-wave Doppler ultrasonography in 500 asymptomatic patients with carotid bruits. The patients were observed prospectively and followed for a mean of 52 months.

Forty patients had transient ischemic attacks during follow-up, and 11 had ischemic stroke. Vertebrobasilar events were not included. Carotid ischemic events were significantly more frequent in patients with carotid stenosis of 75% to 90% than in those with either lesser or greater steno-

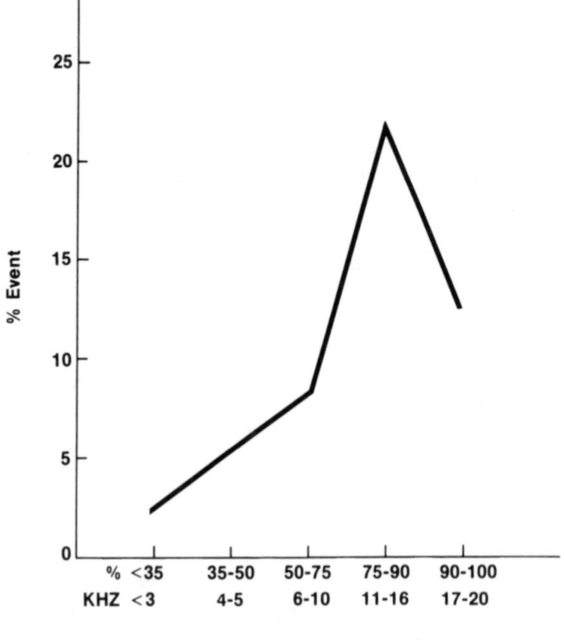

Fig 11–8.—Distribution of ischemic cerebral events according to severity of carotid stenosis. (Courtesy of Norris JW, Zhu CZ: *J Neurol Neurosurg Psychiatry* 53:235–237, 1990.)

sis (Fig 11–8). Carotid stenosis progressed more in patients with ischemic events than in other patients, including those having cardiac events.

These findings support the existence of a critical degree of cartoid stenosis when the risk of a stroke is maximal. This may represent a "therapeutic window," or decision-making point. Treatment at this stage is especially critical if the carotid lesion is progressing rapidly. Once carotid stenosis exceeds about 90%, the collateral supply is adequate and the threat to the cerebral circulation lessens appreciably.

▶ Knowledgeable vascular surgeons will say that this abstract has confirmed the obvious. That is, carotid stenosis of 75% to 90% confers a risk of stroke to those patients who are as yet asymptomatic. However, it isn't the facts of this presentation that is important, it is the origin of the presentation from the Stroke Research Unit in Toronto. These conclusions, then, are derived from an experienced and well-informed neurologist and his fellow and corroborate the previous reports of Strandness and others.

Directed Embolization Is an Alternate Cause of Cerebral Watershed Infarction

Pollanen MS, Deck JHN (Toronto Gen Hosp; Univ of Toronto)

Arch Pathol Lab Med 113:1139–1141, 1989 11–19

Systemic hypotension is the most frequently recognized cause of border zone or watershed infarcts, but an embolic mechanism may sometimes be responsible. In 3 patients thromboembolism was the only reasonable cause of watershed infarction. A cardiac embolism was likely in 2 cases and a carotid artery embolism was likely in the third. On clinical grounds decreased cerebral perfusion caused by hypotension or carotid stenosis was not a probable cause of infarction in these cases.

Apparently, small thromboemboli may be preferentially distributed to small terminal arterial branches in the border zones between major arterial territories. The sharp angle at which small penetrating vessels branch from parent arteries may be part of the explanation, but the unequal size of branches at most bifurcations of subarachnoid arteries probably is a more important factor. This type of infarction may occur only in the cerebral circulation with emboli of a limited size range.

▶ Vascular surgeons know that emboli tend to recur and follow the same pathway as prior emboli.

Pentoxifylline Increases Cerebral Blood Flow in Patients With Cerebrovascular Disease

Bowton DL, Stump DA, Prough DS, Toole JF, Lefkowitz DS, Coker L (Wake Forest Univ, Winston-Salem, NC)

Stroke 20:1662–1666, 1989 11–20

Pentoxifylline is a methylxanthine approved for use in relieving intermittent claudication secondary to peripheral vascular disease. The drug promotes cerebral blood flow. Ten patients who sustained an acute vascular neurologic insult at least 3 months previously received a single oral dose of either 400 mg or 800 mg of sustained-release pentoxifylline. Regional cerebral blood flow was measured by the radioxenon clearance technique.

An immediate dose-dependent rise in global cerebral blood flow was observed that was significant after the larger dose and persisted after 6 hours. The lowest regional flow value did not decline in any case. Cerebrovascular reactivity to carbon dioxide was not significantly altered by either dose of pentoxifylline despite the increase in cerebral blood flow.

Pentoxifylline augments cerebral blood flow in patients with cerebrovascular disease and is not associated with an "intracerebral steal" phenomenon. Further experience will show whether the increase in flow correlates with better neuropsychological function.

▶ Rheologic agents may increase cerebral blood flow, but do they prevent stroke or, as suggested in this abstract, will they improve mentation? It is unlikely that they will decrease the frequency of embolization from the carotid bifurcation to the cerebral cortex.

Patterns of Failure of Aspirin Treatment in Symptomatic Atherosclerotic Carotid Artery Disease

Chyatte D, Chen TL (Yale School of Medicine; West Haven VA Med Ctr, New Haven, Conn)

Neurosurgery 26:565–569, 1990 11–21

Aspirin is widely used to reduce the risk of stroke, but it fails to prevent most strokes in patients at risk. Of 291 patients admitted consecutively in 2 years with new ischemic neurologic symptoms, 90 (31%) experienced ischemic symptoms while taking aspirin. Sixty-six of these patients had ischemic symptoms in the carotid distribution.

Aspirin administration failed in 21 patients who had more than 75% carotid stenosis. Eleven of these patients had cerebral infarction, 7 of them without previous transient ischemic attacks. Aspirin also failed in 45 patients who had less marked carotid stenosis. Transient ischemic attacks without permanent ischemia were the most frequent form of failure in these patients (Fig 11–9). Twelve patients had infarction, 4 of them without warning from transient ischemic attacks.

Patients with symptomatic high-grade carotid stenosis in whom aspirin fails are likely to have a cerebral infarct as the first sign of treatment failure. Alternative measures should be considered for these patients.

▶ It is clear from other work and from this abstract that a carotid stenosis of 75% diameter narrowing or greater is a risk factor for stroke. This presentation suggests that aspirin treatment will not prevent the ultimate stroke, and that a

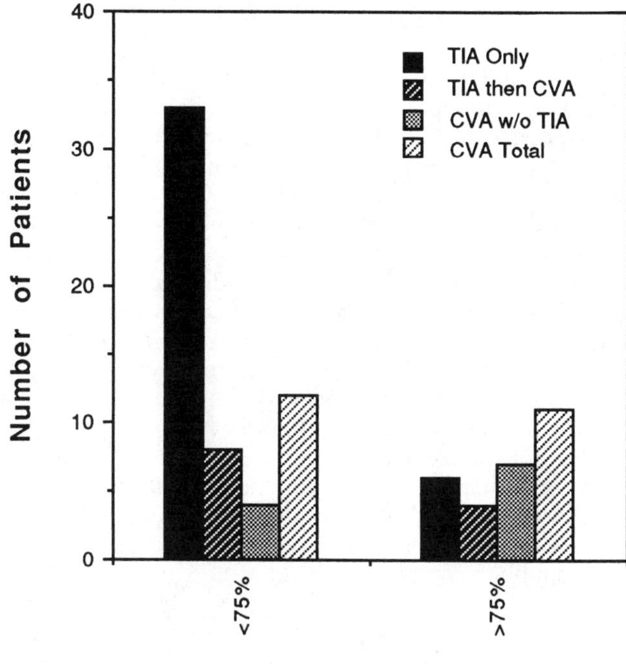

Fig 11–9.—Pattern of aspirin treatment failure varies as a function of degree of carotid stenosis. In patients with high-grade stenoses the most common manifestation of treatment failure was cerebral infarction and, in particular, infarction without warning. In patients with lesser degrees of stenosis, a transient ischemic attack was the most common manifestation of treatment failure. *TIA,* transient ischemic attack; *CVA,* cerebral infarction. (Courtesy of Chyatte D, Chen TL: *Neurosurgery* 26:565–569, 1990.)

cerebral infarct may be the first sign of such treatment failure. The obvious conclusion is that carotid stenosis of 75% diameter narrowing or greater should be marker for surgical intervention in symptomatic as well as asymptomatic patients. It is clear from this series of abstracts that neurosurgeons and neurologists have joined vascular surgeons in a unanimity of opinion that is most unusual in vascular medicine.

Balloon Test Occlusion of the Internal Carotid Artery With Monitoring of Compressed Spectral Arrays (CSAs) of Electroencephalogram

Morioka T, Matsushima T, Fujii K, Fukui M, Hasuo K, Hisashi K (Kyushu Univ, Fukuoka, Japan)

Acta Neurochir (Wien) 101:29–34, 1989 11–22

The balloon Matas test allows occlusion of the common, external, or internal carotid arteries (ICAs) with an inflatable balloon catheter. Brain function during these procedures is frequently monitored by electroencephalography (EEG). The introduction of compressed spectral arrays

(CSAs) has made continuous monitoring possible by converting the EEG into a graphic output.

Nine patients underwent permanent carotid occlusion surgically or with a detachable balloon subsequent to the balloon Matas test monitored by CSAs. Six patients had an unclippable ICA aneurysm, 2 had cervical tumors, and 1 had a carotid-cavernous fistula. Satisfactory CSA recordings were obtained in all 9 patients. In 7 no definite change in the CSA was noted during the procedures. Complications occurred in 3 patients. One, in whom no CSA change was observed who awakened from anesthesia without neurologic deterioration, died of a fatal embolic complication 8 days after ligation of the cervical carotid artery. Two patients had marked or mild slow changes in the CSA during the balloon Matas test. In these 2 patients CSA change always preceded clinical deterioration. One patient had nearly full recovery, but the other had only minimal recovery from sensory aphasia and right hemiparesis.

The complications in these 3 patients were probably related to thromboembolic events. Changes in brain functions attributable to inadequate blood flow can be detected with the balloon Matas test monitored by CSAs. The test does not appear to be reliable, however, for predicting delayed thromboembolic complications.

▶ Rarely is it necessary to occlude the internal carotid artery except for certain well-defined indications. This test occlusion and EEG monitoring is a logical form of testing. However, distal thrombosis and a washout of the most distal thrombus into the cerebral circulation flaws interpretation of the results.

A New Method to Predict Safe Resection of the Internal Carotid Artery

de Vries EJ, Sekhar LN, Horton JA, Eibling DE, Janecka IP, Schramm VL Jr, Yonas H (Univ of Pittsburgh; Wilford Hall USAF Med Ctr, San Antonio; St Luke's Hosp, Denver)

Laryngoscope 100:85–88, 1990 11–23

Treatment of lesions at the skull base often requires translocation, embolization, or resection of the internal carotid artery, but most patients require a patent carotid artery. Tests of collateral flow have not proved to be consistently accurate. In a series of 136 patients referred for elective carotid occlusion, temporary balloon occlusion of the internal carotid was performed and cerebral blood flow was measured by xenon-enhanced CT.

Neurologic function was altered during trial balloon occlusion in 11 patients. Of the 120 patients in whom blood flow was measured, 13 exhibited a significant, chiefly unilateral reeducation in flow. Internal carotid stump pressures had no predictive value. Hemiparesis developed in 2 patients with neurologic dysfunction during trial balloon occlusion. One of the patients with reduced cerebral blood flow had temporary hemiparesis, and 1 who was operated on before accurate interpretation of the CT studies had permanent hemiparesis. Of the patients judged to be at minimal risk, 21 underwent permanent balloon occlusion or resection of the vessel without CNS sequelae.

The combination of temporary balloon occlusion of the internal carotid artery and cerebral blood flow estimation enhances the safety of resection or permanent embolism of this vessel.

▶ Using xenon-enhanced CT, test occlusion by balloon seems quite valid.

Stroke-Related EEG Changes During Carotid Surgery

Krul JMJ, Ackerstaff RGA, Eikelboom BC, Vermeulen FEE (St Antonius Hosp, Nieuwegein, The Netherlands)

Eur J Vasc Surg 3:423–428, 1989 11–24

It is not known how electroencephalographic (EEG) changes that develop after carotid clamping are related to intraoperative stroke during carotid endarterectomy. To investigate this relationship, EEG recordings from 230 carotid endarterectomies performed in a 3-year period with an automatic EEG monitoring system were analyzed. Patients were selectively shunted, based on EEG changes after carotid cross-clamping.

Transient EEG asymmetry, which reversed after placement of a shunt, occurred in 32 of 230 endarterectomies (13.9%); this was not associated with intraoperative stroke. Persistent EEG asymmetry ipsilateral to the operated-on artery occurred in 8 of 230 endarterectomies and 4 of these patients had postoperative major stroke. Permanent EEG asymmetry had a positive predictive value of .5, specificity of .99, sensitivity of .80, and diagnostic gain of 47.8%. Minor strokes were missed by EEG monitoring.

Persisting EEG asymmetry during carotid endarterectomy is associated with intraoperative stroke, but transient asymmetry is not. Thromboembolism may account for these strokes as a result of manipulation of the carotid arteries before or during cross-clamping. Automatic EEG monitoring during carotid endarterectomy is beneficial in selecting patients for shunting and detecting intraoperative major stroke.

▶ The tremendous experience of the St. Antonius Hospital presented here provides a definitive answer to the value of EEG monitoring during carotid surgery.

Carotid Endarterectomy in Community Practice: Surgeon-Specific Versus Institutional Results

Gibbs BJ, Guzzetta VJ (San Diego, Calif)

Ann Vasc Surg 3:307–312, 1989 11–25

Because superior results with carotid endarterectomy have been reported from some centers, it has been proposed that surgery might best be limited to these institutions. Data on 566 carotid endarterectomies performed on 464 patients in a 12-year period were reviewed, and the

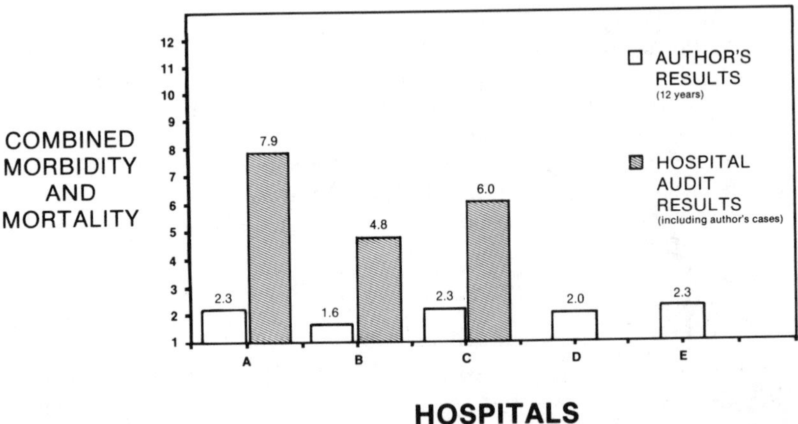

Fig 11–10.—Complication rates in 5 primary hospitals *(A–E)* compared with aggregate audit complication rates in 3 of these hospitals *(A, B, C)*. (Courtesy of Gibbs, Guzzetta VJ: *Ann Vasc Surg* 3:307–312, 1989.)

results were compared with the audit results achieved at 3 hospitals, a cardiac surgery center, and 2 community hospitals.

The 566 operations were performed at 13 different hospitals, 4 of them metropolitan centers with active cardiac surgery programs, and the rest, community hospitals with fewer than 250 beds. Most of the operations were performed with general anesthesia with selective use of a shunt (10%), a short cross-clamp time (average 9 minutes), and loupe magnification. An eversion endarterectomy was performed distally, confining the arteriotomy mostly to the carotid bulb. Patching was unusual. The total operating time generally was less than 1 hour.

Mortality in the 464 patients was .5%, and the rate of permanent stroke was 1.6%. These results did not vary substantially in different hospitals. Overall complication rates, when available from surgical audits at the same hospitals, were significantly higher (Fig 11–10).

These data indicate that it is individual surgeons, not institutions, who determine the effectiveness of carotid endarterectomy in community practice. Monitoring of surgeon-specific surgical results should be encouraged.

▶ This San Diego-based group has shown once again that the results of vascular surgery are literally in the hands of the surgeon.

Relation Between Surgeons' Practice Volumes and Geographic Variation in the Rate of Carotid Endarterectomy

Leape LL, Park RE, Solomon DH, Chassin MR, Kosecoff J, Brook RH (Rand Corp, Santa Monica, Calif; Univ of Los Angeles)

N Engl J Med 321:653–657, 1989 11–26

It has been suggested that inappropriate use of services is not an important factor in explaining regional differences in the use of procedures. Regional differences in the rates of operations may occur because a small number of physicians in high-use areas perform large numbers of operations. To verify this hypothesis, the relationship between the number of operations performed by individual surgeons and variation in the rate of carotid endarterectomy was studied in 1981 Medicare claims in areas of high, average, and low procedure use.

The number of carotid endarterectomies performed per 100,000 Medicare claims was 48 in low-use areas, 129 in average-use areas, and 178 in high-use areas. The larger number of surgeons who performed carotid endarterectomies in high- and average-use areas accounted for a substantial fraction of the higher rates. The number of surgeons performing carotid endarterectomies was twice as great in high-use areas and 33% more in average-use areas than in low-use areas. If the average number of cases per surgeon was similar, the differences in the number of surgeons would have accounted for 36% and 15%, respectively, of the differences in use. Surgeons who performed 15 or more carotid endarterectomies accounted for a major fraction of the differences in rates. These high-volume surgeons represented 15% and 17% of the surgeons in the high- and average-use areas, accounting for 60% and 77%, respectively, of the additional operations. Three fourths of surgeons performing carotid endarterectomies did fewer than 10, and 24% did only 1. These findings indicate that most of the geographic variation in the rate of carotid endarterectomy can be accounted for by a few surgeons in high-use areas who perform a large number of operations.

▶ Or, putting the conclusions differently, the surgeons who get the best results do most of the operations.

Risk of Carotid Endarterectomy in the Elderly

Fisher ES, Malenka DJ, Solomon NA, Bubolz TA, Whaley FS, Wennberg JE
(Dartmouth Med School, Hanover, NH; Yale Univ)
Am J Public Health 79:1617–1620, 1989
11–27

The value of carotid endarterectomy remains uncertain. The Medicare claims for 6 New England states were used to evaluate the effect of age on the operative risk of carotid endarterectomy, the association of low surgical volume with increased risk, and the performance of carotid arterectomy at individual hospitals. The records of 2,089 patients aged 65 and older who underwent carotid endarterectomy in 1984 and 1985 were studied.

Operative mortality increased markedly with age. The risk of death within 30 days of surgery was 1.1% for patients aged 65–69, 2.8% for those aged 70–74, 3.2% for those aged 75–79, and 4.7% for those 80 and older. Nearly 80% of patients underwent surgery at hospitals performing 40 or fewer carotid endarterectomies per year on the Medicare population. Patients who had surgery at these low-volume hospitals had a threefold increased risk of death compared with those who had surgery at high-volume hospitals. The risk of postoperative stroke also increased significantly with age and at lower-volume hospitals. The postoperative complication rates varied widely among individual hospitals.

There is a markedly increased risk of mortality in elderly patients undergoing carotid endarterectomy, particularly in low-volume hospitals. The findings confirm recent reports that a significant proportion of carotid endarterectomies in the United States are performed in clinical settings in which the risk outweighs the potential benefit. Patients should be provided with the best available information on the potential benefits and risks of carotid endarterectomy as well as those of alternative treatments.

▶ The previous abstract (Abstract 11–26), coupled with this one, would suggest that high-volume surgeons obtain the best results, and that a significant portion of carotid endarterectomies in the United States are not performed in clinical settings in which the risk outweighs the benefit.

Hemodynamic Performance of Carotid Artery Shunts

Aufiero TX, Thiele BL, Rossi JA, Miller CA, Neumyer MM (Pennsylvania State Univ, Hershey)

Am J Surg 158:95–100, 1989 11–28

An animal model of contralteral carotid artery ligation was developed that produced ipsilateral carotid blood flows and internal carotid stump pressures in the range often seen in carotid artery surgery. Seven different shunts, including the Javid, 10F and 8F Brener, and 14F, 12F, 10F, and 8F Argyle shunts, were tested in adult goats at ipsilateral carotid flow values of 640 ± 44 mL/min and stump pressures of 52 ± 4 mm Hg.

The larger shunts consistently performed better than those of smaller diameter. Shunt flow correlated closely with the increase in distal pressure caused by shunt placement—indicating that high flow maintains high perfusion pressure. When peak shunt flow and the pressure gradient were related to change in pressure pulse contour, the larger straight shunts were superior to tapered shunts. In contrast, at smaller diameters, the tapered shunts were hemodynamically superior to straight shunts.

Tapered shunts seem preferable when size is restricted, providing higher flow rates with lower pressure gradients than straight shunts of similar minimum diameter. Cerebral function should be monitored to be certain that adequate cerebral perfusion is maintained. If cerebral dysfunction occurs, shunt patency should be checked and, if necessary, cerebral perfusion pressure should be increased by raising systemic pressure. The use of agents (e.g., barbiturates) that protect cerebral function during low perfusion may be considered.

▶ A very clever study providing very useful information.

Salvage After Postoperative Thrombosis of the Carotid Artery
Dooner J, Kuechler P (Greater Victoria Hosp Soc, Victoria, BC)
Am J Surg 159:525–526, 1990 11–29

Most often, patients who experience dense hemiparesis related to an operated-on carotid artery are immediately reexplored, and thrombectomy is done when indicated. During a 5-year period, 4 patients were seen with dense hemiparesis in the recovery room after carotid endarterectomy. A fifth such patient was seen after carotid-subclavian bypass.

All 5 patients had thrombosis of the operated-on vessel. Hemiparesis developed 30 minutes to 10½ hours after the end of surgery. None of the patients had undergone patch closure. Thrombectomy was done as flow was maintained using an indwelling shunt. A saphenous vein patch or interposition graft then was placed. All of the patients survived, and 4 of the 5 were improved postoperatively. One patient had no residual deficit and 3 were left with a mild deficit. The poor outcome was in a patient who had contralateral internal carotid occlusion.

Early reoperation appears to be indicated for salvage in these cases. It is hoped that the liberal use of vein patch angioplasty closure will minimize the risk of carotid stroke after reconstruction of the vessel.

▶ There is no objective proof that reexploration after carotid endarterectomy-induced neurologic deficit confers any benefit. These cases must be taken as anecdoctal, and the outcomes described are exactly as would be expected after a stroke of any kind.

Seizures Following Carotid Endarterectomy
Kieburtz K, Ricotta JJ, Moxley RT III (Univ of Rochester; State Univ of New York, Buffalo)
Arch Neurol 47:568–570, 1990 11–30

It is not clear whether seizures after carotid endarterectomy are secondary to cerebral embolization from the operative site or to disordered cerebral vascular autoregulation. Eight patients with seizures, among about 650 having carotid endarterectomy in 1981–1987, were evaluated.

The average age was 69.5 years, Six patients had anterior transient ischemic attacks, whereas 2 were asymptomatic. Six had a history of hypertension. Angiography showed high-grade stenosis in 7 cases and internal carotid occlusion in 2. Seizures occurred within a mean of 8 days after surgery, usually in conjunction with elevated blood pressure. All of the patients had focal motor seizures contralateral to the site of operation and 6 had tonic-clonic seizures. All patients required anticonvulsant therapy. Five of the 8 patients had CT abnormalities that included diffuse cerebral swelling, cerebral infarction, and intracerebral hemorrhage. Only 1 patient had recurrent seizures requiring long-term treatment.

Patients with seizures after carotid endarterectomy should be screened for metabolic causes and undergo imaging of the internal carotid artery to rule out postoperative thrombosis. Computed tomography will exclude hemorrhage. Anticoagulation should be avoided. The pathogenesis of seizures in this setting remains uncertain; cerebral hyperperfusion and/or cerebral embolization may be involved.

▶ Seizures after carotid endarterectomy are related to elevations in systemic and retinal artery pressures and may be considered a variant of the hyperperfusion syndrome. See Abstract 11–31, which follows.

Hyperperfusion Syndrome After Carotid Endarterectomy: A Transcranial Doppler Evaluation

Powers AD, Smith RR (George Washington Univ; Univ of Mississippi)
Neurosurgery 26:56–60, 1990 11–31

Patients with overabundant cerebral perfusion after vascular surgery may experience seizures and unilateral pain in the head and eye. They are at risk of delayed intracerebral hemorrhage. Two patients were encountered who had increased perfusion velocity after carotid endarterectomy accompanied by symptoms. Flow velocity declined as the symptoms resolved, and initially low vascular resistance increased at the same time.

Woman, 64, a smoker, had recently had several episodes of transient dizziness with visual changes; bilateral carotid bruits were noted on examination. The CT scan was normal, but carotid duplex studies showed bilateral stenotic lesions. Angiography revealed nearly total occlusion of the left internal carotid artery and 50% narrowing of the right carotid. Left hemispheric cerebral vascular resistance was low on transcranial Doppler monitoring.

Left-sided headache occurred after a left carotid endarterectomy was performed, and transcranial Doppler examination showed increased left middle cerebral artery flow velocity. Magnetic resonance imaging showed a high-intensity signal in the ipsilateral thalamic region. There was no focal deficit, and neurologic function remained stable 7 weeks later. At that time transcranial Doppler examination showed normal flow velocities and normal pulsatility in the left hemispheric vessels.

Hyperperfusion was seen in 2 of 14 patients having transcranial Doppler monitoring after carotid endarterectomy. About 10% of patients with hyperperfusion may have more serious complications. Aggressive control of increased blood pressure is appropriate because of the risk of intracranial bleeding. Anticoagulants and antiplatelet agents may increase the risk of serious complications in these cases.

▶ The combination of a very high-grade carotid stenosis (physiologic occlusion) and major ischemic symptomatology sets the stage for postoperative hyperfusion in that, with removal of the stenotic lesion, normal pressure is restored to a circulation that has had its autoregulatory capacity impaired from chronic ischemia. Recognition of this syndrome is important because anticoagulants are contraindicated in that they may precipitate intracerebral bleeding. These patients frequently present with paroxysmal lateralizing epileptiform discharges. They do not have classic grand mal seizures, thus the subtle nature of these seizure discharges may be missed by a casual observer. Because the focus for these discharges is usually in the watershed area of the motor strip, palpation of the pectoralis muscle quite commonly will reveal fine fasciculatory movements that are, in fact, the reflection of a seizure discharge. The treatment is Dilantin. The condition is self-limited, and chronic seizures virtually never result. We see approximately 1 or 2 patients per year with this syndrome from among about 175 undergoing carotid endarterectomy. The frequency, of course, will depend on the particular population of patients undergoing surgery in an individual practice. Fortunately, this syndrome is less common with the use of Forane (isoflurane) anesthesia than with halothane or enflurane anesthesia, agents that have a much more dramatic effect on cerebral blood flow than isoflurane.—Thoralf M. Sundt, Jr., M.D., Chairman, Department of Neurologic Surgery, Mayo Clinic, Rochester

---

Rupture of the Vein Patch: A Rare Complication of Carotid Endarterectomy

Riles TS, Lamparello PJ, Giangola G, Imparato AM (New York Univ)
Surgery 107:10–12, 1990 11–32

Although the saphenous vein patch has been used in carotid endarterectomy, rupture of these patches has occurred during the early postoperative period. To determine whether there might be a correlation between this complication and the use of ankle saphenous vein as patch material, data on saphenous vein patch closure in 2,275 of 2,359 carotid operations performed from 1962 through 1986 were reviewed, Ankle saphenous vein was used in 75 of 240 carotid surgeries from July 1982 to October 1983. In the other 165 patients, saphenous vein from the thigh was used.

In 3 patients in whom saphenous vein from the ankle was used, the patch ruptured within 2–5 days after uneventful carotid surgery. At emergency reoperation, the central portion of the vein was found to be necrotic, but there was no evidence of infection. In all patients, the carotid artery was reclosed with saphenous vein from the thigh, and recovery was uncomplicated. The use of saphenous vein from the ankle was discontinued, and there were no more such complications in more than 600 subsequent carotid endarterectomies.

Rupture of the vein patch is a rare complication of carotid surgery. Although the use of ankle saphenous vein was associated with rupture in a small number of patients in this series, the use of ankle vein should not be condemned solely on the basis of these few experiences. Further study is warranted.

▶ Further studies have confirmed the observations in this report.

Immediate and Long-Term Results of Carotid Endarterectomy

Healy DA, Clowes AW, Zierler RE, Nicholls SC, Bergelin RO, Primozich JF, Strandness DE Jr (Univ of Washington)

Stroke 20:1138–1142, 1989 11–33

Data were reviewed on 200 consecutive patients who had carotid endarterectomy from 1980 to 1987. The mean age of the 123 men and 77 women was 66 years. The stenosis was more than a 50% reduction in diameter of the bifurcation in 88% of sides.

The stroke rate was 6.2% per year for 36 patients who had stroke before surgery, 2.8% per year for 87 who had transient ischemic attacks, and .65% per year for 77 without specific symptoms. The overall annual death rate was 6%, including with 9.2% per year for patients with stroke, 5.5% per year for those with transient ischemic attacks, and 4.6% per year for those without symptoms. One death occurred at operation. Three of the 35 deaths during the average follow-up of 31 months were related to stroke; 13 were secondary to myocardial events.

Duplex scanning revealed 5 occlusions in the internal carotid artery; 1 was perioperative and 3 caused stroke. An early myointimal restenosis occurred in 38 of 152 patients (25%). In 2 patients (5.3%) the lesion regressed.

Long-term survival may not be improved by carotid endarterectomy, but it may be affected by coexisting coronary artery disease. Occurrence of an ischemic event requires a thorough search for causative factors. Myointimal hyperplasia probably can be followed safely by repeat studies.

▶ Although 25% of patients followed carefully with duplex scans had restenosis of more than 50%, some of these lesions regress and others remain smooth and do not cause symptoms.

Long-Term Follow-Up of Surgically Managed Carotid Bifurcation Atherosclerosis: Justification for an Aggressive Approach

Callow AD, Mackey WC (Tufts Univ)

Ann Surg 210:308–316, 1989 11–34

The value of carotid endarterectomy in stroke prevention is controversial. The short- and long-term results of an aggressive surgical approach to carotid bifurcation atherosclerosis in symptomatic and asymptomatic patients were compared with those of medical management.

A total of 619 patients have undergone 993 carotid endarterectomies at 1 center since 1970. After surgery the crude annual stroke incidence including perioperative strokes was 1.9%; this incidence in symptomatic patients was 2.1%. The annual stroke incidence in patients undergoing "optimal" medical therapy reportedly ranges from 2.9% to 8%. In asymptomatic patients undergoing carotid endarterectomy, the crude annual stroke incidence including perioperative stroke was 1.4%. For asymptomatic patients undergoing nonsurgical therapy, such rates have been reported to be 3.4% and 2.7%.

Carotid endarterectomy is superior to "optimal" medical therapy in preventing stroke in patients with symptomatic carotid bifurcation atherosclerosis. This aggressive surgical approach is also superior in selected asymptomatic patients, particularly those with hemodynamically significant stenoses. Surgical series must maintian low perioperative mortality and stroke morbidity to demonstrate superiority over medical treatment. Late death in patients undergoing carotid endarterectomy is mainly caused by coexisting coronary artery disease.

▶ Callow's monumental experience is carefully evaluated in this report given to the American Surgical Association. The report justifies the title.

The Course of Atherosclerotic Diseases After Carotid Endarterectomy in 297 Patients Followed-Up for 21 Years

Salenius J-P (Tampere Univ Central Hosp, Finland)

J Intern Med 225:373–378, 1989 11–35

Overall survival and late results after carotid endarterectomy are influenced by both cerebrovascular disease (CVD) complications and other manifestations of atherosclerosis. The course of atherosclerotic diseases after carotid endarterectomy was defined in 279 patients who underwent 331 consecutive carotid endarterectomies from 1965 to 1984. The patients were followed for 21 years (median, 76 months).

The procedure-combined mortality was 3.9%, all from cerebral causes. The mortality rate was 2% to 3% during the first 3 years, 4% to 6% from the fourth to the seventh year, and 9% to 10% per year thereafter. Of the 101 late deaths, 51% were caused by coronary heart disease (CHD), 17% by CVD, and 32% by other causes. The 3:1 ratio of CHD to CVD deaths is similar to that observed in the normal population. The procedure-combined morbidity was 5.7%. The combined incidence of fatal and nonfatal strokes was 3% during the first and fifth years, and 1% to 2% annually thereafter. Peripheral arterial occlusive disease and CHD occurred in combination with CVD in 68.5% of patients. The incidence of CHD or peripheral arterial occlusive disease was similar during the follow-up. Patients with several manifestations of atherosclerosis had significantly higher serum lipoprotein B and triglycerides, decreased high-density lipoprotein cholesterol levels, and an increased frequency of hypertension than patients with only CVD.

The natural course of CVD is accompanied by disabling cerebral complications and deaths. The development of other manifestations of atherosclerosis, such as CHD and peripheral arterial occlusive disease, are combined with the lipid status and hypertension. Coronary heart disease is the main cause of death after the patient undergoes carotid endarterectomy.

▶ Carotid endarterectomy does not protect the patient from subsequent coronary artery disease, nor is it intended to.

Long-Term Follow-Up and Clinical Outcome of Carotid Restenosis
Healy DA, Zierler RE, Nicholls SC, Clowes AW, Primozich JF, Bergelin RO, Strandness DE Jr (Univ of Washington)
J Vasc Surg 10:662–669, 1989 11–36

The durability of carotid endarterectomy depends on the ability to prevent stroke, the incidence of restenosis, and the frequency with which recurrent stenosis causes neurologic symptoms. Most studies report a low incidence of neurologic symptoms associated with restenosis, whereas others have found that the high rate of postoperative restenosis limits its efficacy because of associated neurologic symptoms.

A 4-year follow-up study was done to assess the long-term results after carotid endarterectomy in 221 men and 80 women. Serial duplex scanning examinations were carried out. Carotid restenosis was defined as a 50% or greater diameter reduction. All patients with more than 50% postoperative stenosis were recalled every 3 months. At each follow-up visit patients were asked about the development of new neurologic symptoms and were classified as asymptomatic or symptomatic.

Of the 301 arteries at risk, recurrent carotid stenosis developed in 78 (26%). Spontaneous stenosis regression occurred in 20 arteries. By life-table analysis, the cumulative incidence of restenosis at 7 years was 31% and the cumulative incidence of restenosis regression was 10%, for a 21% prevalence of recurrent stenosis at 7 years. Nine patients with restenosis experienced hemispheric transient ischemic attacks and 2 patients had a stroke, yielding a 14% incidence of neurologic symptoms. By life-table analysis, at 7 years the cumulative incidence years of ipsilateral transient ischemic attacks in patients with recurrent stenosis did not differ from that in patients without restenosis. Similarly, there was no statistical difference in the cumulative incidence of stroke or survival at 7 years between patients with or without restenosis.

Restenosis after carotid endarterectomy usually occurs early in the postoperative period and tends to regress or remain stable during long-term follow-up. Because there appears to be no obvious difference in the natural history of restenosis with and without stenosis regression, a conservative approach to the treatment of restenosis appears justified.

▶ This study further documents previous observations suggesting that carotid artery restenosis is a benign process. Although this abstract summarizes existing knowledge about postendarterectomy restenosis, it incorrectly identifies aspirin therapy as being effective.

Late Carotid Restenosis: Aetiologic Factors for Recurrent Carotid Artery Stenosis During Long-Term Follow-Up

Salenius J-P, Haapanen A, Harju E, Jokela H, Riekkinen H (Univ of Tampere, Finland)

Eur J Vasc Surg 3:271–277, 1989 11–37

Stenosis recurrence rates after carotid endarterectomy range from 1% to 30%. The results of studies to identify etiologic risk factors for recurrent disease have been inconclusive. The incidence of restenosis after carotid endarterectomy was determined and the risk factors for recurrent stenosis identified.

Between 1970 and 1984, 257 patients underwent 142 carotid endarterectomies; 169 patients were still alive at the time of follow-up. Of the 169 survivors, 116 underwent duplex scanning of 133 carotid arteries during a follow-up period of 28–209 months. These 116 patients, who ranged in age from 30 to 72 years at the time of operation, had undergone 142 operations. Indications for carotid endarterectomy included transient ischemic attack in 102, stroke in 24, and asymptomatic carotid disease in 16.

Follow-up duplex scanning of 133 carotid vessels revealed that 97 (73%) arteries were patent, 18 (13.5%) had a hemodynamically insignificant restenosis, 13 (9.8%) had significant restenosis, and 5 (3.8%) had reoccluded. Only 10 (55.6%) of the 18 patients with either high-grade restenosis or reocclusion had been symptomatic before scanning. Fourteen of these 18 patients were men. Analysis of etiologic risk factors for restenosis identified serum cholesterol, triglyceride, and high-density lipoprotein cholesterol levels as important risk factors. The incidence of recurrent stenosis appeared to be unrelated to hypertension, claudication, obesity, smoking, operative factors, or indications for endarterectomy. Patients with diabetes mellitus, coronary heart disease, or stroke had a higher incidence of recurrent carotid stenoses, but the difference did not reach statistical significance. Directional Doppler of the supraorbital artery and clinical auscultation was of little value in diagnosing restenosis, whereas duplex scanning correctly identified its occurrence. Postoperative treatment with aspirin was most effective, whereas the use of anticoagulation therapy or a combination of aspirin and dipyridamole was not beneficial. These findings confirm that the long-term patency of the carotid artery after carotid endarterectomy is acceptable.

▶ Restenosis of an artery either following PTLA or surgery remains a challenge for vascular surgeons. Multiple causes are in play for restenosis. As summarized nicely in the article on restenosis by Lin et al. (1), biology of intimal hyperplasia is a complex process, involving smooth muscle cells, platelet-derived growth factors, and the like. Prevention may be better achieved by antiproliferative agents than by antiplatelet drugs.

Reference

1. Lin, et al: *Circulation* 79:1374, 1989.

Spontaneous Dissection of the Cervical Internal Carotid Artery: Diagnosis by MRI

Wilms G, Marchal G, DeMaerel Ph, DeCrop E, Van Hecke P, Baert AL (Universitaire Ziekenhuizen KU Leuven, Leuven, Belgium)

J Radiol 780:225–227, 1989 11–38

Spontaneous dissection of the cervical portion of the internal carotid artery (ICA) occurs more often than generally has been reported. Angiographic examination provides only indirect evidence of a characteristic, but nonspecific subintimal blood collection at the base of the skull. According to recent studies, MRI can distinguish spontaneous arterial dissection from fibromuscular dysplasia, tumor invasion, and other systemic disorders. In a patient with spontaneous dissection of the cervical portion of the ICA the use of MRI conclusively confirmed the diagnosis.

Man, 66, was seen with amaurosis, intermittent paresis of the right arm, severe pain in the nape of the neck, and tinnitus. The only finding on physical examination was a painful right ICA on palpation. Doppler examination showed a completely patent carotid bifurcation and right ICA. However, blood flow in the ophthalmic artery appeared to be reversed. Cerebral angiographic examination revealed an irregular stenosis in the upper part of the right cervical ICA extending up to the base of the skull. T1-weighted MR images in the axial plane demonstrated a hyperintense mass partially surrounding the narrowed ICA lumen. In the coronal plane T1-weighted MR images confirmed the hyperintense mass was a subintimal blood collection.

Cerebrovascular accidents caused by an embolism traveling from the dissection site are the most common clinical manifestation of spontaneous cervical ICA dissection. An accurate etiologic diagnosis is very important because the subintimal hematoma resulting from spontaneous ICA dissection will resolve without surgical intervention, and the narrowed lumen returns to its normal dimensions. Administration of an anticoagulant usually prevents further embolization from the dissection site.

Hematomas in the subacute phase, 7 or more days after spontaneous dissection, appear as a hyperintense mass on T1-weighted as well as on T1-weighted images. No other lesions have these characteristics. Fatty deposits also may appear as a hyperintense area on T1-weighted images, but they always appear as hypointense areas on T2-weighted images. Therefore, the MR findings can be considered pathognomonic for spontaneous dissection of the cervical portion of the ICA.

▶ As MRI appears to be a valuable tool in the diagnosis of carotid dissection, one can expect that magnetic resonance angiography (MRA) will be even more useful.

High-Resistance Doppler Flow Pattern in Extracranial Carotid Dissection
Hennerici M, Steinke W, Rautenberg W (Univ of Düsseldorf, Germany)
Arch Neurol 46:670–672, 1989

11–39

Ultrasonography is especially helpful in investigating carotid dissections before arteriography and during follow-up. Ultrasound analysis of 22 patients admitted since 1982 with a diagnosis of internal carotid dissection was performed. The chief initial manifestation was focal cerebral ischemia, seen in 19 patients. Only 27% of the patients had persistent neurologic deficit, and all remained ambulatory and independent. Two thirds of the patients had headache and neck pain, and half had signs of an oculosympathetic lesion.

Continuous-wave Doppler spectrum analysis and duplex examination showed typical signs in the internal carotid artery in three fourths of the patients. A high-amplitude Doppler signal was noted, with much reduced systolic Doppler frequencies and alternating flow direction. The alternating signal consisted of a small early systolic component and a second component directed toward the brain, on which a further component was

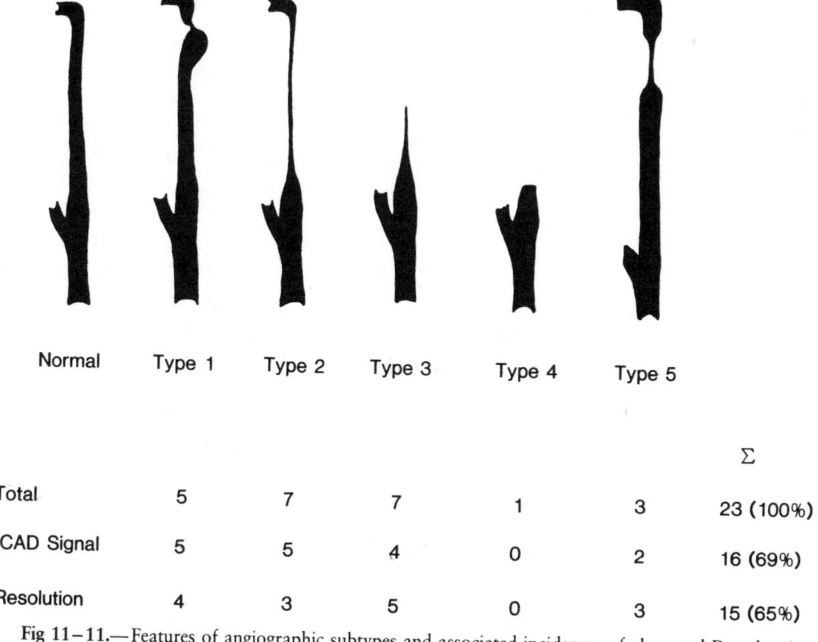

	Normal	Type 1	Type 2	Type 3	Type 4	Type 5	Σ
Total	5	7	7	1	3		23 (100%)
ICAD Signal	5	5	4	0	2		16 (69%)
Resolution	4	3	5	0	3		15 (65%)

Fig 11–11.—Features of angiographic subtypes and associated incidences of abnormal Doppler signals and resolution in cases with internal carotid artery dissection (ICAD). (Courtesy of Hennerici M, Steinke W, Rautenberg W: *Arch Neurol* 46:670–672, 1989.)

superimposed backward. It occurred in cases of severe stenosis at the entry of the carotid canal or in a tapered vessel (Fig 11–11). Vascular obstruction decreased or resolved in two thirds of the patients during follow-up. The Doppler spectrum consistently improved or became normal. Improvement was noted a mean of 6 weeks after diagnosis.

Extracranial dissections of the carotid artery can be usefully evaluated by Doppler ultrasonography, and improvement or resolution of the process can be detected in this way.

▶ Doppler ultrasonography provides the best method for following the natural history of carotid dissection.

Dissection of the Extracranial Internal Carotid Artery: Sixty-Two Cases

d'Anglejan Chatillon J, Ribeiro V, Mas JL, Bousser MG, Laplane D (Hôp André Mignot; Hôp de la Salpêtrière; Centre Raymond Garcin; Hôp Saint-Antoine, Paris)

Presse Méd 19:661–667, 1990 11–40

Spontaneous dissection of the cervical and cerebral arteries accounts for 2% to 4% of all ischemic strokes, and approximately 20% of these occur in young individuals. Extracranial dissections occur more frequently than intracranial dissections, and the carotid artery is more often involved than the vertebrobasilar artery. The case histories of 62 patients diagnosed with dissection of the extracranial internal carotid artery (EICA) during a 16-year period were studied retrospectively.

The study population consisted of 37 men (mean age, 45.5 years) and 25 women (mean age, 40 years) who were treated for a total of 69 dissections of the EICA. Predisposing risk factors and disorders included migraine (34%), hypertension (30%), current cigarette smoking (29%), past cigarette smoking (21%), athletic activity (40%), and oral contraceptive use (48%). Twenty-nine patients had spontaneous onset of EICA dissection, 11 patients had experienced minor head or neck trauma before EICA dissection, and 6 patients had sustained major trauma. One patient had Marfan's syndrome, 2 patients had Ehler-Danlos syndrome, and 13 patients had fibromuscular dysplasia. The most common initial local symptoms were one-sided headache, neck pain, Horner's syndrome, and tinnitus. Ten patients were asymptomatic. Thirty-five patients had a stroke, and 2 patients had ischemic optic neuritis resulting in blindness. Angiographic examination demonstrated a stenotic EICA in 48 patients, 11 of them with an associated aneurysm, EICA occlusion in 17 patients, and an isolated aneurysm in 4 patients. Of the 62 patients, 6 received no special treatment, 13 were treated with antiplatelet agents, and 43 had anticoagulant therapy.

After a follow-up of 2–188 months, 30 patients were cured without neurologic sequelae, 11 had minor neurologic sequelae without disability, and 18 had major neurologic sequelae with severe disability. Three men died during follow-up, 1 of suicide. Forty-one of the 59 surviving patients were able to resume their normal activities. Three patients had a second dissection of the EICA during follow-up.

▶ Although there is not much that vascular surgeons can do to treat carotid dissection, they can withhold surgical exploration and they can emphasize to colleagues who see patients with trauma that carotid dissection may be induced by blunt injury to the neck.

Long-Term Follow-Up of Occlusive Cervical Carotid Dissection
Pozzati E, Giuliani G, Acciarri N, Nuzzo G (Bellaria Hosp, Bologna, Italy)
Stroke 21:528–531, 1990 11–41

Little is known about the long-term course of spontaneous dissection of the cervical carotid artery. Frank occlusion, a severe form of carotid dissection, is reported by some to be relatively uncommon. Nineteen patients with occlusive dissection of the cervical carotid artery diagnosed between 1974 and 1984 were followed for 5–13 years.

In all but 2 patients the string sign was observed on angiograms; this is considered highly suggestive of a carotid dissection. Five patients had transient ischemic attacks, 7 had a minor stroke, 6 had a major stroke, and 1 had epileptic seizures. Five patients wre treated surgically. Medical therapy consisted of antiplatelet drugs in most cases; anticoagulation was never used.

The overall mortality and major morbidity rate was 32%. Three patients died within a month of onset. Three others require total care, 5 have permanent deficits (1 is unable to resume previous activities), and 7 are asymptomatic. One patient was lost to follow-up. Ten of the 16 survivors had control angiography and subsequent yearly Doppler ultrasonography. Occlusion was unchanged in 2 patients, but in the remaining 8 recanalization was seen. Six of the 8 are asymptomatic and 2 have permanent neurologic deficits. The healed artery was completely normal in 3 patients.

Prognosis was less favorable in those older than age 50 years, suggesting a role for concomitant atherosclerotic disease. Long-term outcome and overall carotid reopening rate was better in younger patients. Residual vascular abnormalities occur, however, even with recanalization.

Doppler Color Flow Imaging of Carotid Body Tumors
Steinke W, Hennerici M, Aulich A (Universität Düsseldorf, Germany)
Stroke 20:1574–1577, 1989 11–42

Doppler color flow imaging is a new ultrasonic technique for simultaneous display of tissue and vessel morphology, by B-mode echotomography, and color-coded flow velocity data by Doppler-mode analysis. The method is especially helpful in the neck, both to evaluate cerebral arteries and to identify carotid paragangliomas safely. These tumors are difficult to detect clincially at an early stage because they often occur sporadically and symptoms are absent for some time.

Two patients had Doppler color flow imaging using an angiodynograph. One had a hypervascular tumor that was highly suggestive of a carotid body tumor. The tumor was removed without complications after confirmation by intra-arterial digital subtraction angiography. The other patient had a heterogeneous echo-poor tumor on B-mode study and a diffuse vascularity near the carotid bifurcation. Digital subtraction angiography confirmed the diagnosis.

Even small paragangliomas can be diagnosed by Doppler color flow imaging. The study can be used to follow up patients who have small asymptomatic tumors, resection being reserved for cases in which growth occurs. Angiography should be done only in patients who are to undergo operation.

▶ Doppler imaging has now reached the point where a definitive diagnosis of carotid body tumor can be made if the study is of high quality and shows the bifurcation in profile.

Carotid Body Tumor: Flow Sensitive Pulse Sequences and MR Angiography

Rippe DJ, Grist TM, Uglietta JP, Fuller GN, Boyko OB (Duke Univ)
J Comput Assist Tomogr 13:874–877, 1989 11–43

A carotid body paraganglioma was visualized by both conventional MRI, with and without intravenously administered gadolinium-diethylenetriamine pentaacetic acid (Gd-DTPA) contrast, and flow-sensitive techniques, including MR angiography (MRA).

Woman, 59, had a slowly enlarging painless right neck mass for 2 years. In addition to MRA, multiplanar gradient recalled acquisition in the steady state (GRASS) images were obtained. Carotid body tumors typically are highly vascular, well-circumscribed lesions that separate the external and internal carotid arteries. Hypointense foci are seen on T1-weighted images, whereas T2-weighted images demonstrate a "salt and pepper" pattern. Magnetic resonance angiography showed abnormal morphology of the carotid bifurcation, but intrinsic tumor vascularity was not well visualized. The axial GRASS images showed evidence of blood flow within the tumor.

Magnetic resonance imaging can demonstrate specific features of carotid body paragangliomas. Contrast studies and flow-sensitive MR sequences, including MRA, are of further use in characterizing these tumors.

▶ Similar to the duplex scan experience, MRA will provide sufficient information to allow surgery to proceed without arteriography.

12 Visceral Circulation

Etiologic Factors in Renovascular Fibromuscular Dysplasia: A Case-Control Study

Sang CN, Whelton PK, Hamper UM, Connolly M, Kadir S, White RI, Sanders R, Liang K-Y, Bias W (Johns Hopkins Med Insts)

Hypertension 14:472–479, 1989 12–1

The role of several etiologic factors in renovascular fibromuscular dysplasia (FMD) was evaluated in a case-control study of 33 patients with angiographically documented FMD and 61 renal transplant donor controls with normal renal arteries.

The risk of FMD was significantly increased among cigarette smokers and patients with 5-year histories of hypertension. There was a significant dose-response relationship between FMD and cigarette smoking, with the risk increased by more than eightfold among those who smoked more than 10 pack-years of cigarettes. Markers of HLA-DRw6 antigen were more common in patients with FMD than in controls; the risk of FMD increased by fivefold after adjustment for cigarette smoking. A positive family history of cardiovascular disease was also more common in cases, but the difference between cases and controls was not significant. There was no significant association between FMD and previous contraceptive use, endogenous sex hormone abnormality, or increase in renal mobility.

Genetic predisposition and personal history of cigarette use may play important etiologic roles in FMD. Previous reports suggesting an association between FMD and oral contraceptive use and excessive renal mobility were not supported.

▶ Arterial dysplasias are difficult to analyze. Renal ptosis has always been suggested, but such arterial stretch has not been implicated in FMD affecting arteries elsewhere in the body. The finding of a high prevalence of FMD in premenopausal multiparous women suggests an estrogen or progesterone cause. Other arterial dysplasias described in this volume also implicate a hormonal cause of arterial dysplastic lesions, including nodular intimal thickening and dysplasia of the media and adventitia. It could be that the hormonal effects are not direct but indirect, perhaps by inhibiting T suppressor cell activity.

Can Quantitative Renography Predict the Outcome of Treatment of Atherosclerotic Renal Artery Stenosis?

Gruenewald SM, Collins LT, Antico VF, Farlow DC, Fawdry RM (Westmead Hosp, Westmead, Australia)

J Nucl Med 30:1946–1954, 1989 12–2

Clinically successful renal artery angioplasty requires careful selection of patients. To assess the functional nature of the atherosclerotic stenosis and the likelihood of successful treatment in 31 patients, quantitative gamma camera renography was used before and up to 6 years after vascular surgery or angioplasty.

Before treatment 9 patients had no prolongation of parenchymal transit time in the affected kidney, although they had reduced perfusion and function on the side of the stenosis. After angioplasty, none of the 9 had improved control of blood pressure and 6 had a decreased glomerular filtration rate.

Of 22 patients with prolonged parenchymal transit time, treatment produced complications in 3. Hypertension was improved or cured in the other 19. The glomerular filtration rate improved in 12 but was stable or reduced in 7. Quantitative renography identified the 3 significant recurrent stenoses and the 1 renal artery occlusion.

Renal arterial reconstruction or dilation is effective only in patients who have functionally significant stenosis demonstrated by prolonged parenchymal transit times. Prediction of such patients can be made with quantitative renography. The technique also permits demonstration of recurrent functionally significant stenosis.

▶ The search continues for a reliable preoperative test that will predict the results of renal artery reconstruction or remodeling in treatment of hypertension. It could be that captopril-enhanced scintigraphy will contribute to the accuracy of this method of testing. Whatever technique ultimately emerges will need to combine the anatomical information provided by arteriography with the physiologic information derived from testing.

Symptoms and Signs of Thrombotic Occlusion of Atherosclerotic Renal Artery Stenosis

Weibull H, Bergqvist D, Andersson I, Choi DL, Jonsson K, Bergentz S-E (Malmö Gen Hosp, Malmö, Sweden)

Eur J Vasc Surg 4:159–165, 1990 12–3

To determine the symptoms and signs when a stenotic renal artery occludes and whether such an occlusion can be predicted, 24 patients with an occluded renal artery demonstrated at angiography or operation in whom previous angiography demonstrated atherosclerotic renal artery stenosis (occluded group) were compared with 67 patients with stenosis but no occlusion at the time of reangiography or treatment (nonoccluded group).

Significant differences between the groups included age, degree of stenosis, and advanced generalized atherosclerosis. The median age was 55 years in the nonoccluded group and 65 years in the occluded group. Patients with occlusion were more likely to have ischemic heart disease (90%) than patients without occlusion (70%). However, a third of the patients in each group had renal insufficiency based on a serum level of creatinine higher than 149 μmol/L, and most patients in both groups had hypertensive retinal lesions. Bilateral stenoses were more common in the occluded group (50%) than in the nonoccluded group (9%). All patients in the occluded group had multifocal atherosclerosis, which involved the aorta or iliac arteries, or both; this condition appeared in less than a third of the nonoccluded group.

Flank pain was experienced by only 21% of the patients with occlusion. Other symptoms appeared equally in the patients who did not have occlusion. A tight stenosis (no more than 1.5 mm) was an important risk factor for occlusion. The most consistent sign of occlusion was a sudden rise in the serum level of creatinine in a patient known to have a narrow stenosis.

▶ This article demonstrates the difficulty of following the progression of renal artery stenosis. No doubt, clinical symptoms are often unreliable. Possibly, duplex scan may help.

Percutaneous Transluminal Renal Angioplasty: Initial Results and Long-Term Follow-Up in 202 Patients

Baert AL, Wilms G, Amery A, Vermylen J, Suy R (University Hospitals KU Leuven, Leuven, Belgium)

Cardiovasc Intervent Radiol 13:22–28, 1990 12–4

Most reports on the results of percutaneous transluminal angioplasty for the treatment of renal artery stenosis (PTRA) involve small groups of patients. Few publications provide long-term follow-up.

A total of 250 PTRAs were done in 202 patients. The procedure was successful in 83%. Results were better for postostial atherosclerotic lesions, fibromuscular lesions, and transplant kidneys, compared with ostial atherosclerotic lesions. Overall, 61% of the patients had decreased blood pressure after the procedure, and 31% were cured. At a mean follow-up of 25.8 months the cure rate was 21% in bilateral atheromatous lesions, 30% in unilateral atheromatosis, 65% in unilateral fibromuscular disease, and 40% in bilateral fibromuscular dysplasia. Sixty percent of the patients undergoing transplant were cured. Eleven percent of the patients had complications. Recurrence of stenoses was noted in 8% of the lesions; 80% recurred within the first year.

In technical success of PTRA depends on the skill and experience of the angiographers and on the characteristics of the stenosis. The technical success rate of PTRA appears to be higher in patients with fibromuscular lesions. In this series only 1 lesion was resistant to dilation. The presence of branch artery stenoses caused failure in 1 bilateral attempt and perforation in another.

▶ The development of renal artery PTA has encouraged the early diagnosis of renovascular hypertension. The nonsurgical alternative is understandably popular. Just as in other aspects of vascular surgery, the early enthusiasm needs tempering by long-term observation, as this report shows. Nevertheless, the overall benefits gained by early diagnosis remain.

Intraluminal Angioplasty in Renovascular Arterial Hypertension: 104 Cases

Jeunemaître X, Julien J, Raynaud A, Pagny JY, Gaux JC, Plouin PF, Ménard J, Corvol P (Hôp Broussais, Paris)

Presse Méd 19:205–209, 1990 12–5

Renovascular stenosis is the most common cause of secondary arterial hypertension. Until recently, surgical revascularization of the ischemic kidney was the only available treatment for drug-resistant hypertension. Percutaneous transluminal angioplasty (PTA) has now become the first-line treatment for this indication. The etiology of renovascular hypertension may be atherosclerotic or fibrodysplastic. The immediate and long-term outcomes after PTA were compared in 104 patients with renovascular hypertension of varying etiologies treated between 1985 and 1987.

Fibrodysplastic renal disease was diagnosed in 38 patients, who underwent 42 PTA procedures; 50 patients with atherosclerotic renal disease and normal renal function underwent 52 PTA procedures; and 16 patients with atherosclerotic disease and renal insufficiency underwent 18 PTA procedures. Patients were treated under local anesthesia and remained in the hospital for a mean of 48 hours. Access was via the femoral artery. Each patient was evaluated for control of arterial hypertension and patency of the dilated renal artery immediately after PTA and after a mean follow-up of 7.5 months.

Percutaneous transluminal angioplasty was immediately successful in 35 procedures (83%) performed in patients with fibrodysplastic disease, in 48 procedures (92%) done in patients with atherosclerotic renal disease and normal renal function, and in 11 procedures (61%) performed in patients with atherosclerotic kidney disease and renal insufficiency. After a mean follow-up of 7.5 months, arterial pressures were normal in 65% of the patients with fibrodysplastic disease and in 13% of those with atherosclerosis and normal renal function, but in none with atherosclerosis and renal insufficiency. Angiographic follow-up revealed a patent renal artery in 91% of the fibrodysplastic disease patients, 70% of the patients with atherosclerosis and normal renal function, and 33% of those with atherotic renal disease and renal insufficiency. Two patients in the latter category required chronic hemodialysis after PTA had failed to revascularize the ischemic kidney, but renal function was improved in 3 others after PTA. The results confirm that PTA is effective in the treatment of renal stenosis caused by either fibrodysplastic or atherosclerotic renal hypertension, with or without renal insufficiency.

▶ Certainly, PTA is the favored procedure in patients with fibromuscular dysplasia of the renal arteries. Early and late success is achieved with these lesions.

Transluminal Angioplasty in Patients With Bilateral Renal Artery Stenosis or Renal Artery Stenosis in a Solitary Functioning Kidney

Kim PK, Spriggs DW, Rutecki GW, Reaven RE, Blend D, Whittier FC (Northeastern Ohio Univs, Canton)

AJR 153:1305–1308, 1989 12–6

Renal angioplasty is contraindicated in patients with bilateral renal artery stenosis or renal artery stenosis in a solitary functioning kidney. The results of transluminal angioplasty in 10 patients with severe bilateral renal artery stenosis and 8 with severe renal artery stenosis in a solitary kidney were evaluated.

Overall, 89% of 28 procedures were successful. Patients had a mean improvement of the degree of stenosis from 85% to 18% after angioplasty and restoration of renal blood flow. There was a significant drop in mean blood pressure from admission to follow-up 1 year later. As a result of the reduced blood pressure, 11 patients decreased or stopped taking diuretics and 15 decreased or stopped taking antihypertensive drugs. There was no significant change in renal function according to measures of mean serum creatinine levels over time, but none of the patients had an increased serum creatinine level at follow-up visits, indicating preservation of renal function. One major complication occurred—cholesterol embolization to the bowel.

Transluminal angioplasty was recommended as the procedure of choice for patients with severe bilateral renal artery stenosis or severe renal artery stenosis in a functioning solitary kidney. This procedure restored blood flow, reduced blood pressure, and was associated with minimal side effects.

▶ Renal artery angioplasty is not without its complications. The availability of reconstructive surgery is terribly important, and the value of such surgery must be recognized by the radiologist. In the text of this article, "spontaneous dissection that could not be repaired by angioplasty" is described, as is recurrence of the stenosis in a solitary functioning kidney; "angioplasty was not repeated because of the severity of the lesion."

Pregnancy and Mesenteric Venous Thrombosis

Engelhardt TC, Kerstein MD (Tulane Univ)

South Med J 82:1441–1443, 1989 12–7

Mesenteric venous thrombosis (MVT) during pregnancy is a rare but well-recognized cause of bowel infarction that may lead to acute abdomen. Factors associated with MVT include stasis in the mesenteric bed caused by portal hypertension, intra-abdominal infection, postoperative state, hypercoagulable states such as pregnancy and oral contraceptive use, and smoking.

Woman, 32, at week 10 of pregnancy by ultrasound study, had peritoneal signs of inflammation. She was afebrile and normotensive. She was a nonsmoker and had not used oral contraceptives for 2 years. Abdominal roentgenography showed nonspecific ileus. Exploratory laparotomy showed an infarcted small bowel segment, which on pathologic examination revealed thrombotic occlusion of the mesenteric veins with hemorrhagic infarction. Ultrasonography on discharge showed a viable fetus and portal vein thrombosis of unknown cause. The coagulation profile showed increased factor VII and a fibrinogen level consistent with pregnancy. The patient was discharged with subcutaneously self-administered heparin. She delivered a normal infant.

Mesenteric venous thrombosis during pregnancy in a patient who is nonsmoker and not taking hormones presents a challenge. It appears that the combination of pregnancy and stasis in the mesenteric bed caused by the portal vein thrombosis may have caused the MVT in this patient.

▶ Unfortunately, MVT enters into the differential diagnosis of mesenteric ischemia. The increased recognition of this condition brought on by dynamic CT scanning has focused the attention of surgeons on the benefits of early anticoagulation and the fact that such patients need not always be subjected to laparotomy. Although stasis in the mesenteric venous bed is postulated as a causative factor in this case, it is more likely that a coagulopathy existed and, of course, the successful management of such cases is dependent on immediate anticoagulation and long-term continuation of this modality of treatment.

The Role of Second-Look Procedure in Improving Survival Time for Patients With Mesenteric Venous Thrombosis

Levy PJ, Krausz MM, Manny J (Hadassah Univ Hosp, Jerusalem)

Surg Gynecol Obstet 170:287–291, 1990 12–8

Data on 21 patients with mesenteric venous thrombosis who were treated at 1 institution since 1978 were reviewed to determine factors that contribute to an improved survival rate. Mesenteric venous thrombosis was diagnosed preoperatively in 8 patients. The decision to perform surgery was based on the extent of the ischemic process, the viability of infarcted intestine, and the general condition of the patient. Surgery was performed in 19 patients. A second-look procedure was performed in 10 patients. No additional bowel resection was needed after initial limited resection in 4 patients.

A limited bowel resection was performed in 6 patients, with primary anastomosis in 3, double ostomy in 1, and additional resection with primary anastomosis in 2. The overall survival rate was 60% but was 71% in those treated surgically. Only 2 patients who underwent a second-look procedure died.

The incidence of intestinal infarction resulting from venous thrombosis has increased. Successful management includes a high degree of suspicion for the diagnosis, aggressive surgical intervention, and anticoagulation therapy. When the extent of necrosis is questionable, resection of ischemic intestine should be postponed for a second-look procedure. Anticoagulation therapy retards the thrombotic process and recurrence of thrombosis, thus decreasing the extent of resected intestine.

▶ Although this abstract states that the incidence of intestinal infarction resulting from mesenteric venous thrombosis has increased, in fact, the reverse is true. Mesenteric venous thrombosis is being diagnosed increasingly with CT scanning, and the need for surgery because of infarction is thus decreasing. Anticoagulant treatment early prevents progression of the process.

13 Upper Extremity Ischemia

Subclavian and Axillary Involvement in Temporal Arteritis and Polymyalgia Rheumatica

Ninet JP, Bachet P, Dumontet CM, Bureau du Colombier P, Stewart MD, Pasquier JH (Hôp Edouard Herriot, Lyon, France)
Am J Med 88:13–20, 1990 13–1

Diffuse arterial involvement can occur in temporal arteritis (TA) or polymyalgia rheumatica (PMR). Data on 10 women aged 60–73 years

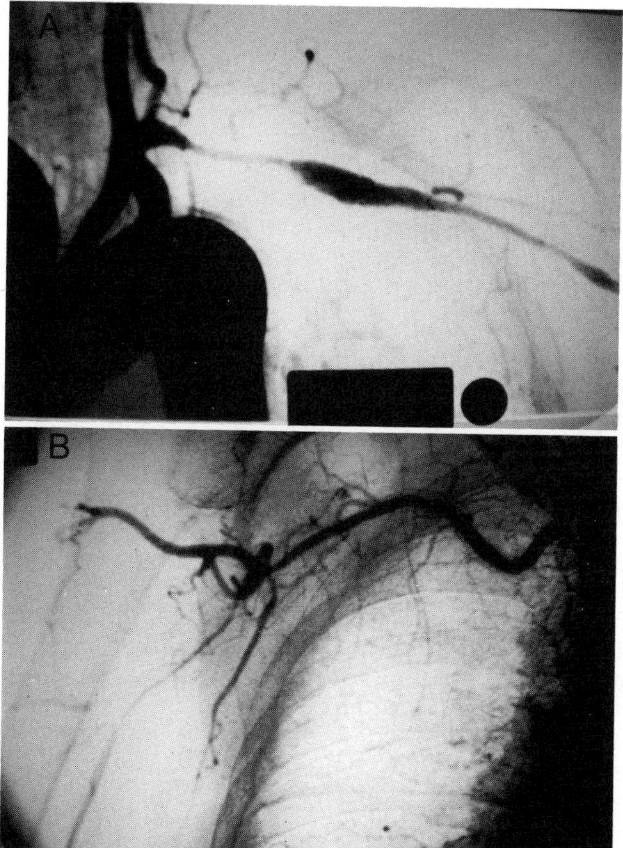

Fig 13–1.—**A,** long stenotic segments with poststenotic ectasia of the left subclavian artery. **B,** high-grade stenosis of right axillary artery. (Courtesy of Ninet JP, Bachet P, Dumontet CM, et al: *Am J Med* 88:13–20, 1990.)

(mean age, 66.7 years) with TA and/or PMR with large-vessel involvement of the upper extremities were reviewed.

The most frequent symptom was arm claudication. Ischemic manifestations were the initial symptoms in 4 patients, appeared with the classic manifestations of TA in 1, and occurred during decreasing corticosteroid therapy in 5. Temporal artery biopsy specimens revealed giant cell arteritis in 7 of 9 patients. Angiography showed bilateral involvement in all patients, with multiple bilateral smooth stenoses or obliteration of the postvertebral subclavian and/or axillary arteries (Fig 13–1). During a mean follow-up of 21 months, all patients improved with corticosteroid therapy, with symptoms of upper-limb ischemia regressing after 3–4 weeks of treatment. None of the patients underwent reconstructive surgery, but revascularization of occluded vessels after stabilization or interruption of treatment did not occur despite clinical improvement.

Large vessel involvement of the upper extremity in TA and PMR affects the subclavian and axillary arteries. This disorder should be differentiated from Takayasu's disease because of similarities in female predominance and angiographic findings. The response to high-dose steroid therapy is rapid, making reconstructive surgery unnecessary.

▶ Although the changes in the subclavian and axillary arteries described in this abstract are very much like atherosclerosis, in fact, the fundamental cause is immunologic injury, which in turn initiates plaque formation. It is well for us to understand that large vessel involvement as described here is common in the systemic arteritides. Perhaps reconstructive surgery can be avoided in early cases, but certainly in those persons in whom the stenosis has progressed to total occlusion, reconstruction is a viable alternative to no therapy.

Induction of Vasospastic Attacks Despite Digital Nerve Block in Raynaud's Disease and Phenomenon

Freedman RR, Mayes MD, Sabharwal SC, Keegan DM (VA Med Ctr, Detroit; Wayne State Univ, Detroit)

Circulation 80:859–862, 1989 13–2

Raynaud hypothesized that the vasospastic attacks of Raynaud's disease and phenomenon were caused by sympathetic hyperactivity, whereas Lewis postulated a "local fault" in which precapillary resistance vessels were hypersensitive to local cooling. To investigate further, vasospastic attacks of Raynaud's phenomenon were induced by a combination of environmental and local cooling in 11 patients with idiopathic Raynaud's disease and 10 with scleroderma. For each patient 2 fingers on 1 hand were anesthetized by local injections of lidocaine, and the effectiveness of the nerve blocks was verified by plethysmography.

Vasospastic attacks, defined as the presence of 2 of 3 possible color changes (pallor, cyanosis, and rubor) and documented by serial photographs, occurred in 9 of 11 patients with idiopathic Raynaud's disease and 8 of 10 with scleroderma. The frequency of vasospastic attacks in nerve-blocked fingers did not differ significantly from that in contralateral intact fingers for either patient group.

Vasospastic attacks in Raynaud's disease and phenomenon can occur without the involvement of efferent digital nerves. These findings argue against the etiologic role of sympathetic hyperactivity. Further studies are needed to define the pathophysiologic mechanisms that underlie these attacks.

▶ The effects of sympathetic stimuli are not excluded by this study, only that a local fault phenomenon in the distal arteriolar bed, as proposed by Lewis in 1929 (1), is probably coexisting.

Reference

1. Lewis T: *Heart* 15:7, 1929.

International Study of Ketanserin in Raynaud's Phenomenon

Coffman JD, Clement DL, Creager MA, Dormandy JA, Janssens MM-L, McKendry RJR, Murray GD, Nielsen SL (Boston Univ; Akademisch Ziekenhuis Gent, Gent, Belgium; Brigham and Women's Hosp, Boston; St James Hosp, London; Janssen Research Found, Beerse, Belgium; et al)

Am J Med 87:264–268, 1989 13–3

A double-blind, placebo-controlled study of ketanserin was carried out at 21 centers in 10 countries to determine its efficacy in treating Raynaud's phenomenon. Outpatients with typical symptoms for 2 years or longer and at least 1 episode weekly in the cooler months were admitted to the study. Patients received ketanserin, 20 mg, 3 times daily for 2 weeks and then 40 mg 3 times daily for 10 weeks. There were 112 patients with primary Raynaud's disease and 110 with secondary Raynaud's phenomenon, 79 of whom had scleroderma.

Vasospastic episodes decreased by 34% with ketanserin and by 18% with placebo, a significant difference. Neither the duration nor the severity of episodes differed significantly in the ketanserin and placebo recipients. In addition, there was no significant difference in finger blood flow in a warm or cool environment in the 41 patients studied. Side effects were not significantly more frequent with ketanserin than with placebo.

Ketanserin significantly lessened symptoms of Raynaud's phenomenon, whether primary or secondary, in this large placebo-controlled study. Ketanserin therapy is appropriate when conservative measures fail. Because the drug may prolong the QT interval it should be avoided in patients with hypokalemia, ventricular arrhythmia, or second- or third-degree heart block and those taking potassium-losing drugs.

▶ Ketanserin, acting as a specific serotonin inhibitor, can certainly relieve vasospastic phenomena. It should have no effect on organic arterial occlusions except when these are accompanied by distal vasoconstriction.

Quantitative Measurements of Finger Blood Flow During Behavioral Treatments for Raynaud's Disease

Freedman RR (Lafayette Clinic, Detroit)

Psychophysiology 26:437–441, 1989 13–4

Finger blood flow has not been measured quantitatively during finger temperature biofeedback and autogenic training for Raynaud's disease. Therefore, venous occlusion plethysmography was used to record finger blood flow in 16 men and women with Raynaud's disease assigned at random to 10 sessions of 1 of these 2 behavioral treatments. Finger temperature, heart rate, blood pressure, and skin conductance levels also were measured.

A maximum vasodilation test showed no differences between groups. Blood flow for the temperature feedback group averaged across training sessions increased during training, reaching significance 6 minutes into the training period (Fig 13–2). It was significantly higher than in the autogenic training group throughout training. Finger temperature was significantly lower in the feedback group than in the autogenic groups between minutes 1 and 10, and then became significantly higher. The skin conductance level was significantly higher in the feedback group than in the autogenic group during both baseline and training and increased significantly during training.

Finger temperature biofeedback induces active vasodilation in patients

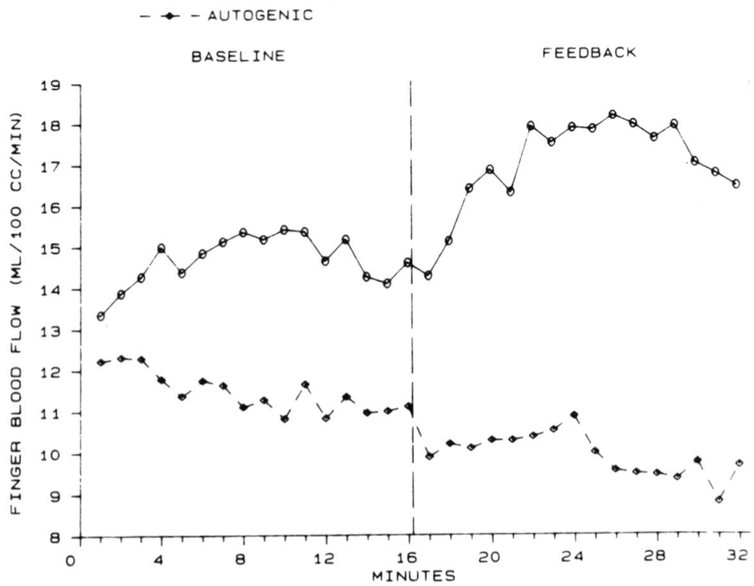

Fig 13–2.—Finger blood flow in temperature feedback and autogenic training subjects averaged across 10 training sessions for both hands. (Courtesy of Freedman RR: *Psychophysiology* 26:437–441, 1989.)

with Raynaud's disease. The vasodilation does not appear to result from a general decline in sympathetic activity.

▶ It is clear that vascular control of digital blood flow does not derive entirely from sympathetic-mediated α-adrenergic constriction and passive withdrawal of this activity. A vasodilating mechanism has been identified, and this study suggests activation of that mechanism by biofeedback.

Fibrinolytic Therapy for Upper-Extremity Arterial Occlusions
Widlus DM, Venbrux AC, Benenati JF, Mitchell SE, Lynch-Nyhan A, Cassidy FP Jr, Osterman FA Jr (Johns Hopkins Univ)
Radiology 175:393–399, 1990 13–5

Because excellent results have been reported with local intra-arterial administration of urokinase in the treatment of lower-extremity occlusions, including those of embolic origin, the efficacy of this approach in the treatment of upper-extremity ischemia was assessed in 6 men and 2 women aged 30–69 years who underwent fibrinolytic therapy for arterial occlusion in an upper extremity during a 6-year period.

One patient was treated twice. Streptokinase was used in only 1 procedure, and urokinase was used in the other 8. Physical examination confirmed the absence of pulses at the wrist in all patients. There was evidence of sensory loss in 6 patients and decreased motor function in 2. All patients underwent diagnostic arteriography to identify the occlusion site. Fibrinolytic drugs were administered directly into the subclavian, axillary, or brachial clot, and either directly into the occluded forearm vessel, or proximally into the brachial artery. The duration of thrombolytic therapy ranged from 30 minutes to 72 hours.

Angiography performed after fibrinolytic therapy revealed that 3 patients had excellent flow through all arm vessels, although in 1 patient minimal residual laminar brachial clot was observed on the arteriogram (Fig 13–3). There were small residual proximal ulnar artery occlusions in 2 patients, and a focally occluded radial artery, which was recanalized in 1. Adjunctive percutaneous transluminal angioplasty was performed in 3 patients after thrombolysis, which proved helpful. Pulses became normal after therapy in 5 patients, 2 of whom regained normal radial pulses within 12–72 hours after fibrinolysis. None of the patients died, no strokes occurred, and none of the patients required amputation of an upper extremity. All patients had at least 1 artery that was continuously patent to the wrist after fibrinolytic treatment. The only significant complication was a puncture-site groin hematoma that required evacuation. Urokinase infusion may be considered a first-line treatment for brachial artery emboli and other upper-extremity arterial occlusions.

▶ Again, thrombolytic therapy aids in uncovering the etiology of the acute arterial occlusion, thus allowing definitive therapy to proceed.

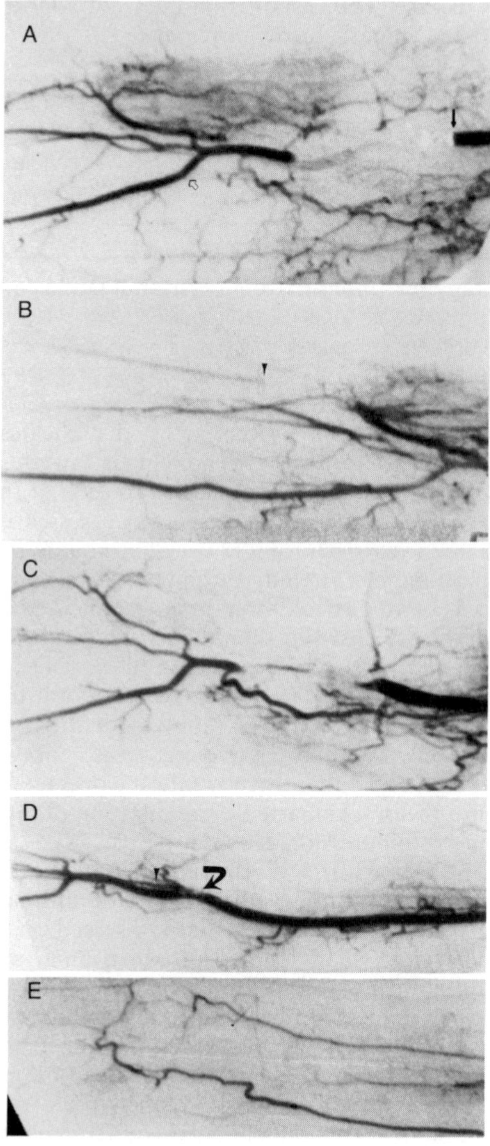

Fig 13–3.—Urokinase administration for brachial artery embolus in a 69-year-old woman with atrial fibrillation/flutter and a cold, numb, painful right arm. **A,** initial arteriogram shows brachial artery occlusion *(solid arrow)* with a patent ulnar artery *(open arrow)*. **B,** proximal radial artery occlusion and reconstitution *(arrowhead)*. **C,** after 2 hours of urokinase administration (500,000 U) selectively into the brachial embolus, some increased flow is seen. **D,** after 12 hours of urokinase administration (900,000 U), minimal residual laminar brachial clot *(curved arrow)* can be appreciated, with good flow through a patent radial artery *(arrowhead)*. **E,** radial and ulnar arteries are open to the hand. (Courtesy of Widlus DM, Venbrux AC, Benenati JF, et al: *Radiology* 175:393–399, 1990.)

Percutaneous Transluminal Angioplasty Versus Surgery for Subclavian Artery Occlusive Disease

Farina C, Mingoli A, Schultz RD, Castrucci M, Feldhaus RJ, Rossi P, Cavallaro A
(Creighton Univ, Omaha; Univ of Rome La Sapienza, Rome)

Am J Surg 158:511–514, 1989 13–6

Percutaneous transluminal angioplasty (PTA) is an attractive alternative to surgical reconstruction for subclavian artery occlusive disease. The results of PTA for proximal stenosis of the subclavian artery in 21 patients were compared with those in 15 patients who underwent carotid subclavian reconstruction. The mean follow-up period was 30 months after PTA and 40 months after surgery.

Early actuarial patency rates were 91% and 86% for the PTA and surgical groups, respectively. Complications included intimal dissection at the puncture site in 1 patient who underwent PTA and transient laryngeal nerve injury and Horner's syndrome in 2 surgical patients. The mean blood pressure difference between the arms was 3.3 mm Hg in the PTA patients and 1.6 mm Hg in the surgical patients. There were no significant differences between treatment groups in these parameters. However, 5-year actuarial patency rates were significantly lower in the PTA group, 54%, as opposed to 87% in the surgical group. Furthermore, the mean systolic blood pressure difference between arms increased progressively with PTA (Fig 13–4).

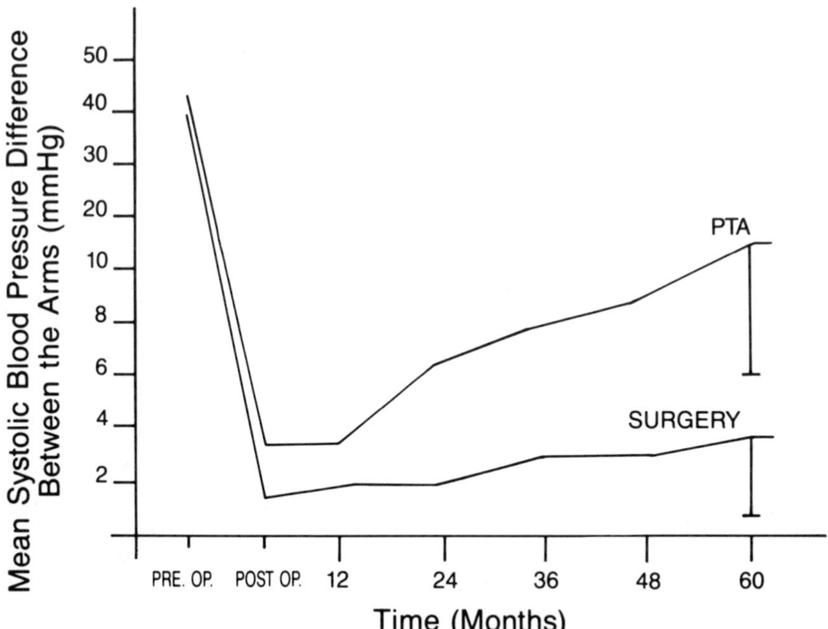

Fig 13–4.—Preoperative, postoperative, and long-term follow-up data on the mean systolic blood pressure difference between the arms after PTA and carotid subclavian reconstruction. (Courtesy of Farina C, Mingoli A, Schultz RD, et al: *Am J Surg* 158:511–514, 1989.)

Subclavian artery occlusive disease is a relatively benign disease, with most patients experiencing remission of symptoms within 2 years. Although symptoms may be temporary, patients may still seek treatment and a temporizing, less invasive procedure such as PTA may be acceptable. Better early results are achieved with PTA, but there is continuous deterioration of the artery's hemodynamic status after PTA, resulting in a relatively high late failure rate. Hence, PTA should be reserved for patients with mild arm claudication or arm weakness, whereas surgical revascularization should be performed in patients with severe arm ischemia, rest pain, or distal embolization.

▶ In the text of this presentation, as in others, no cerebroembolic complications of PTA were reported. Local dissections and occlusions do occur, however, and long-term hemodynamic benefit is not obtained in all patients. Nor are surgical reconstructions free of complications. The authors of this article are wise in saying that PTA is a temporizing therapeutic measure, and such palliation is effective in relieving cerebrovascular ischemia as well as upper extremity ischemia. Further, stroke has been reported after subclavian PTA.

Subclavian Artery Revascularization: A Comparison Between Carotid-Subclavian Artery Bypass and Subclavian-Carotid Transposition
Sterpetti AV, Schultz RD, Farina C, Feldhaus, RJ (Creighton Univ, Omaha)
Surgery 106:624–632, 1989 13–7

Despite its many theoretical advantages, subclavian-carotid transposition (SCT) has not gained wide acceptance in the surgical treatment of symptomatic subclavian disease. The results of SCT or carotid-subclavian artery bypass (CSB) performed during a 15-year period were compared in 46 patients with symptoms referable to occlusion of the subclavian artery. Associated risk factors and angiographic parameters did not differ between treatment groups. The mean follow-up was 46.9 months (range, 2–148 months).

The 7-year actuarial patency rate was 100% for the 16 patients who underwent SCT and 86% for the 30 who underwent CSB (Fig 13–5). Because of the small number of cases, the difference in patency rates was not significant. The mean operative time (75 minutes vs. 134 minutes) and intraoperative blood loss (140 mL vs. 232 mL) were significantly reduced after SCT in comparison with CSB. With CSB, significant progressive deterioration of the hemodynamic status of the reconstruction was noted during follow-up, with a significantly increasing difference in systolic brachial pressure between the arms. Systolic pressures between arms remained stable after SCT.

Subclavian-carotid transposition, whenever feasible, should be the procedure of choice for patients with symptomatic severe subclavian artery disease. The single autogenous end-to-side anastomosis allows physiologic restoration of blood flow to the subclavian and vertebral arteries without using foreign material.

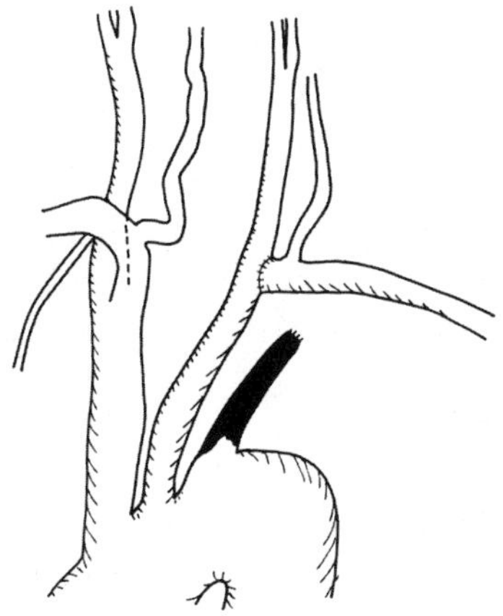

Fig 13–5.—Schematic drawing of the reconstruction. (Courtesy of Sterpetti AV, Schultz RD, Farina C, et al: *Surgery* 106:624–632, 1989.)

▶ For those who are familiar with the technique, autogenous reconstruction of the subclavian artery without bypass has become the favored procedure. Like any operation, there are certain details that ease the performance of the procedure.

Arterial Complications of the Thoracic Outlet Syndrome: Fifty-Five Operative Cases

Cormier J-M, Amrane M, Ward A, Laurian C, Gigou F (Hôp Saint Joseph, Paris; Basingstoke District Hosp, Basingstoke, England)

J Vasc Surg 9:778–787, 1989 13–8

Arterial complications of thoracic outlet syndrome, although not common, are potentially serious. Indications for and methods of surgery were studied retrospectively in 55 operative procedures carried out in 47 patients to correct subclavian-axillary artery lesions caused by compression at the thoracic outlet.

The most common causes of compression were a long cervical rib in 27 instances and an anomalous first rib in 15. Of the 55 arterial lesions, 35 were complicated by distal thromboembolism, most frequently in aneurysms (Fig 13–6). Symptoms reflected the frequency of thromboembolic complications and included claudication, vasomotor phenomena, digital gangrene, and acute limb-threatening ischemia.

A combined supraclavicular and infraclavicular approach was preferred for surgical access. Decompression was accomplished by excision of the cervical rib and the first rib; all soft tissue elements were completely divided. Arterial reconstruction was frequently achieved with either resection anastomosis, performed 23 times, or replacement of vein graft, done on 11 occasions. Axillary emboli were amenable to direct revascularization when the subclavian artery was repaired. If possible,

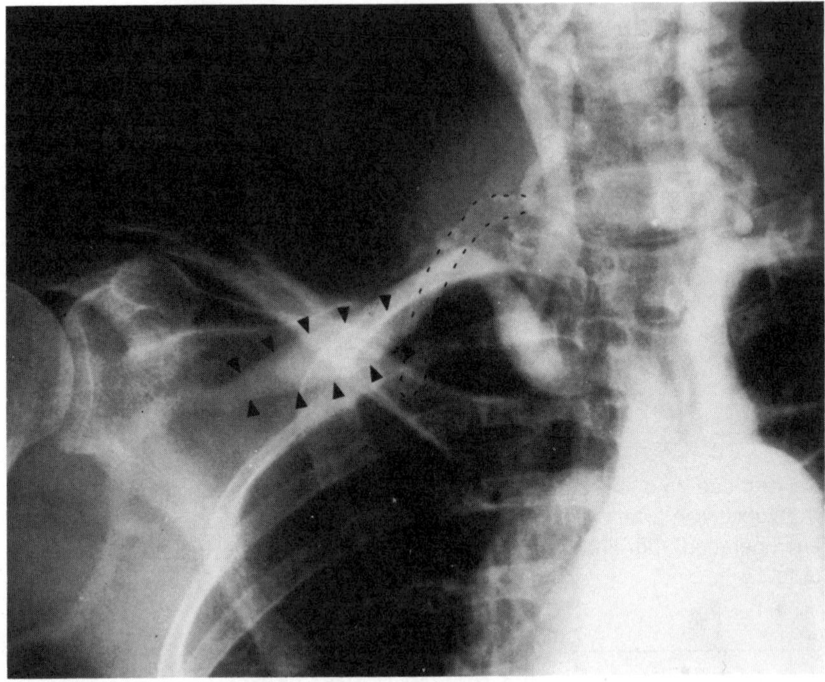

Fig 13–6.—Poststenotic aneurysm with a brachial artery embolus successfully treated by embolectomy. (Courtesy of Cormier JM, Amrane M, Ward A, et al: *J Vasc Surg* 9:778–787, 1989.)

more-distal embolic occlusions were managed without having to use embolectomy catheter manipulations.

No operative deaths resulted. The mean follow-up period was 5 years 8 months (range, 4 months to 16 years). Thirty-nine patients who had 46 arterial procedures were available for late assessment using Doppler ultrasonography, B-mode scanning, and digital subtraction angiography. Of these, 35 had no symptoms and 4 had residual claudication. There was no hemodynamic or anatomical abnormality in the subclavian-axillary segment in the remaining 35 patients. No amputations were necessary.

The classic indications for surgery for the thoracic outlet syndrome seen with thromboembolic complications were confirmed. Furthermore, to prevent further compromise of the distal vascular bed, surgery is recommended as soon as stenosis or poststenotic dilation of the subclavian artery appears.

▶ The large experience of these authors corroborates the impression of others that when a physiologic abnormality is demonstrated (e.g., poststenotic dilation of the subclavian artery), the indications for surgery are clear. The operation itself should consist of arterial reconstruction combined with thoracic outlet depression as described.

First Rib Resection for Vascular Complications of Thoracic Outlet Syndrome

Thompson JF, Webster JHH (Royal South Hampshire Hosp, Southhampton; Princess Margaret Hosp, Wiltshire, England)

Br J Surg 77:555–557, 1990 13–9

The surgical approach to vascular complications of the thoracic outlet syndrome remains controversial. Removing a cervical rib alone has yielded disappointing results. The results were assessed of first rib resection in 20 patients with 29 affected arms treated in a 5-year period (Fig 13–7).

Nineteen patients with uncomplicated subclavian artery compression were cured. Of 6 patients with aneurysm or thrombosis, 5 were improved. Of 12 patients with neurologic symptoms, 9 were cured, and 2 were improved (Fig 13–8). The only late surgical complication was a keloid scar in the axilla of a young Asian patient.

First rib excision is recommended as the essential primary treatment for patients with arterial symptoms caused by thoracic outlet syndrome. There is no significant difference in symptomatic results between the transaxillary and supraclavicular surgical approaches. In a first procedure with no evidence of damage to the subclavian artery, transaxillary resec-

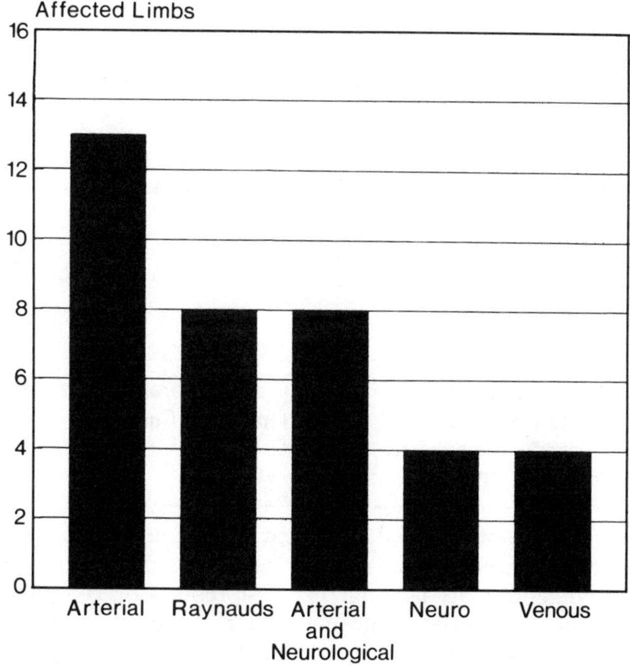

Fig 13–7.—Symptoms at initial presentation. (Courtesy of Thompson JF, Webster JHH: *Br J Surg* 77:555–557, 1990.)

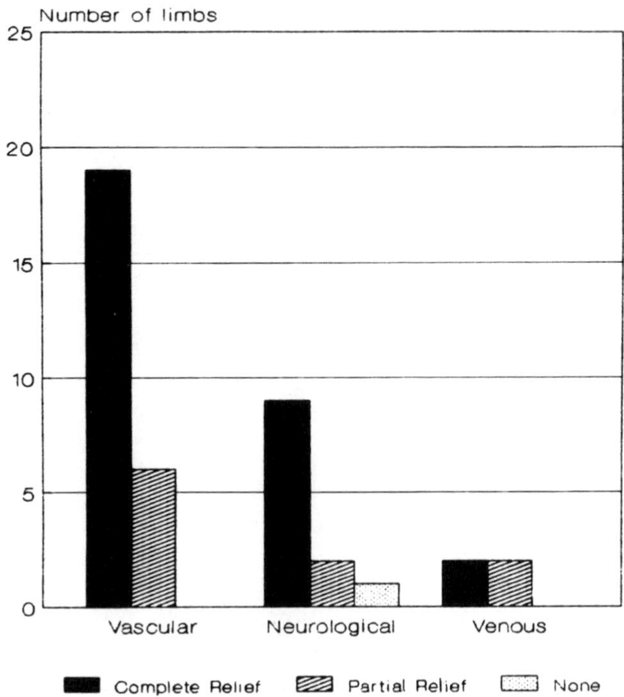

Fig 13–8.—Clinical outcome after surgery. *Solid bars* indicate complete relief; *hatched bars,* partial relief; and *dotted bars,* no relief. (Courtesy of Thompson JF, Webster JHH: *Br J Surg* 77:555–557, 1990.)

tion is recommended. A separate supraclavicular incision is strongly recommended if the subclavian artery is to be reconstructed.

▶ It is refreshing to find, in the experiences of continental surgeons such as in this report and the previous abstract, corroboration of observations made in the United States.

Thoracic Outlet Syndrome: Diagnostic and Therapeutic Approach: Review of One Hundred and Ninety-Four Operated Cases
Bacourt F, Koskas F, Goeau Brissonnière O (Hôp Américain de Paris)
Sem Hôp Paris 65:2895–2902, 1989 13–10

The indications and optimal treatment for the neurologic form of thoracic outlet syndrome remain controversial. Specific neurologic tests to confirm the diagnosis are lacking. The case reports of 148 patients operated on for thoracic outlet syndrome were reviewed.

Between 1977 and 1988, 43 males and 105 females aged 16–55 years underwent 194 operations for thoracic outlet syndrome performed by a single surgeon. Bilateral procedures were performed in 23 patients; 32 patients became symptomatic within a mean of 62 months after sustaining traumatic injury to the neck or shoulder. Another 25% had professions conducive to the development of compressive neurologic syndromes. Overall, 22% had pure neurologic symptoms, 19% had pure vascular symptoms, 53% had neurovascular symptoms, and 6% were asymptomatic.

Diagnosis of the neurologic form of thoracic outlet syndrome was based strictly on clinical findings, which included young age, C8–T1 root involvement, an association between posture and symptoms, and a positive stress test. Neither arteriography nor phlebography was useful in diagnosing the neurologic form of thoracic outlet syndrome, but these studies accurately defined the extent of arterial or venous involvement. Half of the patients had bone abnormalities, most commonly of ribs, hypertrophy of the C7 transverse process, or congenital absence of the first rib. The need to count ribs before initiating operation cannot be overemphasized. Compressive symptoms were attributable to fibromuscular abnormalities in 83% of patients.

Therapeutic indications depend on symptom severity and extent of vascular compression. Asymptomatic patients should be operated on only if there is evidence of compression of a major artery. Which route to use for surgical access remains among the most controversial issues. Although the transaxillary route provides good access to the first rib, the C8–T1 roots, and the subclavicular vein, it does not allow total scalenectomy in patients with C5, C6, or C7 involvement, nor does it enable arterial repairs. The supraclavicular route enables total scalenectomy and resection of the posterior part of the first rib. The transthoracic and the posterior routes are used less often, but the latter route is useful for the treatment of recurrence. In this series, 89% of the operated-on patients had complete resolution of their symptoms or were markedly improved.

▶ This large series of patients with thoracic outlet syndrome is well analyzed and presented. Thirty-two patients experienced symptoms after a mean time of 62 months following trauma to the neck or shoulder, which seems like an unusually long delay. In my experience, patients have immediate pain and muscle spasms in the neck and shoulders that progress into the upper extremities from brachial plexus compression within a few days, weeks, or months of injury. Delay of such neurologic symptoms beyond 1 year may make the association to the previous neck and shoulder trauma suspect. The lack of verification in most cases of neurologic thoracic outlet syndrome with electromyography, Doppler studies, and angiography confirms other authors' experience. The arteriograms and venograms, however, are essential for evaluation of the vascular cases. Half of the patients had bone abnormalities; this is an unusually high percentage, suggesting that many other patients who have principally fibromuscular anomalies with normal x-ray appearances have not been referred for thoracic outlet syndrome or had it diagnosed. The good results these authors obtained in 89% of the surgically treated cases indicate their astute diagnosis, proper selection of patients for surgery, and the appropriate choice of transaxillary first rib resection for lower plexus and total anterior scalenectomy for upper plexus symptoms, combined with careful surgical technique that avoided complications. Overall, this is an excellent presentation of the many complex problems presented by these patients. It should be read in the original form to obtain the greatest benefit of the authors' impressive knowledge and experience.—D.B. Roos, M.D., Denver, Colorado

Two-Year Follow-Up of Patients Operated on for Thoracic Outlet Syndrome: Effects on Sick-Leave Incidence

Lindgren SHS, Ribbe EB, Norgren LEH (Lund Univ, Sweden)

Eur J Vasc Surg 3:411–415, 1989 13–11

There are no objective parameters to compare the results of surgery for thoracic outlet syndrome. In a retrospective analysis of 175 episodes of this syndrome in 165 patients who underwent resection of the first rib, results of surgery were compared with the duration of postoperative sick-leave obtained from regional social insurance offices. Patients were followed for 2 years postoperatively.

Clinical evaluation showed good or fair results in 59% of patients, whereas surgery failed in 41%. During surgery an anomaly causing compression at the thoracic outlet was significantly more common in patients having a good outcome postoperatively. Both groups had long periods of sick leave because of thoracic outlet syndrome at 2 years pre- and postoperatively. However, only the duration of postoperative sick leave correlated with the outcome of surgery; patients with good or fair results had a duration of postoperative sick leave of 180 days compared with 353 days in those with poor results.

The outcome of surgery for thoracic outlet syndrome correlates well with the duration of postoperative sick leave. The only variable that predicts the outcome of surgery is the presence of an anomaly restricting the thoracic outlet. Because of the difficulty in establishing the diagnosis, a conservative attitude to surgical treatment of thoracic outlet syndrome is recommended.

▶ This method of documenting results of thoracic outlet decompression for neurogenic symptomatology is an interesting one. Just as in arterial complications of thoracic outlet syndrome, the documented presence of an anomaly is predictive of ultimate good results.

The Treatment of Thoracic Outlet Syndrome: A Comparison of Different Operations

Sanders RJ, Pearce WH (Univ of Colorado; Northwestern Univ)

J Vasc Surg 10:626–634, 1989 13–12

Experience with late failures after transaxillary first rib resection and with scalenectomy as treatment for thoracic outlet syndrome has led to the use of combined operations. The results from 111 transaxillary first rib resections done from 1964 to 1972, 279 anterior and middle scalenectomies performed from 1972 to 1979, and 278 supraclavicular first rib resections with scalenectomy carried out between 1980 and 1987 were compared. A history of neck trauma was present in 86% of the patients, and 4.5% had cervical ribs. Symptoms consisted of pain, finger paresthesia, and/or occipital headache. Physical signs were limited to scalene muscle tenderness and symptoms with the arms abducted to 90 degrees in external rotation.

Rates of success, as judged by subjective patient evaluation, were similar for all operations: at 1–2 years, 76% to 79%; at 3–5 years, 70% of 73%; and at 5–10 years, 69% to 72%. The chief complication after rib resection was plexus injury in 2.6% of patients, leaving .5% with partial disability. Temporary phrenic nerve palsy followed scalenectomy in 4.4% of patients.

Thoracic outlet syndrome may be managed conservatively at first. If patients with neck injury fail to improve, scalenectomy provides good results with few serious complications. Rib resection is indicated when symptoms do not have a traumatic origin or recur after scalenectomy.

▶ An explicit plan of therapy, as described in this abstract, should be associated with the fewest complications. However, as Abstract 13–11 has indicated, the objective preoperative demonstration of an abnormality is predictive of good results after surgical decompression.

Diagnosis and Treatment of Subclavian Artery Aneurysms

Salo JA, Ala-Kulju K, Heikkinen L, Bondestam S, Ketonen P, Luosto R (Helsinki Univ Central Hosp)

Eur J Vasc Surg 4:271–274, 1990 13–13

Thirteen subclavian artery aneurysms were treated between 1974 and 1988. There were 9 men and 4 women whose mean age was 60 years. Seven patients had symptoms related to the aneurysm. Eleven patients had a mass in the upper mediastinum. The diagnosis was made angiographically in all cases (Figs 13–9 and 13–10). Five of 6 CT studies clearly demonstrated a subclavian artery aneurysm.

Nine patients underwent direct unilateral subclavian or aorticosubclavian reconstruction, and 4 had a caroticosubclavian bypass after exclusion of the aneurysm. Dacron was used in 7 reconstructions and autogenous saphenous vein in 5. In 9 patients the aneurysm was at least 5 cm in diameter. Five intraoperative ruptures occurred.

One patient with very poor lung function died postoperatively of pneumonia. Complications occurred in 45% of the patients, but not in any of those undergoing aneurysmal exclusion and extrathoracic caroticosubclavian bypass. On follow-up for 6 months to 14 years, all patients had a patent vascular graft and a palpable pulse at the wrist. Four follow-up angiograms revealed no problems.

Surgery presentely is recommended for all patients having a subclavian artery aneurysm, even if symptoms are absent. However, the frequency of complications and the lack of knowledge of how asymptomatic aneurysms progress suggest that operative indications need to be defined more clearly.

▶ The problem not addressed by this article or its abstract is what an aneurysm is. It is suggested that the definition is fulfilled with the subclavian artery reaches 2.5 cm in diameter in the area of greatest dilation.

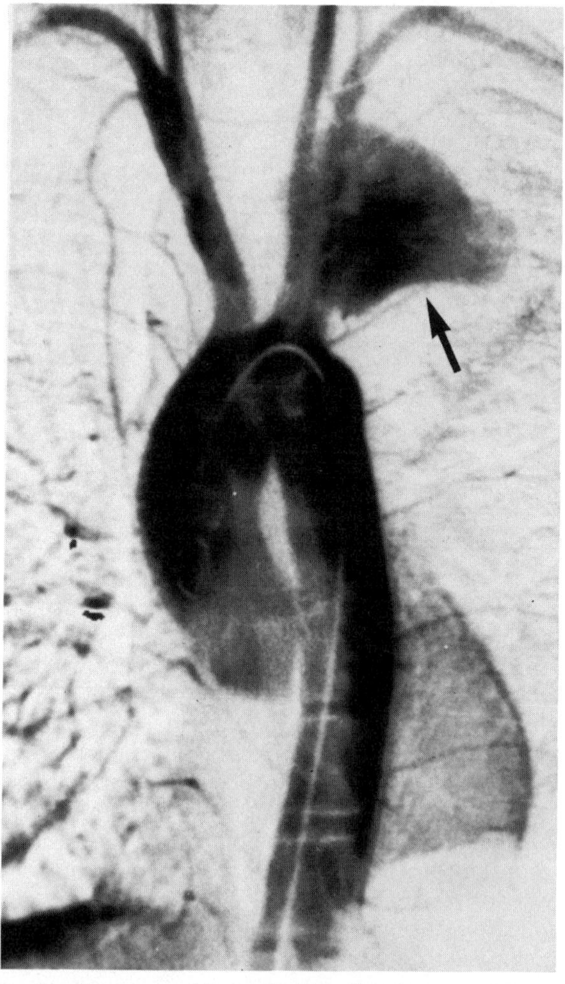

Fig 13–9.—Intrathoracic aneurysm of the proximal left subclavian artery. (Courtesy of Salo JA, Ala-Kulju K, Heikkinen L, et al: *Eur J Vasc Surg* 4:271–274, 1990.)

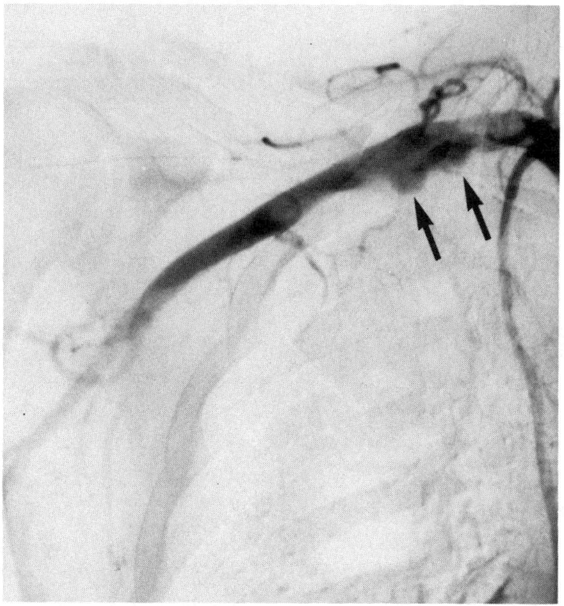

Fig 13–10.—Extrathoracic multilocular aneurysm of the right subclavian artery. (Courtesy of Salo JA, Ala-Kulju K, Heikkinen L, et al: *Eur J Vasc Surg* 4:271–274, 1990.)

Surgical Treatment of Distal Ulnar Artery Aneurysm

Harris EJ Jr, Taylor LM Jr, Edwards JM, Mills JL, Porter JM (Oregon Health Sciences Univ, Portland)

Am J Surg 159:527–530, 1990 13–14

Ulnar artery aneurysms are an infrequent cause of digital ischemia, usually secondary to digital artery embolization. Six patients who had digital ischemia as a result of digital artery occlusion from a distal ulnar artery aneurysm were seen in 7 years.

Each of the patients underwent angiography from the aortic arch to the fingertips (Fig 13–11). After mobilization and excision of the aneurysm, autogenous vein was interposed in an end-to-end manner. Patency was confirmed by repeat angiography (Fig 13–12), or by duplex scanning.

The patients, all men, engaged in activities predisposing the distal ulnar artery to injury. The mean age was 29 years. All patients had acute onset of cool, painful digits in an ulnar distribution. Five patients had ischemia of the third through the fifth fingers; in 1, ischemia was limited to the third digit. Multiple proper and common digital arteries were occluded. All patients improved symptomatically after surgical treatment and no tissue losses occurred. All remained improved during a mean follow-up of 2 years.

Surgery is warranted when an ulnar artery aneurysm produces symp-

Fig 13–11.—Preoperative arteriogram illustrating the irregular lumen characteristically identified in patent distal ulnar artery aneurysms *(large arrow)*. There is a poorly developed superficial palmar arch *(medium arrow)*, and there is diffuse embolization of the proper digital arteries of the third, fourth, and fifth fingers, as well as the ulnar aspect of the second finger *(small arrows)*. (Courtesy of Harris EJ Jr, Taylor LM Jr, Edwards JM, et al: *Am J Surg* 159:527–530, 1990.)

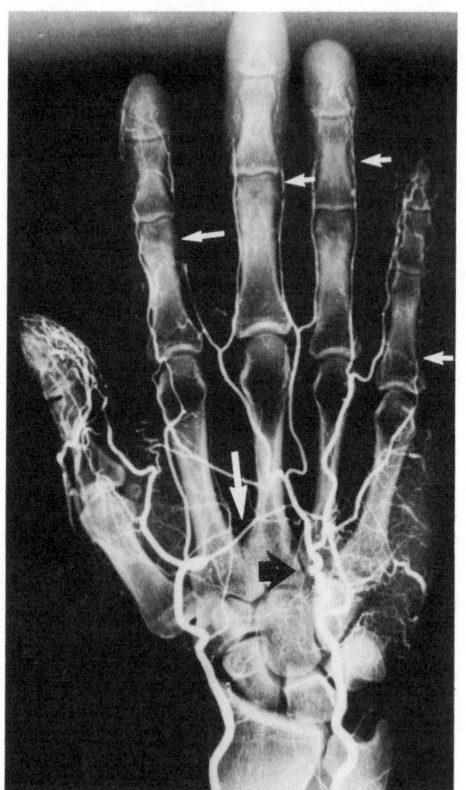

Fig 13–12.—Postoperative arteriogram of the repair of the aneurysm shown in Figure 13–11. A short segment of reversed vein graft is identified *(arrow)*, extending from the hook of the hamate to the superficial palmar arch. (Courtesy of Harris EJ Jr, Taylor LM Jr, Edwards JM, et al: *Am J Surg* 159:527–530, 1990.)

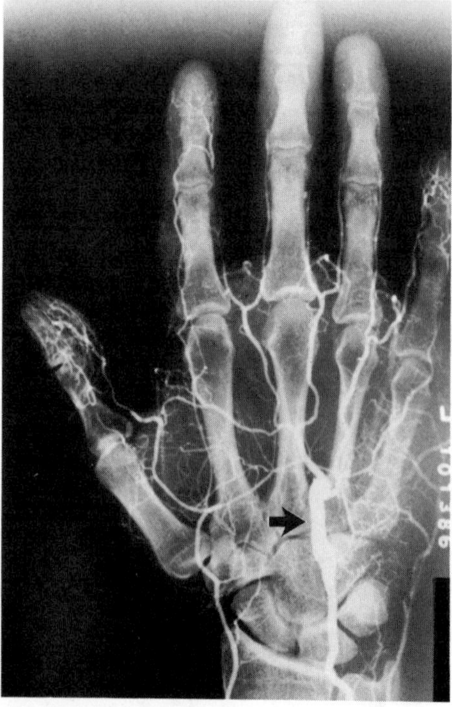

tomatic digital ischemia. Symptoms from the hypothenar hammer syndrome can be disabling and can interfere with occupational tasks.

▶ As illustrated, trauma induces the corkscrew arteries that are associated with palmar aneurysms, and histology discloses medial injury, which leads to aneurysm formation. Even if the aneurysm is rather small, embolization remains a dominant feature.

14 Miscellaneous Aneurysms

Throbbing Buttocks Syndrome

Natali J, Jue-Denis P, Kieffer E, Merland JJ, (Hôp de la Salpétrière; Hôp Lariboisière, Paris)

J Mal Vasc 14:183–189, 1989 14–1

A persistent sciatic artery (PSA) is a rare congenital vascular malformation; only 53 cases of PSA have been reported in the literature. Aneurysm formation in a PSA may cause the throbbing buttocks syndrome, characterized by a large, painful swelling in the buttocks region. However, the same syndrome may also develop as a consequence of congenital or traumatic aneurysm or arteriovenous (AV) fistula formation of the internal iliac artery. The throbbing buttocks syndrome was observed in 7 new patients. In 1, an aneurysm of the PSA was diagnosed; the other 6 patients had AV fistulas of the internal iliac artery. Five of the fistulas were caused by congenital vascular malformations; 1 was caused by trauma.

Woman, with an aneurysm in a PSA, had been treated for 7 years with corticosteroids for chronic polyarthritis. She had severe pain in the lower right leg, intermittent claudication, and painful swelling of the buttocks of approximately 10 cm in diameter. On admission the patient was acutely ill with fever and dyspnea, and she had a recent history of rapid weight loss. Arteriography demonstrated a voluminous aneurysm of a PSA, complicated by what appeared to be a large embolism. The external iliac artery and both femoral arteries were small. The patient underwent urgent operation during which a large, atheromatous, fissured aneurysm was found. Incision of the aneurysm revealed a large mural thrombosis, which was excised. Because the exact location of the sciatic nerve was not known, the 2 arterial openings were simply sutured and the aneurysmal cavity was drained and dried. The postoperative course was uneventful, and there were no neurologic sequelae. The patient has remained well during 2 years of follow-up. The pain in the buttocks gradually disappeared.

The other 6 patients had large angiodysplasias caused by AV fistulas of an internal iliac artery. All 6 first underwent preoperative embolization of the interior iliac artery in an effort to minimize blood loss during later excision of the malformation. None had an isolated aneurysm of the internal iliac artery. Three patients had previously undergone ligation of an interior iliac artery, which had not prevented recurrence. Moreover, the previous ligation rendered embolization extremely difficult or impossible. Transabdominal incisions were required in 2 patients in whom percutaneous vascular access was not possible. Results in 5 of the 6 patients were satisfactory. One patient who underwent arterial embolization only was somewhat improved, but she refused to undergo excision of the malformation and did not return for further follow-up.

▶ French vascular surgeons have taught us a great deal. Uncovering this marvelously named syndrome is not only amusing but practical. Early diagnosis of the persistent sciatic artery may disclose the aneurysms that form in such abnormalities before distal atheromatous embolization occurs. When such complications develop, they are uniformly tragic.

Embolization of Large Saccular Aneurysms With Gianturco Coils

Rao VR, Mandalam RK, Joseph S, Satija V, Gupta VK, Gupta AK, Jain SK, Unni MN, Rao AS (Sree Chitra Tirunal Inst for Med Sciences and Technology, Trivandrum, India)

Radiology 175:407–410, 1990 14–2

The use of Gianturco spring coils for therapeutic endovascular occlusion of arteries and arteriovenous fistulas has been expanded to aneurysms involving major arteries in the neck, legs, and even the aorta. However, obliteration of saccular aneurysms at inoperable sites still presents a special problem. Transfemoral catheter embolization of inoperable saccular aneurysms using Gianturco coils was attempted in 5 patients.

Man, 42, had progressively enlarging and pulsatile swelling of the left popliteal fossa. Angiography confirmed the presence of a large saccular aneurysm arising from the popliteal artery (Fig 14–1). Few collateral vessels were observed and these had poor runoff into the distal artery. Catheterization was attempted 10 days after surgical repair failed. The femoral artery was catheterized and a coronary catheter was introduced into the aneurysmal sac. Five Gianturco coils were then released into the aneurysm. Repeated angiography showed a considerable reduction of flow into the aneurysm. The pain resolved and the swelling regressed. Two months later the patient returned in severe pain with a much larger swelling in the popliteal fossa. On angiography, the popliteal artery was seen tapering into the enlarged aneurysm. Previously implanted coils had scattered into the corners of the enlarged sac. As a limb-saving and life-saving measure, a coronary catheter was advanced distal to a large collateral vessel branch that was contributing to the distal flow. A single Gianturco coil was released into the segment of the artery, preserving the proximal collateral branch. Immediate angiography showed occlusion of the parent artery and no opacification of the aneurysm. The pain subsided within 48 hours; the swelling started to regress and eventually resolved. Movement of the knee was restored.

The other 4 patients had large, nonresectable saccular aneurysms involving the common carotid artery, aortic arch, and abdominal aorta. Although maximal packing was attempted, delayed follow-up angiography revealed displacement of the coils away from the parent vessel, with fur-

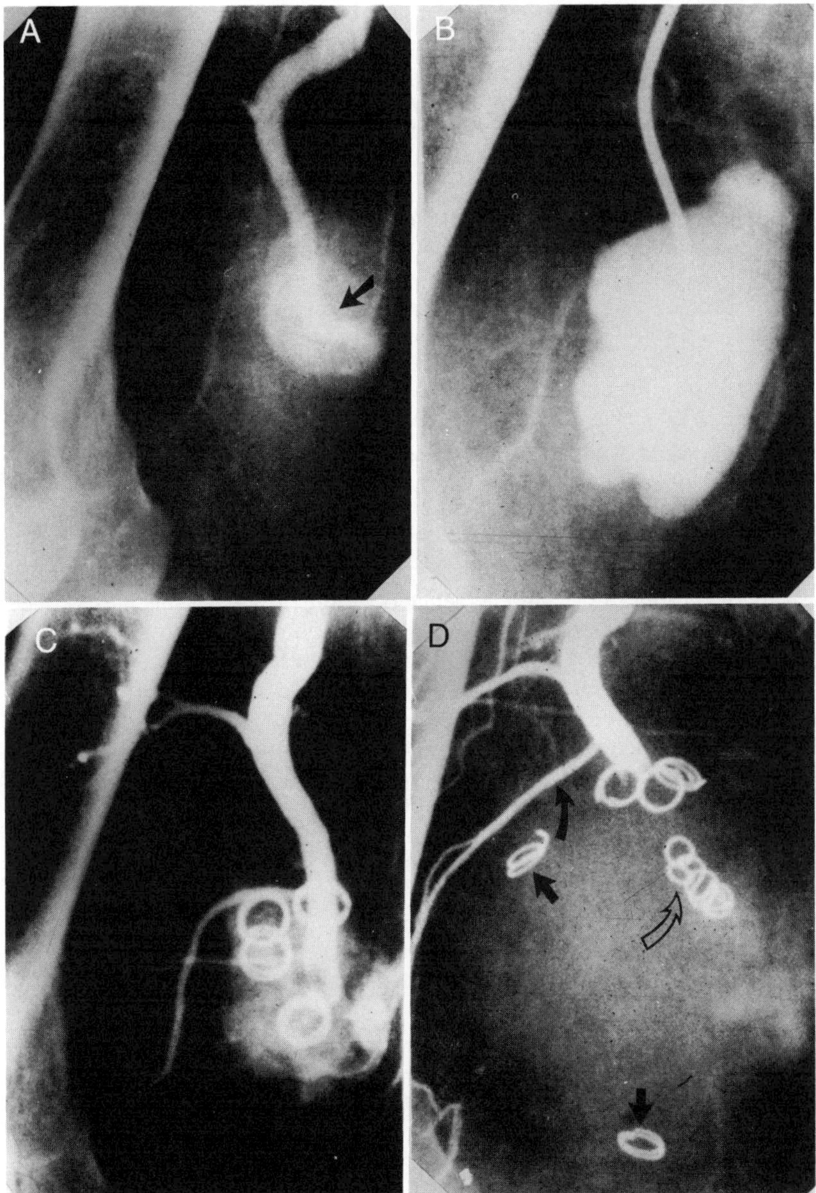

Fig 14–1.—Femoral angiogram. Lateral view. **A,** femoral artery is seen terminating into the aneurysmal sac in the popliteal fossa *(arrow)*. **B,** the extent of the aneurysmal sac is seen after introduction of the 7-F Judkins right coronary catheter. **C,** closely spaced coils with significant reduction of flow are noted. **D,** angiogram obtained 2 months later shows the coils dispersed into the corners of the enlarged aneurysm *(solid arrows)*. The last of the coils that deposited in the arterial lumen *(open arrow)* is seen beyond the large collateral vessel *(curved arrow)*. (Courtesy of Rao VR, Mandalam RK, Joseph S, et al: *Radiology* 175:407–410, 1990.)

ther expansion of the residual aneurysmal sac. Complete embolization of the aneurysmal sac was not possible without first obstructing the parent artery. Despite successful embolization of an aneurysmal cavity, large saccular aneurysms cannot be obliterated effectively because of the aneurysm's continuous growth caused by systolic pressure exerted by the aorta.

▶ Gianturco achieved fame in the United States because of his startling innovations. There is no doubt that the devices he developed have proven useful. However, the lessons of intrasaccular wiring learned before the days of reconstructive aortic surgery are being relearned in the present era. Palliative treatment of aneurysms means that they must be totally removed from the arterial circulation.

The Incidence of Popliteal Aneurysms in Patients With Arteriomegaly

Chan O, Thomas ML (St Thomas' Hosp, London)

Clin Radiol 41:185–189, 1990 14–3

Popliteal aneurysms may cause serious complications, e.g., occlusion leading to amputation. The incidence of popliteal aneurysms was studied in 65 patients with arteriomegaly observed on angiography. Ultrasound or contrast-enhanced CT was used in 58 of these patients.

Popliteal aneurysms, with localized dilatation of 1 segment of an artery, were found in 55% of the patients studied. They were bilateral in 64%. Of 38 patients who had abdominal aortic aneurysms in addition to arteriomegaly, popliteal aneurysms were found in 55%. In 19 patients suspected clinically of having 30 popliteal aneurysms, only 15 aneurysms were confirmed by imaging and 3 unsuspected aneurysms were detected. Twenty-five of the 46 patients not suspected of having an aneurysm had them.

Patients with arteriomegaly shown on angiography have a high incidence of popliteal aneurysms. They should undergo ultrasound or CT scanning to detect such aneurysms. Serial follow-up with ultrasound is also recommended.

▶ The St. Thomas Hospital group has contributed a great deal of knowledge on arterial dilation and the aneurysmosis syndrome. Their experience has led us to consider major artery aneurysm to be a systemic disease process, not an isolated phenomenon.

Pregnancy in a Renal Transplant Recipient Complicated by Rupture of a Transplant Renal Artery Aneurysm

Richardson AJ, Liddington M, Jaskowski A, Murie JA, Gillmer M, Morris PJ (Univ of Oxford, England)

Br J Surg 77:228–229, 1990 14–4

A patient was encountered with what may be the first case reported of transplant renal artery aneurysm rupture taking place during pregnancy.

Woman, 20, conceived for the first time and did well until presenting at 32 weeks' gestation with postcoital back and suprapubic pain. The serum creatinine was 90 micromoles/L. Possible mild toxemia was managed by bed rest. The patient collapsed 3 days after being admitted and a dead infant was delivered at emergency cesarean section. Bleeding was from a ruptured pelvic artery aneurysm, either the internal iliac or renal artery near the site of anastomosis or from the anastomosis itself. End-to-end anastomosis was carried out after excising the aneurysm. The patient was well 8 months postoperatively.

Nonmycotic aneurysm of a transplant renal artery is a rare disorder. It should be considered in a pregnant renal transplant recipient who collapses with abdominal pain. More extensive pelvic ultrasonography may be appropriate in these women.

▶ This case is disturbing. The fact of arterial dysplasia rupturing during pregnancy is accepted, as illustrated in other abstracts in this volume. Immunologic injury to the transplant renal artery may have contributed to wall weakening in this case and, if so, this is a complication to be guarded against. Within the text and not abstracted is the fact that in the years between 1967 and 1982, there were 24 maternal deaths in England and Wales as a result of rupture of visceral aneurysms, most of which occurred in the last weeks of pregnancy.

Sequential Development of Multiple Aortic Aneurysms in a Neonate Post Umbilical Arterial Catheter Insertion

Kirpekar M, Augenstein H, Abiri M (Columbia Univ; St Luke's-Roosevelt Hosp Ctr, New York)

Pediatr Radiol 19:452–453, 1989 14–5

Multiple aortic aneurysms developed in a neonate as a result of umbilical arterial catheterization. Progression from an aorta of normal caliber to one with multiple saccular aneurysms was demonstrated by serial ultrasound examinations.

Infant, 1 day old, had signs of respiratory distress and sepsis. On day 2, an umbilical arterial catheter was inserted to monitor blood gases. On day 4, blood cultures were positive for *Staphylococcus aureus* and antibiotics were changed. The catheter was removed on day 8. Renal ultrasound was performed on day 13 because of increased blood pressure (Fig 14–2). The kidneys and aorta were normal. A repeated ultrasound on day 20 demonstrated a saccular aneurysm of the abdominal aorta just above the origin of the superior mesenteric artery (Fig 14–3); 2 days later, the aneurysm had increased in size, and a second aneurysm had developed at the level of the aortic bifurcation. Surgery was ruled out because of the multiple nature of the aneurysms. Ultrasound examinations performed on day 36 (Fig 14–4) and day 56 (Fig 14–5) showed progressive increases in the size

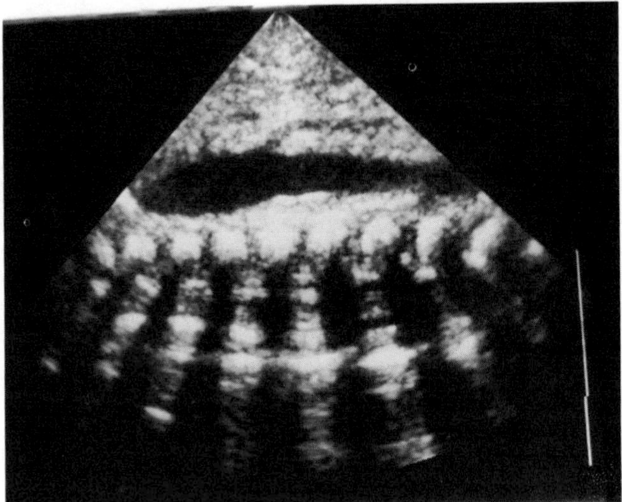

Fig 14–2.—Day 13 of life. Longitudinal scan to the left of midline showing slight bulge *(arrow)* in proximal abdominal aorta. (Courtesy of Kirpekar M, Augenstein H, Abiri M: *Pediatr Radiol* 19:452–453, 1989.)

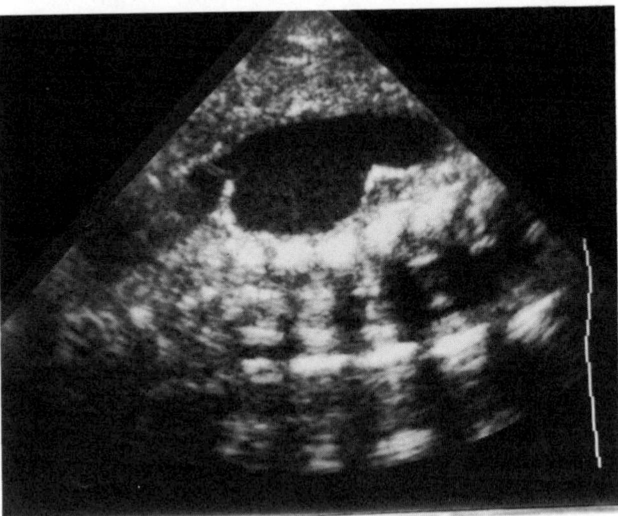

Fig 14–3.—Day 20 of life. Longitudinal scan shows a large aneurysm measuring 1.2 cm. The bulk of the aneurysm is posterior to the origin of the superior mesenteric artery. (Courtesy of Kirpekar M, Augenstein H, Abiri M: *Pediatr Radiol* 19:452–453, 1989.)

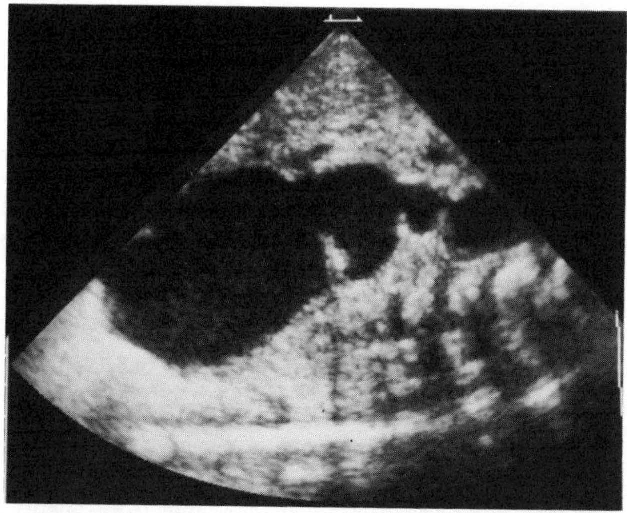

Fig 14–4.—Day 36 of life. Longitudinal scan now demonstrates multiple saccular aneurysms (*arrow* shows origin of superior mesenteric artery). (Courtesy of Kirpekar M, Augenstein H, Abiri M: *Pediatr Radiol* 19:452–453, 1989.)

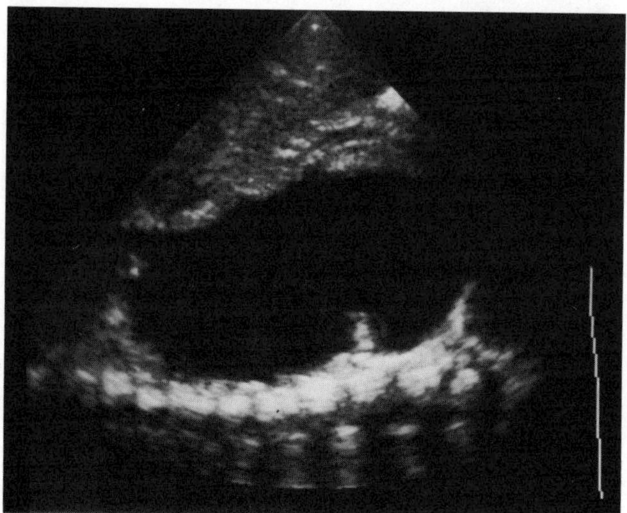

Fig 14–5.—Day 56 of life. Longitudinal scan showing the progressive increase in size of aneurysm. It now measures 3.8 cm in anterior-posterior dimension. (Courtesy of Kirpekar M, Augenstein H, Abiri M: *Pediatr Radiol* 19:452–453, 1989.)

and number of aneurysms. The infant was asymptomatic when discharged on day 56. Adequate blood pressure control has been achieved with captopril. Ultrasound follow-up was performed on an outpatient basis.

Aortic aneurysms are a complication of umbilical catheterization thought to arise from mechanical injury or sepsis. Other predisposing factors include coarctation of the aorta, bicuspid aortic valve, and bacterial endocarditis. In this infant the aneurysms were all thought to have a mycotic basis.

▶ The aortic complications of umbilical artery catheterization come to the attention of vascular surgeons and pediatric surgeons interested in vascular reconstruction. They are difficult to manage and devastating to the infant, but marvelously rewarding if a successful outcome can be achieved.

Spontaneous Rupture of a Renal Artery Aneurysm in Polyarteritis Nodosa: Critical Review of the Literature and Report of a Case

Smith DL, Wernick R (Oregon Health Sciences Univ; VA Med Ctr, Portland)

Am J Med 87:464–467, 1989 14–6

Polyarteritis nodosa (PAN) is a rare cause of perirenal hemorrhage. A patient with PAN-induced perirenal hemorrhage from aneurysmal rupture was seen.

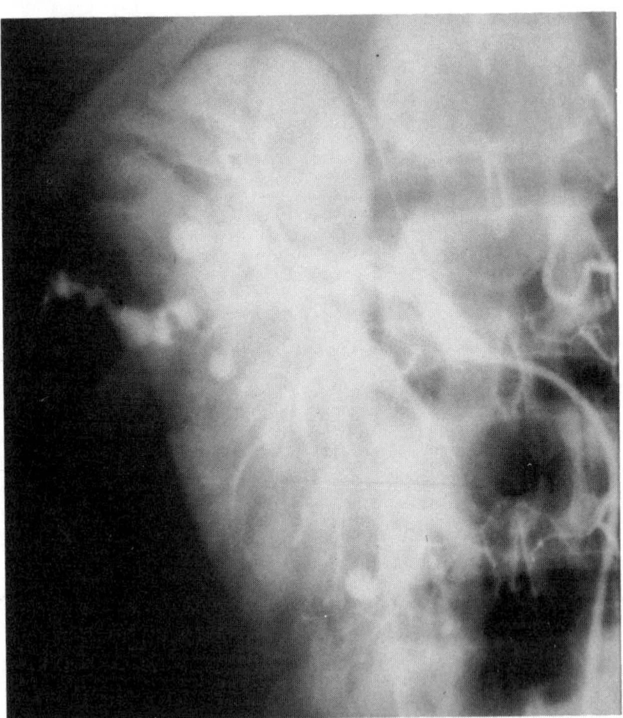

Fig 14–6.—Right renal arteriogram reveals multiple aneurysms and extravasation of contrast along the lateral renal border originating from a ruptured aneurysm just below the cortex at that site. The kidney is compressed and displaced medially by the hematoma. (Courtesy of Smith DL, Wernick R: *Am J Med* 87:464–467, 1989.)

Course of Patients with PAN and a Ruptured Renal Aneurysm

	Number	Percent
Survival with surgery	7/13	54
Survival with medical management	6/15	40
Recurrent bleeding*	5/28	18

*Three patients had been treated surgically, and 2 had combined medical and surgical treatment before recurrence.
(Courtesy of Smith DL, Wernick R: *Am J Med* 87:464–467, 1989.)

Man, 25, had acute severe flank and abdominal pain, hypotension, and anemia. Abdominal CT disclosed a large right perirenal hematoma. Selective renal arteriography revealed multiple aneurysms and extravasation from a ruptured aneurysm (Fig 14–6) along the lateral renal cortex. Gelfoam embolization, performed during arteriography, successfully controlled the aneurysmal bleeding.

A review of 28 previously reported cases of PAN indicates that renal hemorrhage typically is caused by arterial aneurysmal rupture, rarely by renal artery dissection or rupture. Typically, a young man with a history of hypertension would have sudden, severe flank or abdominal pain as an initial symptom, and abdominal mass and anemia would be discovered, sometimes followed by vascular collapse. Arteriography is highly specific in the diagnosis.

The optimal management of PAN-induced perirenal hemorrhage remains to be defined. Despite surgery to control hemorrhage and medical therapy for the underlying vasculitis, mortality remains about 50% with either therapy (table). Therapeutic arterial embolization with gelfoam during arteriography together with aggressive medical management of vasculitis and hypertension is a promising alternative to surgery in the treatment of PAN-induced ruptured renal aneurysm.

▶ Difficulties in treating polyarteritis nodosa begin in patients presenting with acute artery rupture and no previous diagnosis. Fortunately, arteriography, which shows multiple aneurysms in the renal artery bed, is virtually diagnostic. Scanning with CT may have been performed earlier. Although this distinguishes neoplastic from non-neoplastic causes of arterial rupture, the small intrarenal aneurysms cannot be seen by CT.

Visceral Artery Aneurysm: When to Operate?

Mellière D, Becquemin J-P, Kassab M, Souadka F (Centre Hospitalier Univ Henri-Mondor, Créteil, France)

J Mal Vasc 14:206–212, 1989

14–7

The indications for surgical intervention in patients with asymptomatic visceral artery aneurysms are not clearly defined. Both the size and the location of the aneurysm are related to the degree of risk of rupture. A review of the literature indicates that the risk of rupture is greatest for aneurysms of the splenic artery. Between 1978 and 1987, 5 women and 7 men aged 41–83 years were diagnosed with single or multiple visceral artery aneurysms.

Five aneurysms were located on the splenic artery, 1 on the hepatic artery, 3 on the celiac trunk, 2 on branches of the superior mesenteric artery, and 1 on the pancreaticoduodenal artery. Two patients required urgent operation because of a ruptured aneurysm, and 8 patients underwent elective procedures. Two patients did not undergo operation because their aneurysms were small.

One of 2 patients who underwent urgent operation had been operated on 4 years earlier for an abdominal aortic aneurysm. She initially had acute peritoneal hemorrhage. A new aneurysm 8 × 3 cm in size was detected on a branch of the superior mesenteric artery, and colectomy was performed, but the patient died of hemorrhagic shock 2 hours after laparotomy. The other patient who had urgent surgery survived, as did all 8 patients who underwent elective procedures. One of 2 nonoperated-on patients died suddenly 8 years after multiple fusiform aneurysms were diagnosed on branches of the superior mesenteric artery. This patient had a history of severe arterial hypertension complicated by cardiac insufficiency. A ruptured aneurysm could not be excluded. The other nonoperated-on patient was lost to followup.

The data from this series support the published data in that surgical treatment of nonruptured visceral artery aneurysms is associated with low mortality. Surgical treatment is indicated for all symptomatic aneurysms and most asymptomatic aneurysms; it is not indicated for small asymptomatic aneurysms of the splenic artery. Patients not operated on should be monitored at regular intervals.

▸ The findings confirm prejudices but add little new information.

Hepatic Artery Aneurysm

Lal RB, Strohl JA, Piazza S, Aslam M, Ball D, Patel K (Edward Hosp; Univ of Illinois)

J Cardiovasc Surg 30:509–513, 1989 14–8

A patient admitted with a complaint of epigastric pain was found to have an aneurysm of the right hepatic artery.

Man, 67, complained of moderate epigastric pain radiating to the back a month after a similar episode. There was some distention and bowel sounds were hypoactive. A high amylase level was found; after 4 days of improvement and a declining amylase level, it again became elevated when pain recurred. A rounded calcified mass was noted in the mid-upper abdomen during a gastrointestinal series. Cholangiopancreatography revealed an abnormal gallbladder, and a radionuclide scan showed nonfilling. Exploration then revealed a large aneurysm of the hepatic artery. A week later the patient underwent percutaneous transhepatic drainage when jaundice and ascending cholangitis developed. Emergency surgery for the aneurysm followed, with a saphenous vein graft to restore flow to the liver. The patient was well 8 months later.

Because hepatic artery aneuryms are associated with high mortality, aneurysmorrhaphy or direct arterial reconstruction is indicated. Embolization is an alternative if the aneurysm is inaccessible or the patient is unsuitable for surgery. Aneurysms proximal to the gastroduodenal artery may be excised with ligation but more distal lesions require excision and repair, preferably with autogenous tissue. Intrahepatic aneurysms now are being managed by transcatheter embolization with gelfoam.

▶ A concise summary of current practice in treatment of hepatic artery aneurysms.

Aneurysms of the Hepatic Arteries

Salo JA, Aarnio PT, Järvinen AA, Kivilaakso EO (Helsinki Univ Central Hosp)

Am Surg 55:705–709, 1989 14–9

About 20% of visceral artery aneurysms are found in the hepatic artery. Seven patients with hepatic artery aneurysms were treated surgically between 1976 and 1987.

Man, 57, had a history of heart infarction and aortoiliac endarterectomy and femoro-femoral bypass for disabling claudication. He had also had attacks of recurrent pancreatitis for which he underwent a cholecystectomy with choledochotomy. *Pseudomonas* was found by culture after cholangitis developed postoperatively. Fever persisted despite appropriate antibiotic treatment. The patient underwent emergency laparotomy when gastrointestinal bleeding developed. At surgery the common bile duct was found filled with blood. Because of hemobilia and cholangitis, ligature of the common hepatic artery and Roux-en-Y hepaticojejunostomy were performed. Recurrent bleeding developed after 5 weeks. An aneurysm of the right hepatic artery approximately 7 cm from the bifurcation was found at angiography (Fig 14–7). Right hemihepatectomy was performed; however, 2 reoperations were required because of postoperative hematoma and wound rupture. Liver coma with hepatorenal syndrome developed after 3 weeks. The patient died 6 weeks after liver resection.

Of 7 patients who had excision of aneurysms of the hepatic artery, 5 survived, including 2 who had elective surgery. Because hepatic artery aneurysms have a strong tendency to rupture, elective surgery should be performed in all patients with hepatic artery aneurysms.

▶ Because rupture of hepatic artery aneurysms may occur directly into the peritoneal cavity or into the biliary tree, serious consideration should be given to surgical repair in each hepatic artery aneurysm identified.

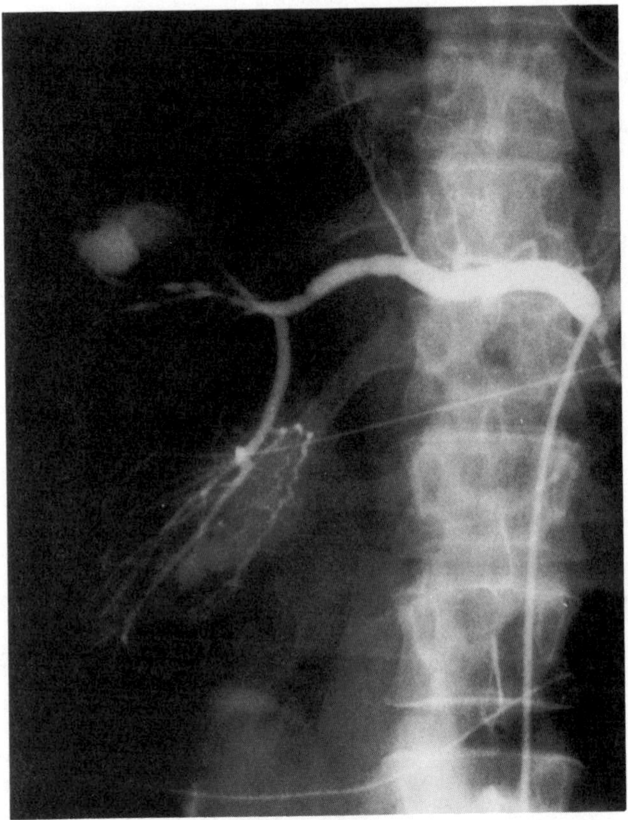

Fig 14–7.—Ruptured intrahepatic aneurysm of the right hepatic artery about 7 cm from bifurcation. (Courtesy of Salo JA, Aarnio PT, Järvinen AA, et al: *Am Surg* 55:705–709, 1989.)

Ruptured Gastroepiploic Artery Aneurysm and Vascular Collapse in a Patient With Thoracic Aneurysm

Rosengart TK, Pass H, Cannon R, Miller DL, Solomon D, Clark RE (Natl Heart, Lung, and Blood Inst; Natl Cancer Inst; Clinical Ctr, NIH, Bethesda, Md)

J Cardiovasc Surg 30:514–516, 1989 14–10

A patient with multiple visceral artery aneurysms, including a ruptured gastroepiploic artery lesion, associated with a thoracic aneurysm was encountered.

Man, 65, known to be hypertensive, had a cough, chest pain, and exertional dyspnea for a year. He collapsed shortly after arriving at the clinic; blood pressure was unobtainable. A large thoracic aneurysm had been detected previously. After a second profound hypotensive episode occurred, the abdomen became progressively distended, and 4–5 L of fresh blood was found in the peritoneal cavity. There was also a moderate retroperitoneal hematoma. Exploration revealed an aneurysm of the right common iliac artery and a ruptured right gastroepiploic artery aneurysm, which was resected. Intraoperative injury necessitated a splenectomy. A week later the tail of the pancreas was resected because of persistent bleeding, and a splenic artery aneurysm was found in the specimen. Elastin staining showed discontinuous and reduplicated elastic fibers. Subsequent angiographic studies demonstrated aneurysms of the left gastric, celiac, and both femoral arteries. A large thoracic aneurysm was later resected; the specimen exhibited myxoid degeneration of the media.

The finding of a single aneurysm calls for a complete vascular examination. Computed tomography is an effective and noninvasive alternative to selective angiography. All visceral artery aneurysms in young subjects at low risk should be resected electively.

▶ In the aneurysmosis syndrome, i.e., major artery aneurysms in the thoracic and abdominal cavities with peripheral arteries, one does not usually think of associated gastroepiploic or pancreaticoduodenal artery aneurysms. As is so well stated in the abstract, the finding of a single aneurysm calls for a complete vascular examination. This can now be achieved with magnetic resonance arteriography.

Ruptured Aneurysm of the Omentum: Case Report

Ambrosetti P, Robert J, Erne M, Rohner A (Hôp Cantonal Univ, Geneva, Switzerland)

Acta Chir Scand 156:187–188, 1990 14–11

Abdominal apoplexy refers to spontaneous and massive hemorrhage in or behind the peritoneum.

Man, 61, was admitted with generalized abdominal pain of 48 hours' duration. The patient was being treated with dicoumarin because of a history of 2 previous cardiac infarcts. Physical examination revealed a tense abdomen sensitive to palpation, guarding around the umbilicus, and generalized peritonism. Selective aortic arteriography visualized several small aneurysms on the omental artery, 1 of which was leaking (Fig 14–8). Laparotomy was performed and a small, ruptured saccular aneurysm was excised. The abdomen contained 2 liters of partially coagulated blood, but there was no active bleeding. The postoperative course was uneventful, and the patient was discharged on the 15th postoperative day. Histologic examination of the aneurysm demonstrated arterial cystic medial necrosis.

This case was unusual for 2 reasons: The small aneurysm was on the lower margin of the omentum, a site not previously reported. However, preoperative arteriography accurately pinpointed the source of bleeding in this patient. Furthermore, cystic medial necrosis usually affects the aorta and its branches, but it is rarely seen in smaller arteries, as it was in this case.

Survival after abdominal apoplexy depends on whether or not the

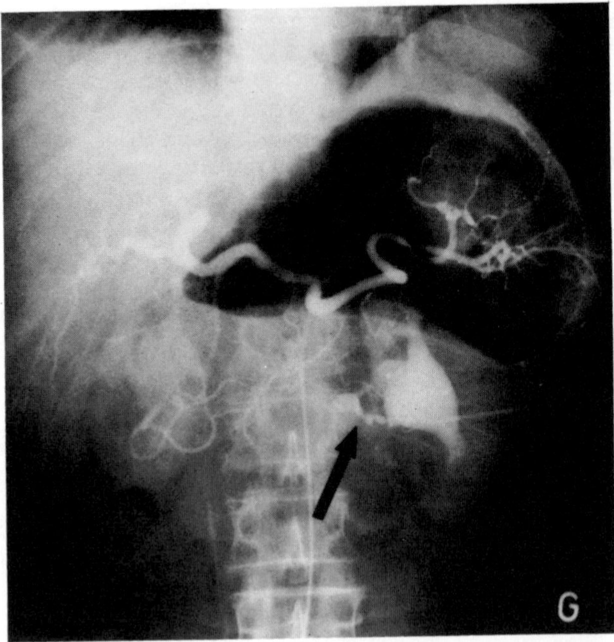

Fig 14–8.—Small saccular aneurysms with extravasation on one *(arrow)*, on a peripheral epiploic branch injected through the celiac axis. (Courtesy of Ambrosetti P, Robert J, Erne M, et al: *Acta Chir Scand* 156:187–188, 1990.)

source of hemorrhage is found at laparotomy. In a previous study the source of hemorrhage was not found in 38% of all patients operated on. To avoid missing the source of the retroperitoneal hemorrhage during laparotomy, patients suspected of having abdominal apoplexy should undergo preoperative arteriography as long as their condition remains stable.

▶ The term abdominal apoplexy should call forth a vision of small visceral artery aneurysms or, as in this case, an artery within the omentum.

Spontaneous Rupture of an Ovarian-Artery Aneurysm in the Third Trimester of Pregnancy

Høgdall CK, Pedersen SJ, Øvlisen BØ, Helgestrand UJV (Hillerød County Hosp, Hillerød, Denmark)

Acta Obstet Gynecol Scand 68:651–652, 1989 14–12

Spontaneous rupture of an intra-abdominal arterial aneurysm in late pregnancy is an unusual occurrence that carries an increased risk for both the mother and fetus.

Woman, 31, reported acute, severe abdominal pain and fainting at 39 weeks' gestation. She had previously been well and had delivered healthy infants uneventfully. When seen the patient was acutely distressed with no recordable diastolic pressure, and there was marked tenderness in the lower uterine segment. A term infant was delivered by cesarean section but could not be resuscitated. A rapidly growing retroperitoneal hematoma then was noted, and exploration after clamping the aorta showed a ruptured aneurysm of the right ovarian artery just before its entry into the broad ligament. The vessel was ligated and the patient recovered despite an estimated operative blood loss of 6 liters.

Only 4 cases of pregnancy-related ovarian artery rupture have been reported. If an asymptomatic aneurysm is found by sonography, it can be monitored by serial examinations, and treated if it grows. Treatment also may be recommended if an asymptomatic aneurysm is more than 2 cm in diameter. Transcatheter embolization is an alternative to resection or ligation in high-risk patients.

▶ Repeatedly, obscure aneurysms are being reported to have ruptured in pregnant women near termination of their pregnancies.

15 Acute Ischemia

Morbidity and Mortality in Acute Lower Limb Ischaemia: A 5-Year Review
Clason AE, Stonebridge PA, Duncan AJ, Nolan B, Jenkins A McL, Ruckley CV
(Royal Infirmary, Edinburgh)
Eur J Vasc Surg 3:339–343, 1989 15–1

Acute ischemia of a lower limb usually occurs secondary to arterial embolism or thrombosis in an already narrowed atherosclerotic artery. Early differentiation between embolism and thrombosis is often difficult. The mortality and morbidity in patients with acute lower limb ischemia who undergo urgent balloon catheter embolectomy remain high. Because of a concern over high hospital mortality after embolectomy, risk factors for morbidity and mortality after treatment for acute ischemia in the lower limb were determined in 204 patients aged 41–98 years (mean, 70 years) treated between 1983 and 1987 for acute ischemia in 234 lower limbs at risk.

Embolectomy was performed in 181 patients, of whom 53 died in the hospital within 30 days. Previously, 23 patients had additional vascular procedures and 27 had undergone fasciotomy. Four of 12 patients who required amputation of a previously operated-on limb died. Nine patients were operated on because of reocclusion. At the time of admission, 132 of the 204 patients had atrial fibrillation. Twenty-two patients had sustained an acute myocardial infarction within 14 days before admission, 13 of whom died in the hospital, compared with a 27% hospital mortality rate among those who had no history of recent myocardial infarction (table). The limb salvage rate among survivors was 95%. Factors adversely affecting mortality in this series were increasing age, proximal occlusion, recent myocardial infarction, grade 3–4 New York Heart Association functional score, and the presence of preexisting peripheral artery

Effect of New York Heart Association Functional Score

Score	No.	Died	Amputation
1	19	0	3 (16%)
2	65	21 (32%)	4 (6%)
3	85	24 (30%)	4 (5%)
4	32	17 (51%)	1 (3%)
Not Recorded	3	–	–
Total	204	62 (30%)	12 (6%)

(Courtesy of Clason AE, Stonebridge PA, Duncan AJ, et al: *Eur J Vasc Surg* 3:339–343, 1989.)

disease. However, the latter did not affect the amputation rate in this series.

▶ Mortality associated with treatment of acute limb ischemia remains extremely high. As outlined here, this is because of the advanced age and coexisting heart disease in most patients. This group from Edinburgh found that acute ischemia superimposed on chronic ischemia was not associated with a high rate of amputation, but this only testifies to the sophistication of the vascular group. Surgeons operating recognized that simple removal of thrombus by balloon catheter would not be effective when such thrombus was superimposed on atherosclerotic stenosing or occlusive disease. They recognized that a full-scale formal arterial reconstruction was necessary.

It is important to recognize that most of the deaths that occurred in this group developed more than 72 hours after surgery. This suggests that a toxin washout during revascularization played very little part in the ultimate outcome. This fact is confused by the patients who die immediately after surgery, most of whom would have died regardless of the success or failure of the surgical intervention.

In dealing with the severe problems of acute arterial occlusion and severe ischemia in the elderly, consideration must be given to thrombolytic therapy, at least to uncover the lesion that caused the acute occlusion and perhaps prepare the patient for the definitive surgical revascularization.

Ischemia–Reperfusion in Humans: Appearance of Xanthine Oxidase Activity

Friedl HP, Smith DJ, Till GO, Thomson PD, Louis DS, Ward PA (Univ of Michigan)

Am J Pathol 136:491–495, 1990 15–2

Reperfusion after ischemia results in tissue injury. This injury may be caused by the generation of toxic oxygen products, perhaps xanthine oxidase (XO), within the ischemic tissue. To investigate the relationship of XO to ischemic injury in humans, 10 adults undergoing reconstructive limb surgery were monitored.

Patients underwent upper extremity exsanguination and tourniquet application, resulting in upper extremity ischemia. After tourniquet release reperfusion occurred. There were immediate increases in the plasma levels of XO activity, uric acid, and histamine in the affected limb, without corresponding increases in the opposite limb. Xanthine dehydrogenase was not detected. The plasma of the treated limb also contained evidence of the formation of oxygen-derived free radicals.

Ischemia–reperfusion events in humans are associated with the appearance of XO activity and its products in the plasma. The pathophysiologic significance of these events remains to be determined.

▶ Observations continue to accumulate regarding ischemia–reperfusion events in humans. Ultimately, these observations may result in therapeutic benefit. However, as pointed out in the previous article and its abstract, 2 classes of patients die following relief of acute ischemia of the limbs. The first group appears to be agonal when they present and the therapy's success or failure plays very little part in the ultimate outcome. The second group succumbs beyond 72 hours after revascularization and, of course, the reperfusion event plays little part in their demise.

16 Grafts and Graft Complications

Dacron Vascular Prostheses in Man: Mechanical Performance, Lesions, and Molecular Stability

Vinard E, Eloy R, Descotes J, Brudon JR, Guidicelli H, Patra Ph, Huc A (Unité 37 INSERM, Bron, France)

Presse Méd 19:709–714, 1990 16–1

Polyethylene terephthalate is a synthetic material that is commonly used in arterial allografts for vascular surgery. Dacron has replaced Orlon and Teflon because it is considered safer and more durable for vascular bypass procedures. However, reports of vascular complications are increasing. The reported incidence of prosthesis failure now ranges from 10% to 28%, but the actual failure rate is thought to be greater. The 4 major indications for graft removal are aneurysmal dilatation (48%), separation of the anastomosis (18%), structural flaws (24%), and hemorrhagic and infectious complications (10%). During a 3-year study period, 212 vascular prostheses had to be removed because of complications; 22 of them were subjected to extensive mechanical, microscopic, and histologic examinations.

Mechanical testing showed that resistance to rupture of the explanted Dacron prostheses was reduced by 2% to 75% when compared with preuse values. Changes in mechanical properties and duration of implantation were not correlated. Similarly, no relationship existed between the structure of the prosthesis (e.g., knitted or woven) and the occurrence of mechanical failure.

Scanning electron microscopy of the interface between blood and prosthesis showed that failed Dacron prostheses were covered to a variable extent with noncellular fibrous tissue. No neoendothelial structures were observed. Microorganisms in contact with Dacron fibers or fibrous tissue could be found in 10 of the 22 explants. Seven of the 12 explants that were not covered with fibrous tissue had polyester fibers with partial or complete ruptures. The ruptured ends of the fibers were either smooth, as in a clean break, or frayed (Fig 16–1). Ruptured fibers were seen in both knitted and woven prostheses. Conventional histologic examination confirmed the absence of new endothelial structures on the luminal surfaces of the prostheses. The tissues around the prostheses contained a mostly collagen-like fibrous substance. Six patients had indications of an inflammatory reaction, as many small lymphocytes and polynuclear neutrophils were present. Reactive giant cells and phagocytosis of polymer debris were seen in 8 explanted prostheses. Examination of explanted, failed

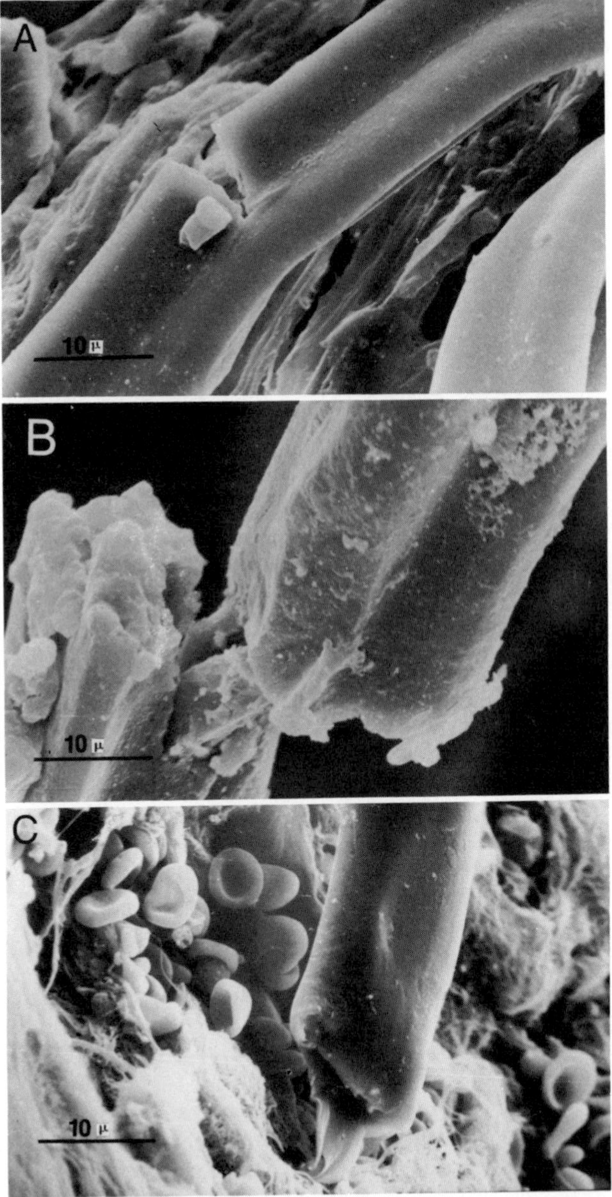

Fig 16–1.—Scanning electron microscopic examination of the lumen of explanted prostheses. A and B, partial ruptures of polyester fibers in a knitted, double-velour prosthesis after 72 months of implantation. C, complete, clean rupture of a polyester fiber in a knitted velour prosthesis after 116 months of implantation. (Courtesy of Vinard E, Eloy R, Descotes J, et al: *Presse Méd* 19:709–714, 1990.)

vascular prostheses is an important part of the ongoing search for suitable biomedical vascular allograft materials.

▶ The finding of ruptured fibers in Dacron prostheses is troublesome. Nevertheless, reports of graft fracture with pseudoaneurysm formation are exceedingly rare. Scientists analyzing properties of vascular grafts after removal must be guided in their studies so that grafts that are infected and removed are separated from those that are mechanically disrupted without infection.

Anaphylactoid Reactions to Vascular Graft Material Presenting With Vasodilation and Subsequent Disseminated Intravascular Coagulation

Roizen MF, Rodgers GM, Valone FH, Lampe GH, Benefiel DJ, Gelman S, Rapp J, Weiler JM, Ota M, Shuman MA, Goetzl EJ (Univ of Chicago; Univ of Utah; Univ of California, San Francisco; et al)

Anesthesiology 71:331–338, 1989 16–2

A previously unreported complication occurred after vascular graft replacement in 5 patients. Immediately after restoration of blood flow across the prosthetic graft, all 5 patients had unusually persistent decreases in blood pressure associated with peripheral vasodilation and erythema, followed by clinically evident disseminated intravascular coagulation (DIC) and bleeding. The graft material was either woven or knitted Dacron. Of 3 patients in whom the graft was replaced, 2 had an uneventful recovery; the other died of complications of DIC. The other 2 patients in whom the graft was not replaced died.

Blood samples obtained during these episodes from 2 patients allowed verification of contact activation and DIC. Both blood samples showed markedly increased plasma kallikrein activity and levels of complement fragment C3a, whereas blood samples from normal controls did not have increased levels of activation products. In addition, plasma obtained from 1 patient 4 months after the reaction generated kallikrein activity when incubated in vitro with the suspected graft material but not control graft material. Rapid recognition of anaphylactoid reactions to vascular graft material presenting as vasodilation, erythema, and subsequent DIC, is essential to patient survival, which appears to depend on rapid replacement of the graft.

▶ This paper was selected for abstracting simply because there is no such report in the literature to date. The fundamental cause of the phenomenon observed and carefully documented is still unsettled.

Magnetic Resonance Imaging of Abdominal Aortic Grafts

Alessi G, Di Renzi P, Farina C, Cisternino S, Pavone P, Sciacca V, di Marzo L, Mingoli A, Passariello R, Cavallaro A (Università di Roma "La Sapienza," Rome)

J R Coll Surg Edinb 34:316–320, 1989 16–3

Magnetic resonance imaging was carried out in 29 patients having abdominal aortic grafting, 19 for chronic obstructive disease and 10 for abdominal aortic aneurysm. Dacron was used in all patients but 1, who received a polytetrafluoroethylene prosthesis. Coronal and axial MR images were acquired using T1-weighted spin-echo sequences and, in a few cases, multi-echo T2-weighted sequences as well. Sagittal images were obtained in 4 cases.

The entire graft and anastomotic sites were identified in all cases. Coronal images were helpful in studying the anteroposterior orientation of the prosthesis and the native aorta. Axial images exhibited abnormalities of the graft wall and the anastomoses. Fourteen grafts were patent, whereas 15 patients had complications of various types, including thrombotic deposits, occlusion, and proximal or distal dilatation.

Magnetic resonance imaging accurately depicts both normal abdominal aortic grafts and complicated cases. The findings are nearly always better than those achieved by ultrasonography or CT. Aortoenteric fistulas are not identified by MR imaging.

▶ As in other situations in science, new techniques must be evaluated against older methods before achieving universal acceptance. There are indeed many advantages of MR imaging and predictably it will achieve an increasing degree of utility. However, a flat statement that aortoenteric fistulas are not identified by MR imaging will undoubtedly be modified by future experience.

Aortoenteric Fistula and Perigraft Infection: Evaluation With CT

Low RN, Wall SD, Jeffrey RB Jr, Sollitto RA, Reilly LM, Tierney LM Jr (Univ of California, San Francisco)

Radiology 175:157–162, 1990 16–4

Although few complications are associated with aortic reconstructive surgery, the most serious are life threatening. Perigraft infection (PGI) occurs in 2% to 6% of patients undergoing aortic graft operations and aortoenteric fistula (AEF) occurs in .6% to 2%. The sensitivity and specificity of CT in detecting PGI and AEF were assessed in a blinded retrospective study.

During the study period 55 patients were referred for CT to detect possible PGI or AEF. The CT scans were examined for the presence of ectopic gas, focal bowel wall thickening, perigraft fluid, perigraft soft tissue, pseudoaneurysm formation, and increased soft tissue between graft and wrap. The CT findings were compared with operative results.

There were 23 patients with AEF, 12 with PGI, and 20 with normal, noninfected grafts. Some scans were clearly abnormal, with large amounts of perigraft soft tissue and ectopic gas, but other scans had more subtle findings with few or no abnormalities.

Although CT was not 100% accurate, it was able to detect either complication with a high degree of sensitivity (94%) and specificity (85%). Early and aggressive operative intervention is essential in the management of AEF and PGI; thus strict criteria must be applied to interpretation of CT scans after aortic surgery. In these 35 patients positive for complications, CT showed only minimal abnormal findings in 4 and no signs of abnormality in 2.

▶ Experience has shown that CT has the highest diagnostic accuracy in identifying graft infection but, like other modalities in these complicated cases, it must be correlated with the clinical findings.

Diagnosis of Synthetic Vascular Graft Infection: Comparison of CT and Gallium Scans

Johnson KK, Russ PD, Bair JH, Friefeld GD (Univ of Colorado; VA Med Ctr, Denver)

AJR 154:405–409, 1990 16–5

Synthetic graft infection complicating peripheral vascular surgery is uncommon but can cause significant morbidity and mortality. Various methods have been used to assess suspected graft infections. Gallium-67 scintigraphy was compared with CT in the diagnosis of synthetic vascular graft infections in 16 patients. Two patients were studied twice, and 25 grafts were examined. The results of the 2 methods of assessment were compared for grafts in specific anatomical locations, including the retroperitoneum, groin, and abdominal wall, and for combined sites.

When considered as a group, CT for all locations had a sensitivity of 100% and specificity of 72%. Gallium-67 scintigraphy had a sensitivity of 78% and a specificity of 94%; it was more specific than CT for combined sites. However, there were no significant differences in sensitivities, possibly because of the small number of infected grafts in the series. None of the differences in sensitivities or specificities were significant when grafts in individual sites were analyzed.

Because CT can be performed immediately, it was recommended as the initial examination in patients with suspected graft infection. Gallium-67 scintigraphy is an important complementary test that adds specificity to the diagnostic workup.

▶ Both indium and gallium have their limitations in detecting perigraft infection. Computed tomography remains the primary method of evaluation and imaging.

Percutaneous Management of Abscesses That Involve Native Arteries or Synthetic Arterial Grafts

Lambiase RE, Dorfman GS, Cronan JJ (Rhode Island Hosp, Providence)

Radiology 173:815–818, 1989 16–6

Generally, abscesses that involve native arteries or synthetic arterial grafts are treated by operative débridement and extra-anatomical vascular reconstruction. Four patients with such abscesses had successful treatment via percutaneous drainage.

Three abscesses involved infection of synthetic arterial bypass grafts (aortic, femoropopliteal, and aortobifemoral grafts) and 1, infection of the abdominal aorta. Percutaneous drainage of the abscess coupled with intravenous antibiotic therapy resulted in resolution of the abscess in 3 patients, whereas the third had a recurrent abscess after an initial resolution. In 2 patients preoperative abscess sterilization allowed subsequent performance of an alternative revascularization procedure of less technical complexity and associated with decreased morbidity. The duration of catheter drainage was 5 weeks to 4.5 months. There were no catheter-induced complications.

On rare occasions when emergent surgery is absolutely contraindicated, percutaneous drainage is an effective palliative therapy (which occasionally may be curative) for abscesses that involve native arteries or synthetic arterial grafts. The goal of percutaneous management is to optimize the preoperative status to allow substitution of a procedure of a lower morbidity.

▶ Interventional radiology has taught surgery a great many lessons. This one—the possibility of clearing up a perigraft infection by percutaneous drainage—is important and has been verified by other groups. It still could not be taken as the treatment of choice. Nevertheless, it certainly is an adjunct to other therapy.

Results of 132 PTFE (Gore-Tex) Bifurcated Graft Implantations

Petrovic P, Lotina S, Djordjevic M, Avramov S, Pfau J, Velimirovic D, Fabri M, Stojanov P, Savic D (Yugoslavia Inst of Surgery, Novi Sad)

J Cardiovasc Surg 30:897–901, 1989 16–7

The results of bifurcation grafting with Gore-Tex polytetrafluoroethylene (PTFE) prostheses were reviewed in 132 patients (mean age, 62 years) who were operated on in 1982–1986. The indication was aortoiliac occlusive disease in 118 patients and abdominal aortic aneurysm in 14. Five patients had undergone surgery previously and had a thrombosed Dacron PTFE prosthesis. A proximal end-to-end anastomosis was made in 94 patients and an end-to-side anastomosis was made in 38. The distal anastomoses were to the common femoral artery in 89 patients, the deep femoral artery in 32, and the iliac artery in 11.

The 30-day mortality rate was 6%. The 3 immediate thromboses resulted from technical errors and were effectively managed by Fogarty thrombectomy. Of 124 grafts that were patent at 30 days, only 2 later thrombosed, both in the first postoperative year. The cumulative 4-year patency rate was 98.4%.

The Gore-Tex PTFE bifurcated graft is an excellent choice for reconstructing occlusive and other aortoiliac or aortofemoral disease. Few subsequent corrective procedures have been necessary.

▶ The Belgrade group that is reporting this study is extremely experienced. Their original article contained beautiful color photographs, which are not reproduced here. They have confirmed the utility of this prosthesis but have not provided detailed information regarding local sepsis or incidence of anastomotic aneurysms.

Aortoenteric Fistulas: A Study of 28 Autopsied Cases Spanning 25 Years
Grande JP, Ackermann DM, Edwards WD (Mayo Clinic and Found, Rochester, Minn)
Arch Pathol Lab Med 113:1271–1275, 1989 16–8

The formation of an aortoenteric fistula is an uncommon but often catastrophic event. The autopsy reports of 23 men and 5 women aged 19–91 years in whom aortoenteric fistulas were diagnosed during a 25-year period were reviewed.

Of the 28 patients, 23 died of exsanguination; the other 5 underwent surgical repair and died of various related complications. Of 16 patients who had previously undergone aortofemoral bypass grafting, fistulas developed at proximal anastomosis sites in 15. Six patients had gastrointestinal tract carcinoma, in 3 of whom fistulas developed in association with radiation injury. A severely retarded 19-year-old woman died of exsanguination after swallowing an opened safety pin that subsequently perforated both the midesophagus and the distal portion of the aortic arch; another patient had idiopathic muscular esophageal hypertrophy.

On the enteric side, the fistulas involved the duodenum in 16 patients, the esophagus in 9, and other gastrointestinal tract sites in 3. On the aor-

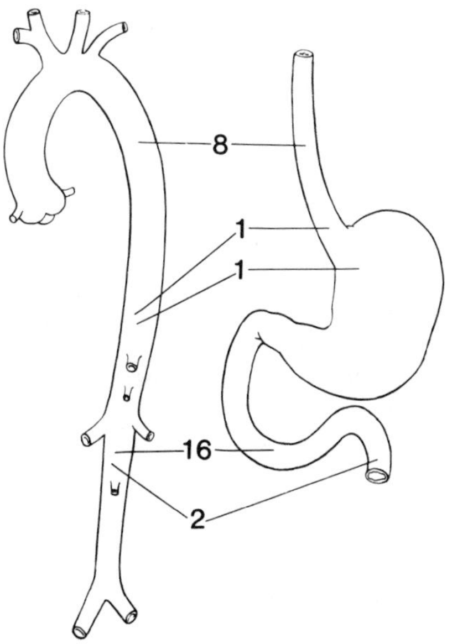

Fig 16–2.—Distribution of sites of aortoenteric fistulas. (Courtesy of Grande JP, Ackermann DM, Edwards WD: *Arch Pathol Lab Med* 113:1271–1275, 1989.)

tic side the fistulas involved the abdominal aorta in 20 patients and the descending aorta in 8 (Fig 16–2). Aortic bypass grafts and gastrointestinal tract carcinomas are the major risk factors for aortoenteric fistulas.

▶ The fascinating aspects of this report are the nongraft causes of aortoenteric fistualization.

Anastomotic Aneurysms: An Underdiagnosed Complication After Aorto-Iliac Reconstructions

Sieswerda C, Skotnicki SH, Barentsz JO, Heystraten FMJ (St Radboud Univ Hosp, Nijmegen, The Netherlands)

Eur J Vasc Surg 3:233–238, 1989 16–9

An anastomotic aneurysm (AA) is a serious late complication after aortoiliofemoral reconstruction (AIFR). The reported incidence of AA after AIFR ranges from 2% to 8%. However, these rates are based mostly on retrospective series; recent studies suggest much higher incidence rates. An attempt was made to determine the actual incidence of AA after AIFR by systematic clinical investigation during long-term follow-up of patients who underwent AIFR.

The original group consisted of 263 men and 40 women aged 30–85 years who underwent primary arterial reconstruction between 1977 and 1981 and who had been followed for 6–10 years. Of these 303 patients, 73% underwent primary arterial reconstruction and 27% had a second operation. Most of the primary reconstructions were bilateral procedures. Sixteen patients had autologous venous grafts and 287 received prosthetic grafts. During follow-up, 158 patients (52%) died and 145 survived. Of the survivors, 122 underwent physical examination, ultrasonography, and intravenous digital subtraction angiography.

In 36 of the 122 investigated patients 52 AAs were diagnosed, for a mean 15.7% incidence per anastomosis. Twenty-two patients had a single AA, 12 had 2 AAs, and 2 had 3 AAs. Fourteen of the 52 AAs (33%) were operated on and the diagnosis was confirmed. Physical examination alone was falsely negative in 67% and falsely positive in 37% of the patients. Thirty-seven AAs were detected in 29 patients based on the combined findings of echography and digital subtraction angiography. Echography alone detected only 8 of these 37 AAs. Five patients had undergone earlier correction of 7 AAs. An additional 7 had already undergone reoperation for 8 AAs before the start of this study. Routine follow-up in the original 303 patients had discovered only 16 AAs.

An anastomotic aneurysm after AIFR is a much more frequent complication than has been assumed previously. Intravenous digital subtraction angiography should be performed at regular intervals during the follow-up of patients who have undergone AIFR.

▶ The increased incidence of anastomotic aneurysms reported by the Nijmegen group is alarming, but their method of follow-up study suggests that their report is accurate. It is well known that anastomotic aneurysms remain an unsolved problem. However, it has been largely unsuspected that the problem was of the magnitude described in this report. It is important, after establishing the frequency of this complication, to look for the cause. In this study only 1 vascular suture was seen to be disrupted. Further research is clearly indicated, and a fruitful area might be comparison of the various types of grafts used in distal end-to-side anastomosis. One would suspect that the stretchier, knitted grafts would be associated with a higher incidence of false aneurysms than the less-giving, woven grafts or PTFE grafts.

Anastomotic Aneurysms of the Femoral Artery: Aetiology and Treatment

Clarke AM, Poskitt KR, Baird RN, Horrocks M (Bristol Royal Infirmary, England)

Br J Surg 76:1014–1016, October 1989 16–10

Data were reviewed on 29 patients seen in a 4-year period with a total of 35 noninfective femoral false aneurysms secondary to arterial anastomoses in the groin. Primary and mycotic aneurysms were excluded. These false aneurysms represented 4% of all femoral artery anastomoses done during the study period. The mean time from primary arterial suture to repair of the false aneurysm was 6 years.

About two thirds of the false aneurysms followed aortofemoral bypass, and most of the rest occurred after iliofemoral bypass. Six patients had bilateral anastomotic aneurysms. Superficial wound infection had been present in one fourth of the cases. All but 3 of the 35 false aneurysms were repaired surgically. Interposition grafting was done in 17 cases (53%) and simple reanastomosis was used in 14 (44%). Six direct repairs have required further revision, but only 1 patient had repair of an interposition graft. Both bleeding and wound infection were more frequent than after primary reconstruction.

Close follow-up is necessary after primary arterial reconstruction, because false aneurysms can cause complications if left untreated. A conservative approach is indicated only for high-risk patients who have small, asymptomatic aneurysms. Care in avoiding superficial wound infections and incorporating a generous amount of arterial wall in the primary repair will limit the risk of an anastomotic aneurysm developing. Femoral false aneurysms are best managed by interposition Dacron grafting.

▶ As usual, the title is deceptive as the etiology is not explained and treatment is elaborately presented.

False Aneurysms After Prosthetic Reconstructions for Aortoiliac Obstructive Disease

Van den Akker PJ, Brand R, van Schilfgaarde R, van Bockel JH, Terpstra JL (Univ Hosp Leiden; Univ Hosp Groningen, The Netherlands)

Ann Surg 210:658–666, 1989 16–11

Anastomatic or false aneurysm after prosthetic vascular reconstruction is considered a rare late complication. However, published incidence rates vary greatly, and its exact incidence is not known. A retrospective review as conducted to determine the cumulative incidence rate of false aneurysm development after prosthetic reconstruction for aortoiliac obstructive disease (AIOD) after a follow-up of 20 years.

Between 1958 and 1980, 471 men and 47 women (mean age, 55.9 years) underwent prosthetic reconstruction for AIOD. Of these 518 patients, 157 had a history of hypertension and 37 had diabetes mellitus. Indications for operation included claudication in 76.8%, rest pain in 14.1%, and nonhealing foot ulcers or gangrene in 9.1%. Angiographic evaluation revealed that 45.8% of the patients had single-level disease and 54.2% had multilevel disease. Surgical procedures included insertion of an aortobi-iliac prosthesis in 63.9% of the patients. Patients were evaluated routinely at 3, 6, 12, and 24 months after operation and then at 2-year intervals for the rest of their lives. Complete follow-up data were available for 369 patients.

A total of 101 false aneurysms—21 aortic, 53 iliac, and 27 femoral—were detected in 69 patients and verified by operation, yielding an incidence of 13.3%. Of all false aneurysms, 47.5% were asymptomatic and were detected by routine follow-up angiography or ultrasonography. Calculations indicated that the chance of being free of a false aneurysm at any site 15 years after operation was 77.2%. These chances were 92.3% for aortic anastomoses, 84.5% for iliac anastomoses, and 76.2% for femoral anastomoses. Development of a false aneurysm was significantly correlated with the presence of hypertension, multilevel disease, type of suture material used, and type of anastomosis. At all sites, end-to-side anastomoses were associated with a higher incidence of false aneurysms than were end-to-end anastomoses. However, the difference was statistically significant only for aortic anastomoses.

The unexpected high incidence of false aneurysm development during long-term follow-up after AIOD justifies the routine use of periodic ultrasound scans and angiography. Patients with prosthetic arterial reconstructions should be included in a life-long follow-up schedule that includes periodic ultrasonography and angiography in addition to clinical evaluation.

▶ This presentation comes closer to explaining the cause of anastomotic false aneurysms. The finding of false aneurysms in association with silk sutures is an echo of the past and its forgotten practices. In the present era, a study of graft material would be more fruitful.

Lower Limb Oedema After Arterial Reconstructive Surgery: Influence of Preoperative Ischaemia, Type of Reconstruction, and Postoperative Outcome

Persson NH, Takolander R, Bergqvist D (Univ of Lund; Malmö Gen Hosp, Malmö, Sweden)
Acta Chir Scand 155:259–266, 1989 16–12

Edema formation of the foot and lower leg after arterial reconstruction is common. Although numerous studies have investigated this well-known phenomenon, most studies do not provide information on how, or how frequently, the swelling was measured. When reported, most studies performed the measurements only once, usually 1 week after operation. Preoperative and daily postoperative circumference measurements have rarely been performed.

To investigate the natural history of early limb edema after various types of arterial reconstructions, 180 patients who were operated on for occlusive or aneurysmatic arterial disease were studied. The leg circumference was measured with a tape on 2 levels on the day before operation. All patients were followed after operation for up to 14 days by daily circumference measurements of the lower limb. The volume of the lower leg was calculated according to the formula for the frustrum of a cone. Patients were mobilized from the first postoperative day. Compression stockings were not worn. Patients were allowed to have their legs hanging down.

Circumference measurements of the lower leg correlated well with water displacement volumetry; thus the frustrum method is suitable for follow-up of volume changes in the lower leg. Femoropopliteal bypass resulted regularly in pronounced edema that was significantly greater than after any of the other procedures. Aortofemoral reconstruction did not result in significant leg edema, but all other reconstructions resulted in a volume increase in the symptomatic leg. The same maximal volume increase developed in patients who had no ischemia before operation as in patients with severe ischemia. The volume increase did not significantly correlate with preoperative ankle blood pressure or the ankle brachial pressure index. Furthermore, both successful and unsuccessful reconstructions were followed by a significant edema, although less so in failed reconstructions. Even exploration of the vessels without reconstruction resulted in postoperative edema.

The pathogenesis of postoperative lower limb edema after arterial reconstruction is clearly multifactorial. The most important risk factor is the type of reconstruction performed, not the indication. The degree of preoperative ischemia and success of operation are both contributory factors.

▶ This study confirms some known factors regarding postoperative edema. That is, the degree of ischemia or success of revascularization are not related; the presence of a groin exploration alone seems unrelated to the edema, but groin exploration plus distal exploration of vessels is associated with edema. All of these factors point toward lymphatic damage being the common pathway of production of the swollen leg after arterial surgery.

Lymphoceles: Percutaneous Treatment With Povidone-Iodine Sclerosis

Gilliland JD, Spies JB, Brown SB, Yrizarry JM, Greenwood LH (Wilford Hall USAF Med Ctr, Lackland Air Force Base, Tex; Univ of Miami)

Radiology 171:227–229, 1989 16–13

Percutaneous transcatheter drainage has gained acceptance as an alternative to surgical treatment of lymphoceles, but success rates have been less than optimal. Transcatheter sclerosis with various agents has been advocated to increase the success rate of percutaneous therapy. Eight patients with 9 pelvic lymphoceles were treated with percutaneous transcatheter drainage and sclerosis with povidone-iodine. Four patients had undergone lymphadenectomy for pelvic malignancy and 4 had renal transplantation. The majority of the treatment was performed on an outpatient basis in 3 patients. The minimum follow-up was 3 months.

Eight (89%) lymphoceles resolved completely without complications. The only failure required internal drainage. The average duration of catheter drainage was 25 days (range, 15 to 37 days), and the drainage rate ranged from 25 to 400 mL/day. Four lymphoceles were infected at initial drainage, but this did not alter the duration of catheter drainage.

Percutaneous transcatheter drainage with providone-iodine sclerosis is safe and effective in the treatment of lymphoceles. Its only drawback is the prolonged treatment time. The early results are encouraging and warrant further investigation.

▶ The intrapelvic lymphocele is quite different from the groin lymphocele. The former has no method of achieving resorption of the fluid extravasated through ruptured lymphatics. Marsupialization of the lymphocele, allowing lymph to be absorbed by the peritoneum and underside of the diaphragm, is an effective therapy. Infected lymphoceles, of course, are a different problem, and groin lymphoceles surrounding prosthetic grafts are yet another.

Sartorius Muscle Coverage for the Treatment of Complicated Vascular Surgical Wounds

Kaufman JL, Shah DM, Corson JD, Skudder PA, Leather RP (Albany Med College; VA Med Ctr, Albany, NY)

J Cardiovasc Surg 30:479–483, 1989 16–14

The outcome of sartorius muscle flap surgery in 14 patients—the largest series reported to date—was evaluated. The patients had complicated groin wounds that followed vascular surgery and, in 8 cases, had risk factors for poor wound healing such as diabetes, past radiotherapy, or poor nutrition. The indications for flap coverage included hemorrhage, groin wound sepsis, graft sepsis, wound necrosis, and exposure of a reconstruction. Eleven patients had multiple indications.

Nine patients had a proximal sartorious segment rotated into the groin (Fig 16–3). Four others had a distal muscle flap—proximally based—

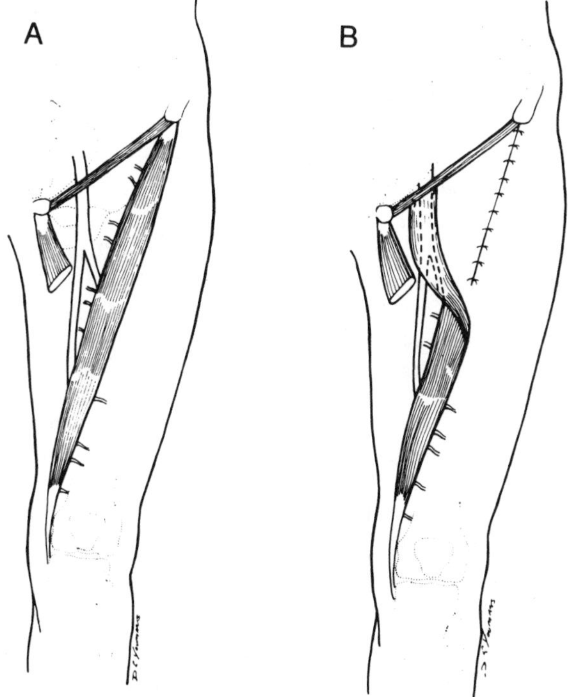

Fig 16–3.—**A,** anatomical relationship of the sartorius muscle to the arterial structures of the groin; **B,** mobilization and rotation of the proximal portion of the sartorius muscle into the groin with fixation at the inguinal ligament. Because of deep and medial segmental blood supply to the muscle, it is often necessary to turn the muscle over itself in achieving its position in the groin. (Kaufman JL, Shah DM, Corson JD, et al: *J Cardiovasc Surg* 30:479–483, 1989.)

reflected into the groin, and 1 patient received a mobilized midportion of sartorius muscle. Primary wound closure was achieved in 7 patients, whereas 7 had delayed closure and 4 of those required a skin graft. Hemorrhage was controlled in all cases, and all patent reconstructions were salvaged. One patient had infection of the proximal sartorius muscle bed and 1 had a late recurrence of groin infection. No patient had a long-term functional deficit as a result of transposition of the sartorius muscle.

A sartorius muscle flap may be considered if the healing ability of a groin or thigh wound is in question. The sartorius flap is well tolerated and provides excellent wound coverage.

▶ The sartorius flap is a marvelous addition to vascular surgery techniques. The procedure must be performed carefully so as to preserve the blood supply to the sartorius.

Implantation of Vascular Grafts Lined With Genetically Modified Endothelial Cells

Wilson JM, Birinyi LK, Salomon RN, Libby P, Callow AD, Mulligan RC (Massachusetts Inst of Technology; Tufts Univ)

Science 244:1344–1346, 1989 16–15

If the vascular endothelial cell can serve as a target for gene replacement therapy, then the luminal surface of prosthetic vascular grafts can be lined by endothelial cells genetically modified to promote repopulation, prevent thrombosis, or secrete therapeutic proteins. To test this hypothesis, dogs received vascular grafts seeded with autologous retrovirus-transduced endothelial cells. Recombinant retroviruses were used to transduce the *Escherichia coli lacZ* gene into endothelial cells harvested from dogs. The product of expression of this gene, β-galactosidase, can be detected in situ by enzymic histochemical assay. Seeded carotid interposition grafts were placed in the dogs from which the original cells were harvested.

Analysis of grafts 5 weeks after placement showed that genetically modified endothelial cells lined their luminal surfaces. Cells that expressed viral-directed β-galactosidase were found in all cultures established from genetically modified grafts.

This technology has potential uses for treating atherosclerotic disease and in the design of drug delivery systems. Endothelial cells may be modified genetically to secrete proteins that prevent thrombosis or inhibit neointimal smooth muscle cell hyperplasia, both common mechanisms of graft failure. Applications of drug delivery can include the secretion of vasodilators or angiogenic factors and the delivery of antineoplastic agents to sites of metastatic tumor.

▶ This is a most interesting report, opening a window into the future when endothelial cells can be specifically modified, as indicated in the last paragraph of the abstract.

Growth Factor Gene Expression by Intimal Cells in Healing Polytetrafluoroethylene Grafts

Golden MA, Au YPT, Kenagy RD, Clowes AW (Univ of Washington)

J Vasc Surg 11:580–585, 1990 16–16

Smooth muscle cell (SMC) proliferation contributes to many forms of vascular abnormalities and is a major cause of late graft failure. To examine the regulation of intimal SMC proliferation, a baboon model of prosthetic arterial graft healing was studied. The porous polytetrafluoroethylene (PTFE) vascular grafts in this model heal by transmural invasion of capillaries from the surrounding granulation tissue. The intimal cells were examined for evidence of mRNA for growth factors known to be mitogenic for SMCs.

Two-year-old male baboons received PTFE vascular grafts. Six weeks later the graft and the thoracic aorta were freed from surrounding tissues and removed. Endothelial cells were scraped from the luminal surface of the graft and aorta. The remaining intima was removed from the lumen of the graft material. The cell types were identified by morphological studies and immunocytochemistry with monoclonal antibodies.

The grafts had formed an intima containing mainly SMCs by 6 weeks. An endothelial monolayer was observed to line the luminal surface. Occasional macrophages were also observed in the intima from the PTFE. Occasional endothelial cells, SMCs, and numerous macrophages were noted in the interstices of the graft material.

The finding of intimal SMC proliferation underneath an intact endothelium, without platelet adherence, suggests that intimal cells rather than platelets may provide the growth factors regulating SMC proliferation. Graft intima produce mRNA for growth factors known to regulate SMC growth in vitro in a pattern different from that of native artery. The SMCs cultured from these 2 tissues are capable of expressing growth factor genes.

▶ It is fascinating to see that intima is necessary to regulation of SMC proliferation.

Histological Appearances of the Long Saphenous Vein

Milroy CM, Scott DJA, Beard JD, Horrocks M, Bradfield JWB (Bristol Royal Infirmary, England)

J Pathol 159:311–316, 1989 16–17

The long saphenous vein is the conduit of choice as a graft in femorodistal and coronary artery bypass operations. Although the pathologic changes that occur in saphenous vein grafts after implantation have been well studied, the histologic appearance of the donor long saphenous vein before grafting has received little attention.

The histologic appearance of the long saphenous vein was examined in 25 patients who were undergoing femorodistal bypass operation in treatment of critical ischemia caused by peripheral vascular disease. Portions of the long saphenous vein in excess of that required for operation were submitted for histologic examination. None of the veins was clinically varicose. The examined sections were from .5 cm to 8 cm in length.

None of the veins examined had a histologic appearance resembling that of a normal long saphenous vein (Fig 16–4). All vein portions showed evidence of intimal fibrosis, elastosis, and hypertrophy of the muscle layers (Fig 16–5). Intimal lesions were composed of fibrous tis-

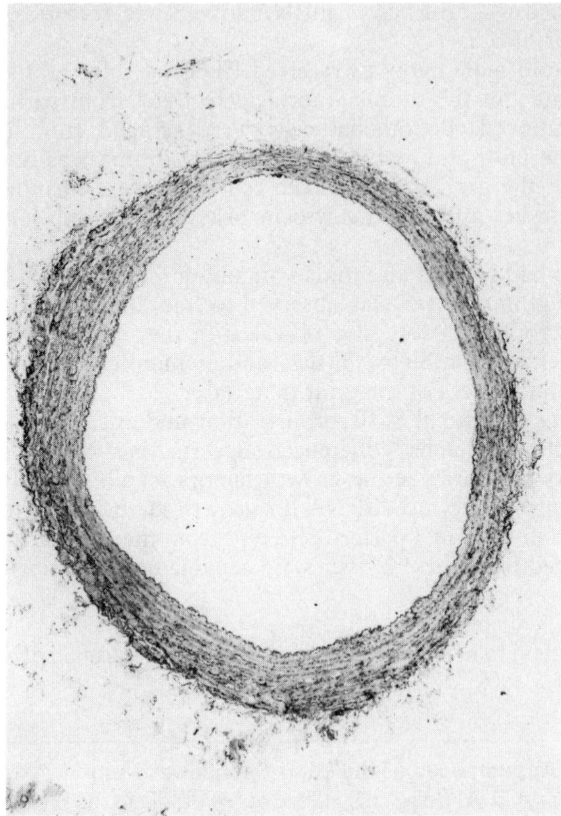

Fig 16–4.—Normal long saphenous vein (elastic van Gieson). (Courtesy of Milroy CM, Scott DJA, Beard JD, et al: *J Pathol* 159:311–316, 1989.)

sue, elastic tissue, and longitudinally arranged smooth muscle, and appeared identical to lesions seen in arteries, except that no lipid-laden cells or calcification was noted in any of the vein segments. Longitudinal and circular muscle layers showed evidence of muscle cell hypertrophy with an increase in intervening connective tissue.

The changes that occur in veins after implantation may have important consequences once the vein is used as a graft, and they may well be contributing factors in early and late graft failure.

▶ One would have hoped that the authors of this report would have differentiated ankle vein from proximal vein and provided us with an explanation for the observation that vein patch rupture is associated with veins taken from the ankle.

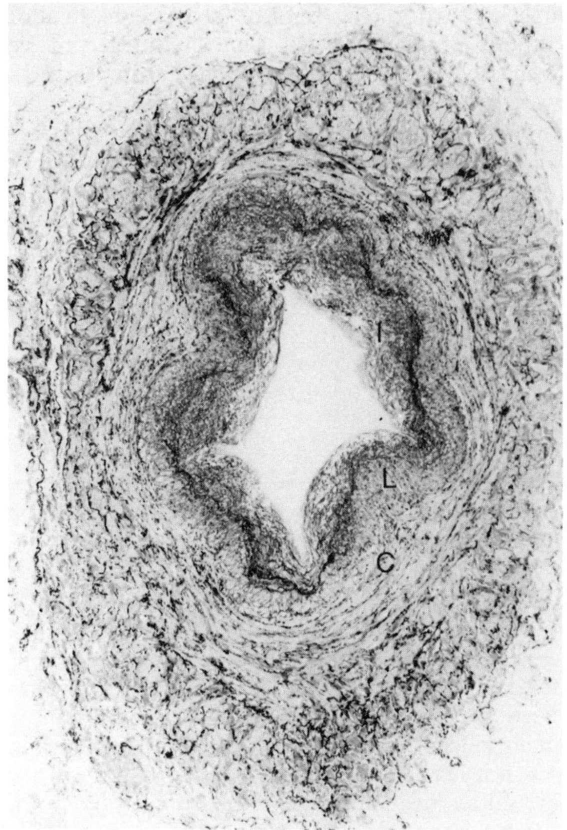

Fig 16–5.—Low-power view of vein showing intimal fibrosis *(I)* and hypertrophy of the longitudinal *(L)* and circular muscle *(C)* layers. (Courtesy of Milroy CM, Scott DJA, Beard JD, et al: *J Pathol* 159:311–316, 1989.)

Functional Analysis of Cryopreserved Veins: Preliminary Report

Brockbank KGM, Donovan TJ, Ruby ST, Carpenter JF, Hagen P-O, Woodley MA (CryoLife Inc Marietta, Ga; Hartford Hosp Research Lab, Conn; Univ of Connecticut, Farmington; Duke Univ)

J Vasc Surg 11:94–102, 1990 16–18

A study was undertaken to assess the viability of veins after cryopreservation and thawing. The endothelial, smooth muscle, and fibroblast functions of cryopreserved and fresh canine saphenous, cephalic, and jugular veins were compared.

Morphometric analysis showed that vein procurement and cold ischemia before cryopreservation resulted in 18% loss of endothelial integrity. There was no significant loss of endothelial integrity as a result of cryopreservation, with 80% to 100% of the remaining endothelial cells forming clones in tissue culture. In vitro isometric tension studies in response to norepinephrine showed that cryopreserved veins retained 52%

of smooth muscle function relative to fresh segments. In addition, in vitro collagen synthesis studies showed that cryopreserved veins retained 43.5% of connective tissue functions. Eight cryopreserved cephalic vein autografts were placed as femoral artery grafts. All grafts were patent within 1–8 weeks after transplantation. Light and electron microscopic studies showed complete restoration of the mild endothelial damage, similar to that described previously for fresh autologous veins.

Cryopreserved veins retain much of their cellular and tissue functions on thawing. When transplanted, cryopreserved vein segments display a sequence of histologic events similar to that associated with the use of autologous fresh vein as an arterial substitute.

▶ Although cryopreservation may not alter the sequence of histologic events after vein implantation into the arterial system, the fact of rejection of allograft veins remains with us.

Axillopopliteal Bypass Grafting: Indications, Late Results, and Determinants of Long-Term Patency

Ascer E, Veith FJ, Gupta S (Montefiore Med Ctr-Albert Einstein College of Medicine, New York)

J Vasc Surg 10:285–291, 1989 16–19

During the past 3 decades several extra-anatomical bypass graft procedures have been devised to treat patients who are in imminent danger of limb loss but in whom limb salvage by standard abdominal arterial reconstruction is not feasible. The benefits and limitations of conventional axillofemoral and femorofemoral extra-anatomical operations have been well studied, but extra-anatomical axillopopliteal bypass grafting has received limited attention. A 12-year experience with axillopopliteal bypass grafting for limb salvage in patients at high risk for limb loss was evaluated.

The study population comprised 30 men and 20 women aged 49–88 years who underwent 55 axillopopliteal arterial bypass operations with 6-mm standard nonringed polytetrafluoroethylene grafts. Indications included severe atherosclerotic disease of the common, superficial, and deep femoral arteries; failed aortofemoral bypass grafting with disease progression in the deep femoral artery; insufficient clinical improvement after axillofemoral bypass grafting; and sepsis in the groin from a previously infected graft. All patients had preoperative arteriographic evidence of severe lower limb ischemia.

The 30-day operative mortality rate was 8%. All 4 patients died of myocardial infarction. The 5-year cumulative patient survival was 40%. Overall cumulative primary graft patency rates were 58% at 1 year, 45% at 3 years, and 40% at 5 years. Comparable limb salvage rates were 83% at 1 year, 68% at 3 years, and 58% at 5 years. Although at 1 year the mean graft patency for the 28 bypass grafts to the above-knee popliteal artery was superior to that for the 27 reconstructions to the below-knee popliteal artery, the difference did not reach statistical significance after 2 years and 3 years of follow-up. The overall graft infection rate was 3.6%. Twelve limbs required amputation, 9 above the knee and 3 below the knee. Fourteen (77%) of the 18 patients who died in the late follow-up period had functional limbs at the time of death. Axillopopliteal bypass grafting is an effective and durable limb salvage operation for patients at high risk for limb loss in whom more standard arterial reconstructions are not feasible.

▶ Because axillary popliteal grafts must be used in certain complex situations, it is well to know that their half-life is short. Definitive, intracavitary reconstructions can be performed before multiple extra-anatomical graft failures.

Exertional Disruption of Axillofemoral Graft Anastomosis: "The Axillary Pullout Syndrome"

White GH, Donayre CE, Williams RA, White RA, Stabile BE, Wilson SE (Harbor-UCLA Med Ctr, Torrance, Calif)

Arch Surg 125:625–627, 1990 16–20

Disruption of the axillary anastomosis of an axillofemoral graft occurred in 5 patients, with resultant pseudoaneurysm formation. The patients were seen in a 2-year period in 3 vascular practices. Each prosthesis was made of polytetrafluoroethylene (PTFE) supported by plastic ribbing. The prostheses were sutured in place with 5–0 or 6–0 propylene using standard technique.

The patients had axillary pain, anterior chest wall hematoma, or pseudoaneurysm formation 13–30 days after axillofemoral graft surgery. Two patients were amputees who became symptomatic when performing weight transference using an overhead bar with the arm abducted and the torso flexed. Reconstruction required either lengthening of the graft or replacement. Brachial plexus neuropathy occurred transiently after surgery, but no patient had significant hand ischemia.

During a 2-year period, 22 patients with axillary anastomotic disruption were reported to the Food and Drug Administration. A manufacturer of PTFE grafts provided information on 10 cases occurring in a 7-year period. Surface measurements in controls indicated that arm abduction and torso flexion increase the distance between the axillary and femoral arteries by about 15%. This complication can be avoided by allowing several centimeters of extra length and by placing the axillary anastomosis medial to the pectoralis minor muscle. These measures are especially important in amputees.

▶ The last paragraph of this abstract captures the essence and the wisdom of the presentation.

17 Vascular Trauma

The Widened Mediastinum: Diagnostic and Therapeutic Priorities
Richardson JD, Wilson ME, Miller FB (Univ of Louisville; Humana Hosp Univ, Louisville)
Ann Surg 211:731–737, 1990 17–1

More and more patients are seen with multiple injuries and mediastinal widening, but little attention has been given to the sequential assessment and management of those with potential aortic disruption. Data were reviewed on 408 patients seen from 1981 to 1989 with mediastinal widening who underwent aortography. All had incurred significant blunt trauma with the potential for causing multisystem injuries. No absolute diagnostic or therapeutic protocol was followed.

The 318 male and 90 female patients had an average age of 39 years and a mean Injury Severity Score of 21. Sixty-eight percent of these patients required diagnostic peritoneal lavage (DPL) and 18% required celiotomy. Injury to the CNS occurred in 68% of the group and 40% had orthopedic injuries. Thirty-five patients had thoracic aortic injuries and 17 had branch injuries; 15 of these patients died. The chief causes of death were bleeding, neurologic injury, and multisystem organ failure.

In 7 cases there was a potential triage error or delayed diagnosis. In 5 of these cases DPL was omitted incorrectly. In 2 instances treatment was delayed because of an overriding concern for assessing mediastinal widening. The rate of sequence errors was 1.6%. In no case did aortic injury delay treatment. There were relatively few cases in which abdominal injury was not promptly treated.

An integrated plan is needed for optimal management of patients who present after blunt injury with a widened mediastinum. In selected cases it is appropriate to treat intra-abdominal injuries before repairing aortic rupture, but the lethal potential of blunt aortic injuries must be kept in mind.

▶ This enormous experience displayed by the Louisville group is extremely informative. The very high incidence of CNS injury underscores the severity of the trauma, and the importance of DPL is underscored in this report.

Aortic Ruptures in Seat Belt Wearers
Arajärvi E, Santavirta S, Tolonen J (Univ Central Hosp, Helsinki)
J Thorac Cardiovasc Surg 93:355–361, 1989 17–2

Immediate death in traffic accidents is often caused by rupture of the aorta. To study the effect of seat belt wearing and mechanisms of injury,

68 persons who died in traffic accidents who had rupture of the thoracic aorta were compared with 72 unbelted persons with fatal aortic rupture incurred in similar accidents.

The distal part of the descending aorta was the most common site of injury in seat belt wearers, especially in right-front-seat passengers and those in frontal impact collisions. In unbelted persons the ascending aorta was the usual site of rupture, especially among drivers. Lateral impact collisions caused ruptures in the isthmus region and in the ascending aorta in seat belt wearers. The part of the car thought to cause injury was the seat belt in only 7% of belted persons; usually, some interior portion of the car was the cause. In unbelted persons the most frequent cause was the steering wheel.

The mechanism of injury in rupture of the isthmus region usually was rapid deceleration and in lateral impact collisions, complex body movements. Fracture of the thoracic vertebra often led to rupture of the distal portion of the descending aorta. In unbelted persons, ascending aortal rupture resulted from a blow to the thorax.

Aortic rupture plays a more important role in fatal chest trauma in seat belt wearers than was once thought. Seat belts fail to protect in lateral impact collisions, and steering wheels still cause injury in seat belt wearers.

▶ The emergence of seat belt wearing is changing the location of aortic rupture, as indicated in this report. Lateral impact collisions are especially lethal, as emphasized.

Interventional Neurovascular Treatment of Traumatic Carotid and Vertebral Artery Lesions: Results in 234 Cases

Higashida RT, Halbach VV, Tsai FY, Norman D, Pribram HF, Mehringer CM, Hieshima GB (Interventional Neuroradiology Section, San Francisco; Truman Med Ctr, Kansas City; Univ of California, Irvine; Harbor-UCLA Med Ctr, Torrance)

AJR 153:577–582, 1989 17–3

Surgical techniques for treating arteriovenous fistulas resulting from traumatic injuries to the head and neck are associated with an excessively high risk of complications. Various interventional neurovascular techniques have been used successfully to treat carotid-cavernous sinus fistulas (CCFs) and vertebral arteriovenous fistulas (AVFs). Several of these newer methods were used in the treatment of 234 patients, aged 14–84 years.

There were 206 patients with direct and 7 with indirect CCFs and 21 patients with traumatic vertebral fistulas. Interventional devices included detachable balloons, liquid tissue adhesives, microcoils, and silk suture. Most of the procedures were performed under local anesthesia.

Intravascular detatchable balloon embolization was the treatment of choice for direct CCFs and was also used for the 21 patients with traumatic vertebral AVFs. In 41 patients it was necessary to occlude the carotid or vertebral artery by endovascular techniques because of extensive vascular injury (28 patients) or subtotal occlusion of the fistula (13). Complications included transient cerebral ischemia in 6 patients, pseudoaneurysm formation in 5, stroke in 5, and peripheral nerve injury in 1.

These AVFs often occur in the acute setting, with the risk of uncontrollable hemorrhage. Preservation of vision and of the carotid artery can be achieved by interventional neurovascular techniques. When injuries involve the vertebral artery, effort should be directed toward closing the fistula and preserving the parent vessel.

▶ Surgical approaches to vertebral AVFs are so difficult that it is a welcome relief to find our interventional radiologic colleagues leading us in definitive management of these injuries.

Arterial Injury Complicating Knee Disruption

Varnell RM, Coldwell DM, Sangeorzan BJ, Johansen KH (Univ of Washington; Harborview Med Ctr, Seattle)

Am Surg 55:699–704, 1989 17–4

Dislocation of the knee is accompanied by a substantial risk of injury to the popliteal artery, and the use of arteriography in ruling out occult arterial damage in knee dislocation is well accepted. Because dislocations may occur and then spontaneously reduce, an occult arterial disruption may still be present despite the absence of an obvious knee dislocation. Hence, arteriograms have been performed routinely in all trauma victims who have sustained extensive knee ligamentous disruptions without dislocation. To test the validity of this policy, the records of 19 patients with dislocated knees and 11 with severe ligamentous disruption were reviewed.

The incidence of major (22% versus 18%) or minor (38% versus 36%) vascular abnormalities did not differ significantly between the groups. Doppler measurements of arterial pressure were highly predictive of major arterial injury. No clinically significant arterial injury was discovered among the 17 patients who had arteriography in the angiography suite. In contrast, 4 of 12 patients who had "1-shot arteriograms" in the operating room (33%) had major vascular injuries.

Arterial injury should be ruled out in all trauma victims with severe knee ligamentous disruption, whether or not actual knee dislocation is present. Doppler measurements of pressure in screening injured extremities for occult arterial injury seem promising. Although the "1-shot arteriogram" provides rapid localization of the level of injury in a patient highly suspected clinically of having vascular damage, a combined digital angiographic-surgical suite may be optimal for the management of patients with potential vascular injuries, including knee disruption.

▶ The unstable knee remains a problem frequently associated with vascular injury and, as stated in this abstract, arterial injury should be ruled out whenever an unstable knee is seen. This can be done by direct examination early and sequential determination of distal Doppler ankle pressures later.

Compartment Syndrome in Combined Arterial and Venous Injuries of the Lower Extremity

Shah PM, Wapnir I, Babu S, Stahl WM, Clauss RH (Lincoln Med and Mental Health Ctr, Bronx)

Am J Surg 158:136–141, 1989 17–5

In compartment syndrome, increased pressure within a limited space compromises the circulation, causing ischemic dysfunction and necrosis of tissues. There are 4 limited unyielding spaces in the leg bounded by the tibia, the fibula, the interosseous membrane, and the crural fascia. Many causes have been reported for the development of this syndrome. A series was reviewed in an attempt to better understand the factors responsible for the development of compartment syndrome in patients with combined arterial and venous injuries of the lower extremity and to develop a rationale for prophylactic fasciotomy.

Forty-five patients were treated for dual vascular injuries of the lower extremity. Concomitant fasciotomies were done at the time of initial surgery for associated soft tissue injury, fracture, or prolonged ischemia in 9 patients. In an additional 8 patients compartment syndrome developed postoperatively and delayed fasciotomy was necessary. In 7 of these patients the vein was either ligated or the repaired vein was occluded. In the eighth patient massive swelling of the thigh caused peripheral venous hypertension.

In a study of experimental animals, compartment pressure was monitored by wick catheter in 24 hind legs of 12 dogs with simulated vascular injuries. A significant increase was noted in compartment pressure in animals with arterial and venous injuries managed by arterial repair and venous outflow obstruction.

Obstruction to venous drainage and venous hypertension appear to be major factors in the development of compartment syndrome in dual vascular injuries of the lower extremity. Prophylactic fasciotomy should be performed in such injuries when restoration of the circulation is delayed, venous repair is not adequate, or injuries to the thigh muscles impede venous collateral outflow.

▶ Venous injury concomitant with popliteal arterial injury, as might occur in posterior knee dislocation, is a situation that produces increased risk for distal compartment syndromes. Prophylactic fasciotomy in such situations is not cosmetic, but it is certainly limb saving.

Management of Blunt Injuries of the Axillary Artery and the Neck of the Humerus: Case Report

Laverick MD, Barros D'Sa AAB, Kirk SJ, Mollan RAB (Royal Victoria Hosp, Belfast)

J Trauma 30:360–361, 1990 17–6

Vascular injury in association with fractures of bones of an upper extremity occur infrequently but can result in permanent disability if not treated promptly. One woman had an axillary artery injury that complicated a closed humeral fracture, a particularly rare occurrence.

Woman, 65, was hospitalized after a fall that injured her left shoulder. Her left arm was cyanosed, cold, and pulseless. Radiography revealed a comminuted fracture of the neck of the humerus, with subluxation of the humeral head. Angiography revealed an occluded 4-cm segment of the axillary artery just distal to the fracture site. The head of the humerus was excised and replaced with a 15-mm Neer hemiarthroplasty prosthesis. The damaged section of artery was resected and repaired with a 6-mm thin-walled polytetrafluoroethylene graft. Pulses at the patient's wrist reappeared and arterial perfusion of the whole arm improved dramatically. At 2-year follow-up, the arterial supply to the hand and arm was essentially normal.

Thorough clinical assessment complemented by angiography is necessary when such an injury is suspected. Delay may result in permanent damage or even amputation. Stable fixation of the fracture must be undertaken first to avert anastomotic disruption. The vascular surgeon and orthopedic surgeon should formulate the policy for managing these cases. When 2 prostheses are implanted, as in this case, the potential for infection increases.

▶ Upper extremity blunt injury may produce vascular compromise much as dislocation of the knee does.

The Problem of Vascular Shotgun Injuries: Diagnostic and Management Strategy

Bongard FS, Klein SR (Univ of California, Los Angeles; Harbor-UCLA Hosp, Torrance)

Ann Vasc Surg 3:299–303, 1989 17–7

Shotgun injuries have become increasingly prevalent with the increase in urban violent crime. The spectrum of tissue damage is related to the proximity of the weapon to the victim, pellet size, choke, and barrel length. Data on 11 vascular injuries to the extremities in 10 patients wounded by shotguns during a 5-year period were reviewed.

The 9 males and 1 female, aged 17–25 years sustained injuries to vessels, including the brachial artery, femoral artery, iliac artery, tibioperoneal trunk, and axillary vein. All patients with arterial injuries had distal ischemia at presentation. Physical findings included parethesia, cyanosis, and paresis; 6 patients had an absent palpable pulse distal to the injury. Active hemorrhage occurred in 4 patients; the remainder had a nonbleeding hematoma over the wound site. The only patient with an isolated upper extremity venous injury presented with active bleeding, an expanding hematoma, distended veins on the ipsilateral extremity, and reduced distal artery pulses. Arteriography was performed on 7 hemodynamically stable patients.

Four patients underwent primary repair, 4 received a saphenous vein graft, and 1 had a prosthetic graft. All patients with primary arterial injuries also had associated venous disruption that was either repaired or ligated. There were 7 associated nerve injuries; 3 patients had extensive compartment injuries that necessitated fasciotomy. Most complications were caused by associated nerve damage or soft tissue loss.

Management of patients with vascular shotgun injuries includes hemodynamic stabilization followed by arteriography to define the anatomical origin of complex injuries (Fig 17–1). Surgery is performed for rapid proximal and distal control of disrupted segments. After vessel débridement, continuity is restored by either primary repair or by autogenous grafting. The patency of the grafts is evaluated by on-table arteriography, which also provides evidence of distal arterial emboli. Fractures are then

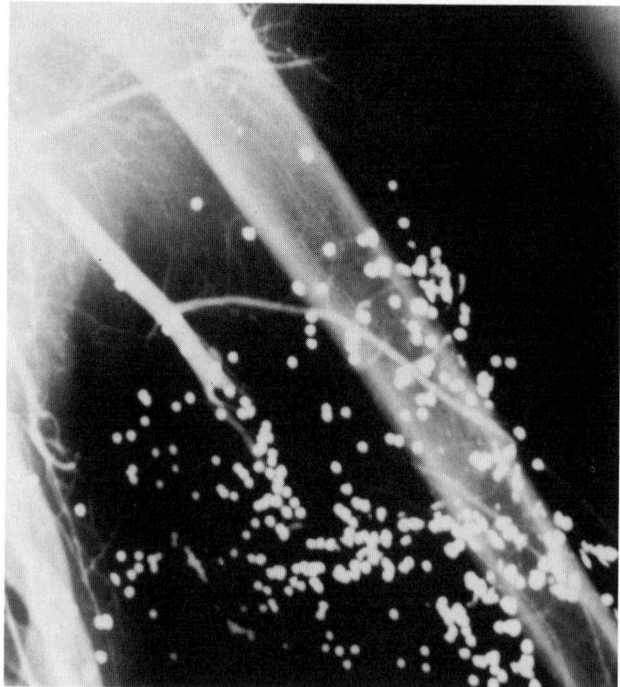

Fig 17–1.—Preoperative arteriogram of close range (3 ft) shotgun blast to brachial artery. This patient had extensive soft tissue damage as well. Operative repair was by reversed saphenous graft. (Courtesy of Bongard FS, Klein SR: *Ann Vasc Surg* 3:299–303, 1989.)

stabilized and disrupted nerves isolated for subsequent repair. If there is prolonged ischemia or distal swelling, fasciotomy is performed.

▶ Emphasis is properly placed in this report on preoperative arteriography. This is done not so much to define the main artery damage as to locate any branch artery injury.

Results of Venous Interposition Grafts in Arterial Injuries
Mitchell FL III, Thal ER (Univ of Texas, Dallas)
J Trauma 30:336–339, 1990 17–8

Repair of arterial injuries has traditionally been accomplished with autogenous vein grafts, although some vascular surgeons advocate the use of polytetrafluroethylene (PTFE) grafts. To assess the problems associated with use of autogenous interposition vein grafts in patients with severe arterial injuries, the charts of 191 patients who received 192 grafts were reviewed. Aspects studied included the type of trauma, location of injuries, associated injuries, and complications. Seventy-six percent of the arterial injuries were the result of penetrating trauma and 51% were in the lower extremities (table).

During follow-up ranging to 9 years, there were no graft-related complications in 168 patients (88%). The 1 death was not related to the interposition graft. Thrombosis occurred in 16 patients (8.3%), usually within 48 hours after operation. No late (more than 30 days) graft thromboses are known to have occurred. Ten patients with thrombosis had sustained penetrating trauma and significant soft tissue injury.

Seven grafts showed signs of infection. Each of these patients had sustained significant soft tissue injury in addition to the vascular injury. The three infected grafts that ruptured were in a femoral artery, 2 were in a

Location of Interposition Grafts

	No. of Injuries		(%)	
1) Upper Extremity		86		(45.0)
Subclavian	6		(3.0)	
Axillary	18		(9.5)	
Brachial	47		(24.5)	
Radial/ulnar	15		(8.0)	
2) Lower Extremity		98		(51.0)
Femoral	38		(19.5)	
Popliteal	41		(21.5)	
Distal	19		(10.0)	
3) Others		8		(4.0)
Carotid	4		(2.0)	
Renal	4		(2.0)	

(Courtesy of Mitchell FL III, Thal ER: *J Trauma* 30:336–339, March 1990.)

popliteal artery, and 2 were in a brachial artery. Eight of the 18 amputations were graft related; 3 resulted from graft thrombosis and 5 from graft infection followed by hemorrhage.

Autogenous vein grafts were associated with a low rate of complications. Because these grafts are safe and readily accessible, synthetic grafts should be used only when autogenous grafts are not available or delay would compromise the patient's outcome.

▶ Autogenous grafts are, in general, preferred everywhere in the repair of vascular problems. Many extremity vascular injuries are associated with large soft tissue defects, and soft tissue coverage is essential. Extra-anatomical routing of the autogenous graft may be necessary.

Vascular Complications Associated With Pelvic Fractures

Vicq Ph, Hajji A, Le Reveillé R, Darrieus H, Chaussard JF (Hôp d'Instruction des Armées du Val de Grâce, Paris)

J Chir (Paris) 126:507–513, 1989 17–9

The frequency of pelvic fractures in patients with multiple trauma has been increasing. Pelvic fractures are always life-threatening, and the mortality associated with them remains high, mainly because concomitant major vascular injuries and abdominal injuries are common. Although there is controversy over the best surgical approach to treatment, surgical vascular repair is always indicated when major hemorrhage occurs.

The records of 11 men and 4 women (mean age, 28 years) were reviewed. Twelve of the 15 patients had been transferred from other institutions and early resuscitation data on them were not available. All patients had sustained multiple trauma, and the mean injury severity score (ISS) was 31.5. Treatment differed for each patient, and a general pattern of injury and treatment could not be established from the record review.

The primary concern in multiply injured patients with pelvic fractures is stabilization. Hemostasis should be initiated, and the patient should be given antibiotics to avoid secondary infection. The clinical signs obtained from physical examination are usually nonspecific. Radiographic examination without proper preparation only visualizes bone fractures and provides little information about the severity of the vascular injuries. When the patient has been resuscitated and hemodynamically stabilized, whole-body CT with contrast medium should be performed to identify the source of hemorrhage. Arteriographic examination should be performed as soon as possible thereafter. Vascular repairs should then be performed as indicated by the radiographic findings. Stabilization of the pelvis can wait until the patient is no longer critical. In general, treatment of these severely injured patients requires a multidisciplinary approach by the resuscitation team, the radiologist, and the surgeon.

▶ Scanning with CT in the stabilized patient is an extremely important adjunct to the routine evaluation of pelvic trauma.

The Role of Duplex Ultrasonography in the Differentiation of Pseudoaneurysm, Hematoma, and Abscess

Montefusco CM, Rhodes BA, Bakal C, Grossman DS, Dietzek A, Veith FJ (Albert Einstein College of Medicine)

J Vasc Tech 14:11–17, 1990 17–10

Of 216 patients referred to a vascular laboratory in 1987 through 1988 with a pulsatile groin mass, 135 had had femoral artery puncture and catheterization. Fifty-four other patients were intravenous drug abusers, and 27 others had had surgery that involved the groin vessels.

A duplex ultrasonography device with a 7.5-MHz B-mode imaging probe showed that 56 of the patients who had femoral puncture had a pseudoaneurysm of the common femoral artery; 19 had confirmatory arteriograms. All patients with a diagnosed pseudoaneurysm underwent corrective surgery. Eight of the drug abusers also had pseudoaneurysms, all confirmed at operation. The other 46 drug abusers had an abscess or hematoma. Ultrasonography showed a pseudoaneurysm in 4 of the patients who had had surgery that involved the groin vessels. Four others had a diagnosed abscess and 19 had a hematoma; 2 abscesses were not confirmed.

Duplex ultrasonography is a rapid, noninvasive means of diagnosing pseudoaneursm in the groin and is accurate if strict criteria are followed. This would seem to be the preferred diagnostic method in patients with a pulsatile groin mass secondary to arterial trauma. The study can be helpful in following the resolution of a hematoma and in detecting a recurrent pseudoaneurysm or abscess.

▶ In evaluating iatrogenic vascular trauma, the duplex scan avoids arteriography and, as indicated in the Abstract 17–11, may guide therapy.

Doppler Sonographic Demonstration of the Progressive Spontaneous Thrombosis of Pseudoaneurysms

Kotval PS, Khoury A, Shah PM, Babu SC (New York Med College, Valhalla, NY)

J Ultrasound Med 9:185–190, 1990 17–11

Pseudoaneurysm of the common femoral or superficial femoral artery complicates about 1% of femoral catheterizations. Three patients in whom surgery was delayed for clinical reasons were followed with Doppler sonography. In 1 patient a new pseudoaneurysmal lobe developed and progressive centripetal thrombus formation occurred in each lobe, culminating in total thrombosis of the pseudoaneurysm.

Woman, 29, underwent angiography after spontaneous rupture of the liver during parturition. A pulsatile mass was noted at the puncture site the next day, and sonography showed an ellipsoidal pseudoaneurysm of the right common femoral artery with a narrow neck. Doppler study showed flow throughout the cavity of the lesion. A small new lobe was present 10 days later, and further studies showed progressive centripetal thrombus formation within the pseudoaneurysm (Fig 17–2). Thrombus ultimately totally occluded the larger lobe of the pseudoaneurysm. The right femoral bifurcation appeared normal on sonographic examination 4 months after the pseudoaneurysm was first seen, as did the arterial wall.

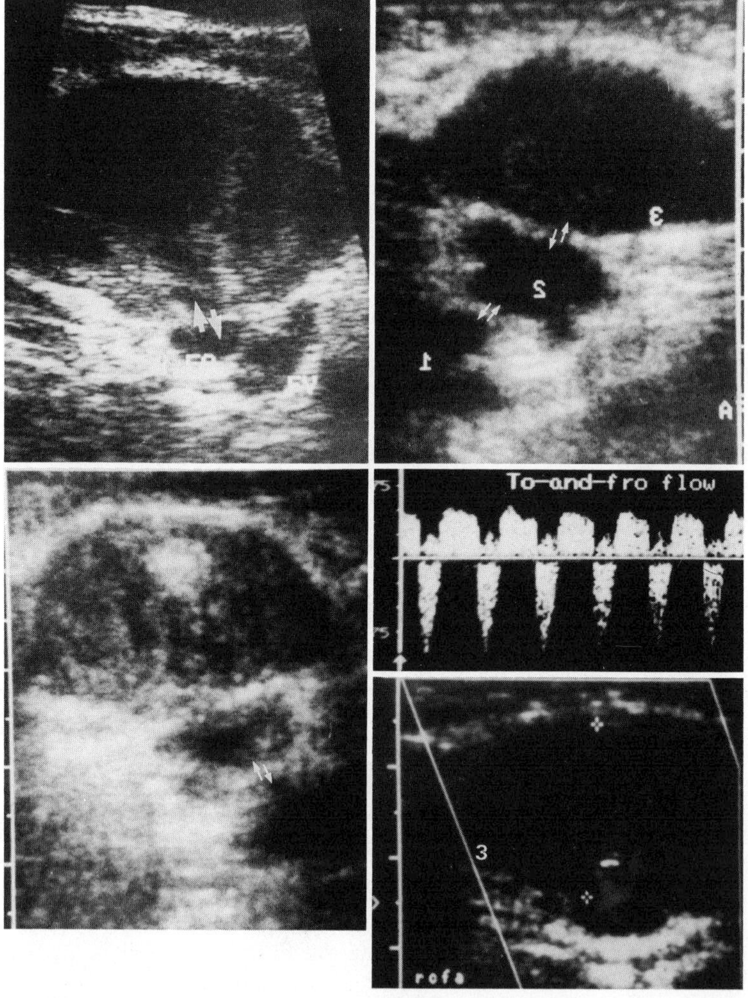

Fig 17–2.—Real-time, color Doppler, and pulsed Doppler images from 5 successive examinations in patient with a pseudoaneurysm of the right common femoral artery. The dates of the examinations are shown at the bottom with the schematic figures. The pseudoaneurysm seen at the initial examination forms a second lobe. Progressive centripetal thrombus formation is seen in the main lobe of the pseudoaneurysm leading to successive thrombosis of both lobes. At 4-month follow-up *(image at extreme right),* a normal-appearing right femoral bifurcation is seen with no sonographic evidence of rebleeding and complete resolution of the pseudoaneurysm. (Courtesy of Kotval PS, Khoury A, Shah PM, et al: *J Ultrasound Med* 9:185–190, 1990.)

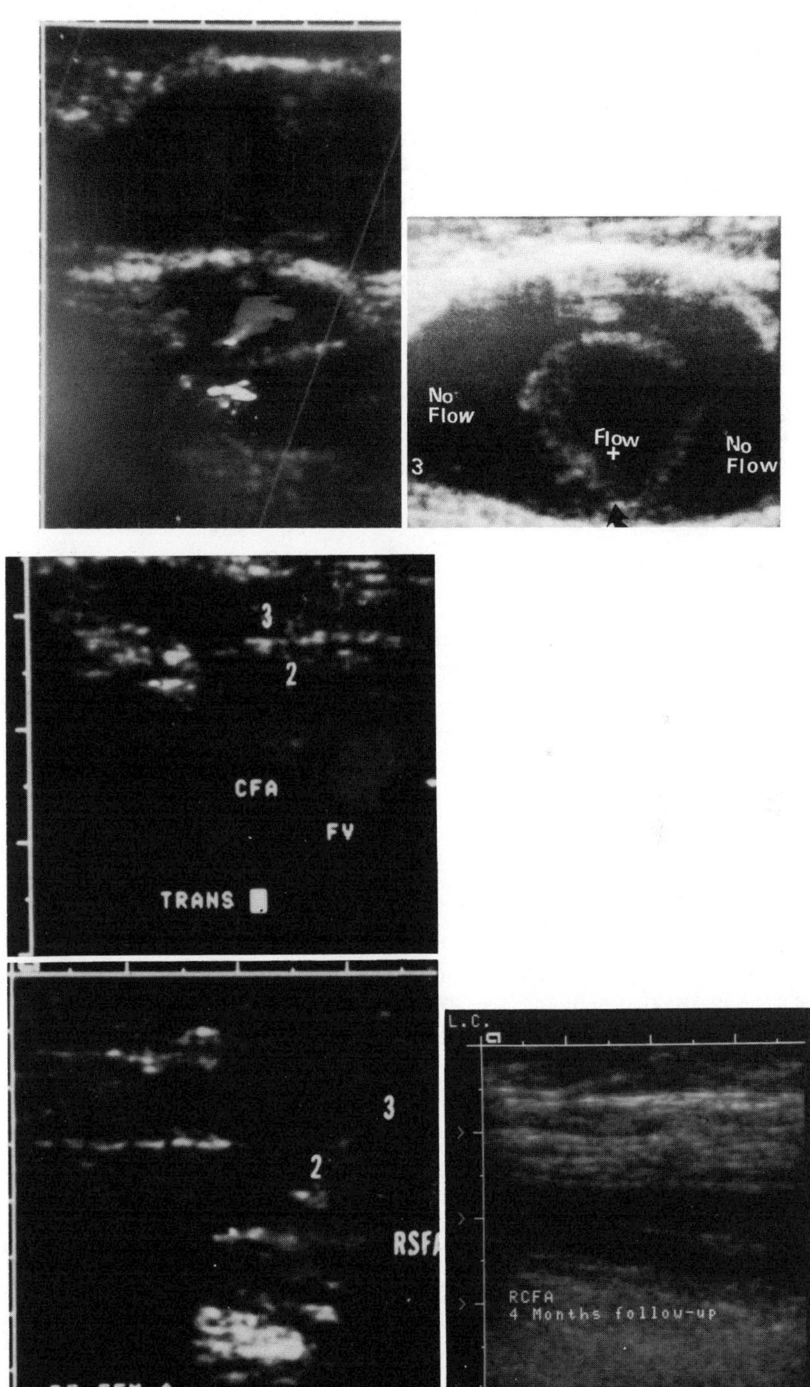

Fig 17–2, *cont'd.*

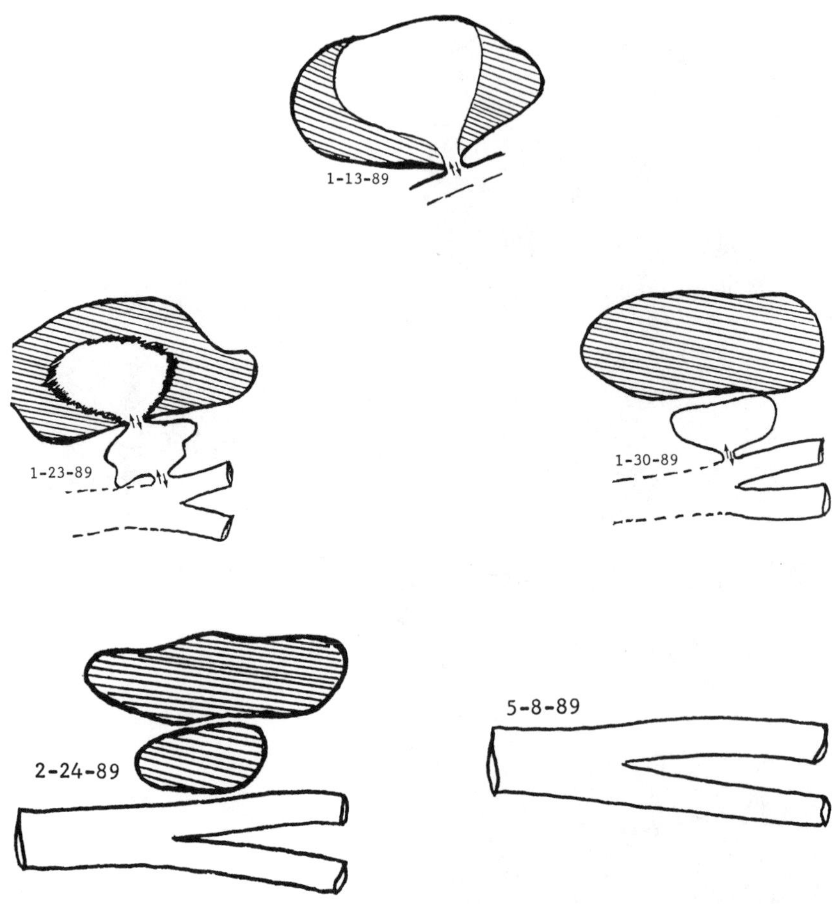

Fig 17–2, *cont'd.*

Color Doppler sonography should prove helpful in predicting which pseudoaneurysms will resolve spontaneously and which are candidates for repair. Progressive centripetal thrombus formation indicates that the pseudoaneurysm will be self-healing, and surgery sometimes can be avoided in such cases.

▶ Occasionally, local pressure may hasten the development of centripetal thrombosis and cure the pseudoaneurysm. This can be monitored by duplex sonography.

Infected False Aneurysms of the Femoral Artery in Intravenous Drug Addicts

McIlroy MA, Reddy D, Markowitz N, Saravolatz LD (Henry Ford Hosp, Detroit)
Rev Infect Dis 11:578–585, 1989 17–12

Data were reviewed on 60 intravenous drug addicts with infected false aneurysms of the femoral artery who were treated from 1977 to 1988. In 56 cases groin swelling or a mass, usually tender or painful, was present. The usual sites for this lesion were the common femoral artery and the bifurcation points. In diagnosis, digital subtraction angiography had a sensitivity of 92% and standard arteriography a sensitivity of 96%. The microorganism identified was *Staphylococcus aureus* in 50 patients (83%); in 21 patients (42%) the strain was a β-lactam–resistant isolate. Anaerobic infection was present in 12 patients (20%). In 23 patients (39%) the infection was polymicrobial. Associated bactermia was present in 36 cases (60%).

Broad-spectrum antimicrobial therapy with anaerobic activity was given to all patients, usually for 2–6 weeks, but a significant failure rate occurred with 15 or fewer days of treatment. Surgical ligation was performed in all cases, with grafts for 12 patients, 6 of which failed. There were no deaths, but 6 patients had to have amputation.

Groin swelling or pain in an intravenous drug addict should raise the suspicion of infected false aneurysm. It is best detected by digital subtraction angiography. Treatment consists of parenteral therapy with broad-spectrum antibiotics for at least 3 weeks, ligation, and packing of the open wound, with a graft in selected cases.

▶ Pus and blood in the groin of an intravenous drug addict are ominous findings.

Infected False Aneurysms in the Groin of Intravenous Drug Abusers
Welch GH, Reid DB, Pollock JG (Glasgow Royal Infirmary, Scotland)
Br J Surg 77:330–333, 1990 17–13

An infected false aneurysm of the common femoral artery is an infrequent but serious complication of intravenous drug abuse. Six patients with infected common femoral false aneurysms (Fig 17–3) were encountered. The findings in a patient whose infected iliofemoral Dacron graft was replaced by polytetrafluoroethylene iliopopliteal graft are shown in Figure 17–4. *Staphylococcus aureus* was isolated in all cases. Three of the patients have viable extremities despite infection and removal of the graft or graft closure.

Treatment of infected false aneurysms involves parenteral antibiotics, extensive débridement, control of bleeding, and, when necessary, restoration of distal circulation. Proximal control by high ligation avoids having to ligate an inflamed, friable vessel. Distal control subsequently is achieved by opening the aneurysm and suture-ligating it from within. Five of the patients had early graft infection, which in 4 cases led to major bleeding.

Surgery should not be delayed in these cases. If the extremity appears nonviable after débridement or becomes nonviable after ligation, revascu-

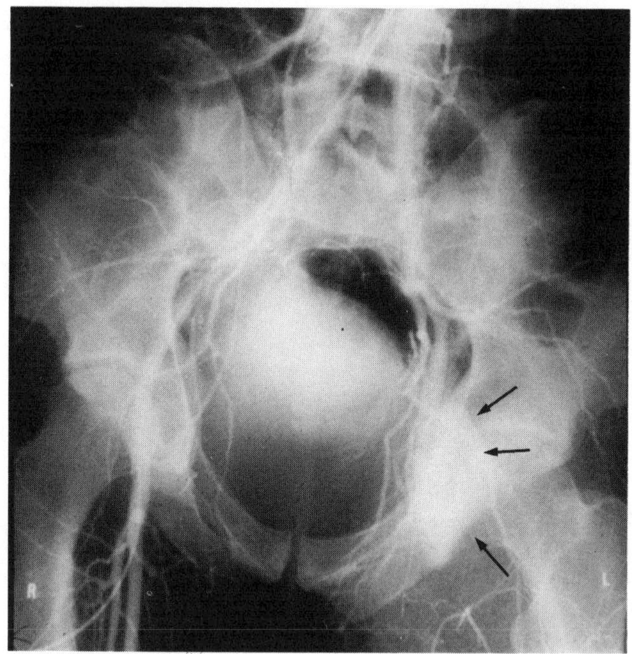

Fig 17–3.—Angiogram showing false aneurysm *(arrows)* arising from the left common femoral artery. (Courtesy of Welch GH, Reid DB, Pollock JG: *Br J Surg* 77:330–333, 1990.)

larization may be necessary. If possible, this should be done by an extra-anatomical route. Otherwise, an in situ graft is the only alternative. In this instance, planned graft occlusion might allow collaterals to develop, making removal of the temporary graft safer.

▶ The infected false aneurysm in the groin of the intravenous drug user requires that therapy be dictated by John Hunter.

Pathogenesis and Changes in the Aetiology of Arterio-Venous Fistulae
Schönbach B, Schlosser V (Univ of Freiburg, Germany)
Eur J Vasc Surg 4:233–237, 1990 17–14

A large artery and venous trunk may be connected when both vessels are injured at the same time. A shunt near the heart leads to cardiac volume loading and an increased preload. Vascular enlargement occurs proximally, whereas the section of the artery distal to the fistula is constricted, as is the distal vein. Previously, most arteriovenous fistulas resulted from shotgun, knife, or glass wounds. Today, most such lesions result from injuries incurred during reconstruction or orthopedic surgery, or during procedures involving catheterization.

Forty-two arteriovenous fistulas were surgically treated in the past decade at 1 institution. Three arose spontaneously and 2 were congenital;

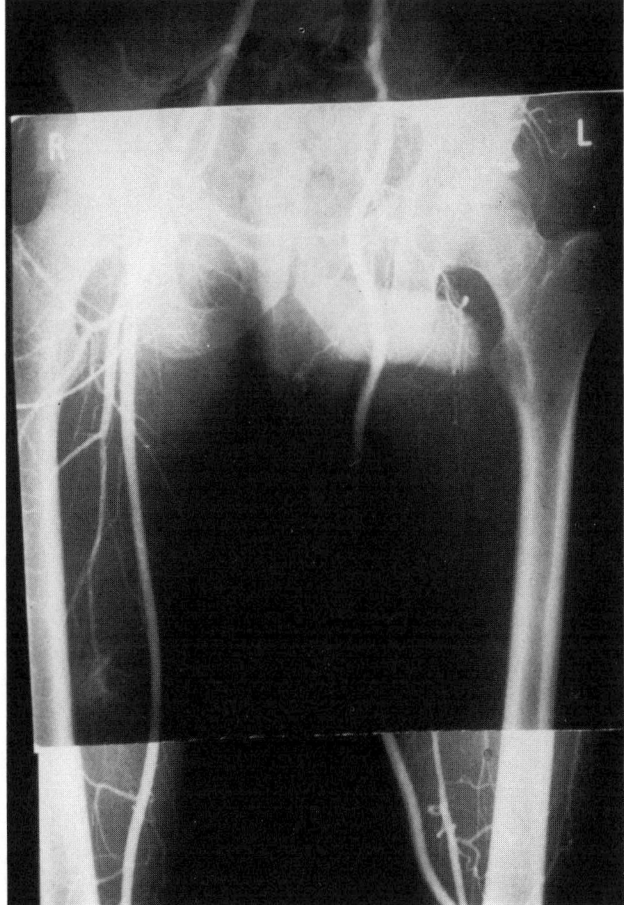

Fig 17–4.—Angiogram showing functioning iliopopliteal obturator graft. (Courtesy of Welch GH, Reid DB, Pollock JG: *Br J Surg* 77:330–333, 1990.)

28 lesions resulted from therapeutic or diagnostic procedures. An old gunshot wound accounted for 4 fistulas, a knife wound for 3, and a glass splinter for 2. Eight fistulas arose in the course of reconstructive skeletal or joint surgery. Catheters used in cardiology, angiology, or neurology accounted for 15 fistulas.

Arteriovenous fistulas resulting from surgical procedures or catheterization should be treated as early as possible. Surgical interruption is a simple approach to recently established fistulas. In operating on a fistula arising from groin catheterization, it may be necessary to repair the walls of the superficial femoral artery as well as a puncture wound in the anterior wall of the deep femoral artery.

▶ Iatrogenic arteriovenous fistulas are almost epidemic. They should be repaired promptly to avoid late complications.

Aneurysmatic Dilatation of Popliteal and Femoral Artery Due to Long-Standing Traumatic Arteriovenous Fistula

Özcan F, Baki C, Pişkin B, Kaptanoğlu M, Yavaş D (Farabi Hosp, Karadeniz Technical Univ, Trabzon, Turkey)

VASA 19:79–81, 1990 17–15

Rupture and thromboembolism are possible complications of arterial dilatations proximal to arteriovenous fistulas (AVFs). One patient experienced complications 24 years after penetrating trauma to her right popliteal fossa.

Woman, 65, had a pulsating mass in the right popliteal fossa. She had sustained penetrating trauma to the fossa 24 years earlier. Her blood pressure was 190/70 mm Hg. Clinical examination revealed irreversible cardiac changes and a continuous murmur at all cardiac focal points. The femoral and popliteal arteries were massively dilated and elongated. The exact location of a long-standing fistula was visible on CT, which also showed a connection between the popliteal artery and vein just above the bifurcation. The patient underwent 10 days of antihypertensive, cardioprotective, and antiaggregation therapy, which reduced her blood pressure to 110/60 mm Hg and improved her cardiac failure. She refused a planned surgical reconstruction, however, and was discharged.

Popliteal aneurysms account for a high proportion of embolic complications in the leg. Traumatic false aneurysms form from the site of trauma or slightly proximally or distally. The development of an aneurysm is facilitated by long duration of an AVF. A solid or pulsatile mass is diagnostic and CT offers the most accurate information about the site of the AVF. Surgical therapy consists of closure of the fistula and repair of the aneurysm. The aneurysmal sac can be bypassed with proximal and distal ligation of the aneurysm. Another option is excision of the aneurysm and end-to-end anastomosis with a saphenous vein or vascular prosthesis.

▶ It is good that our Turkish colleagues call attention once again to the complications that may arise from arteriovenous fistulas and the desirability of their early excision. Cardiac failure rarely occurs immediately after a communication between an artery and vein is established and only when the fistula is very large, but it is a real potential hazard in all save tiniest ones if it is allowed to persist over a period of time. Furthermore, the heart is under stress long before it fails. The development of an aneurysm in the proximally dilated artery is also not common, but the possibility of its occurrence increases progressively with the duration of the fistula. The characteristic continuous murmur and thrill are diagnostic, and the exact site of the shunt can almost always be detected by location of the precise place at which digital compression abolishes these signs. The authors properly call attention to the advisability of closure of the fistula and repair of the vessels and, when an aneurysm or marked arterial dilatation is present, of its excision with interpolation of a graft. Bypassing, with ligation of the aneurysm and fistula, would, however, be a poor choice because the extensive collaterals characteristic of arteriovenous fistulas would probably make this effort unsuccessful in achieving a cure.—Harris B. Shumacker, Jr., M.D., Indianapolis

Retrohepatic Vein Injuries: Experience With 20 Cases
Buechter KJ, Sereda D, Gomez G, Zeppa R (Univ of Miami)
J Trauma 29:1698–1704, 1989 17–16

Improved treatment of liver trauma has decreased mortality, but injuries of the retrohepatic veins continue to be lethal. The records of 185 patients with liver injuries seen in a 5-year period were reviewed. Of these, 20 (11%) had injuries of the retrohepatic veins. There were 17 men and 3 women.

Of the 20 patients with retrohepatic vein injuries, 11 sustained penetrating trauma and 9 blunt trauma. Fifteen patients died; 14 died during surgery of exsanguination, and 1 died of sepsis postoperatively. Nine of 10 patients in whom a shunt was used to bypass the injury died. Six of the 10 patients who did not have shunts also died. Mortality in patients with shunts was 90%; in patients without shunts, it was 60%.

The results support previous reports of a lower mortality with direct exposure and repair of retrohepatic vein injuries. In hypotensive patients total vascular occlusion of the liver may not be well tolerated, but rapid implementation of this approach will probably result in better patient survival than will the use of shunts.

▶ The problems of the retrohepatic caval injury are not resolved.

18 Lymphatics

Long-Term Results After Microlymphaticovenous Anastomoses for the Treatment of Obstructive Lymphedema

O'Brien BMcC, Mellow CG, Khazanchi RK, Dvir E, Kumuar V, Pederson WC (St Vincent's Hosp, Fitzroy, Vic, Australia)

Plast Reconstr Surg 85:562–572, 1990 18–1

Obstructive lymphedema may be treated by microlymphaticovenous anastomosis, either alone or in combination with segmental resection. This treatment was reviewed and measured against treatment objectives of permanent decrease in the size of the affected limb, improved skin texture and consistency, freedom from use of conservative measures, and reduction of episodes of cellulitis.

Eighteen men and 116 women had microlymphaticovenous surgery. The average age of the patients was 52 years. The upper limb was affected in 102 patients and the lower in 32. Edema was bilateral in 4 patients. The average excess volume of edematous limb was 56%. Lymphedema was most commonly caused by surgery and/or radiation treatment for breast cancer. Of patients followed for at least 6 months, 52 had microlymphatic surgery only; 38 also had reduction surgery. In the latter group 30 had segmental reduction and 8 had ablative reduction. The volume and circumference of normal and edematous limbs were measured before surgery and at intervals of 3–6 months thereafter. At follow-up, patients reported the incidence of cellulitis, subjective changes, and requirement for conservative measures.

Subjectively, 75% of the patients were improved, with reduced limb size, better fitting of clothes, softer skin, and decreased incidence of cellulitis. Results were similar in all treatment groups. Objectively, 42% of the microlymphatic group had at least 10% reduction in limb volume, as did 60% of the reduction group (Fig 18–1). The average reduction in limb volume in both groups was 44%. There were no significant differences between those who had segmental reduction and those who had ablative reduction. One third of the patients in both groups had a decrease in circumference of more than 4 cm in the forearm or leg. When lymphedema occurred in the arm or thigh, however, results were better in the reduction group than in the lymphatic group.

Microlymphaticovenous anastomoses should be the treatment of choice in patients with obstructive lymphedema. Reduction surgery may be used as an adjunct, particularly in the posteromedial aspect of the upper arm.

▶ Management of a patient with a swollen leg comes to the attention of vascular surgeons. When the problem is lymphedema, the situation may be frus-

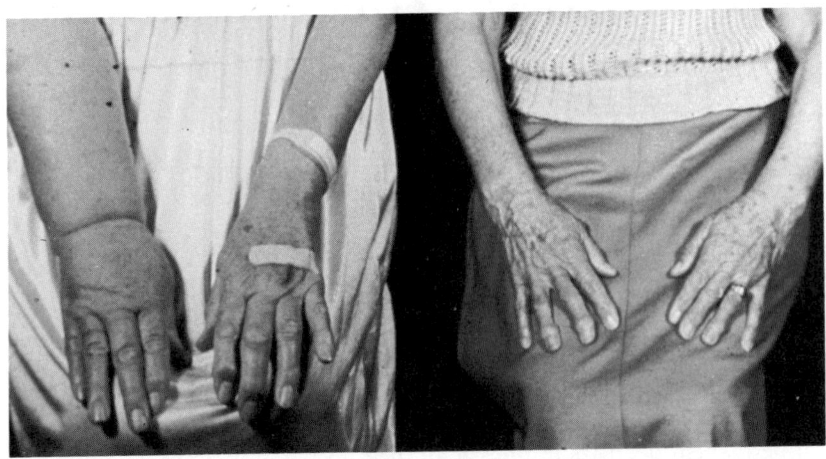

Fig 18–1.—Patient with obstructive lymphedema of right arm. **Left,** before microlymphaticovenous surgery; **right,** 5 years after microlymphaticovenous surgery in the medial upper arm. (Courtesy of O'Brien BMcC, Mellow CG, Khazanchi RK, et al: *Plast Reconstr Surg* 85:562–572, 1990.)

trating because there is little that can be done surgically. On the other hand, patients with disabling lymphedema are enormously grateful for whatever little can be done. O'Brien's work has been looked to for many years and, as indicated in the abstract, his experience is relatively enormous. Most of his patients had acquired lymphedema and a significant number had reconstructive lymphatic surgery as opposed to ablative reduction. His experience now reported with longer-term follow-up suggests that both forms of treatment are palliative but useful.

Treatment of Lymphedemas by Microsurgical Lymphatic Grafting: What Is Proved?

Baumeister RG, Siuda S (Univ of Munich, Munich, West Germany)
Plast Reconstr Surg 85:64–74, 1990 18–2

Lymphedema occurs when there is an imbalance between lymphatic load and lymphatic transport capacity. Lymphatic load is defined as the amount of tissue fluid to be transported from one part of the body to another through the lymphatic system during a given unit of time. The lymphatic system's transport capacity is dependent on the number of available functioning lymphatic vessels. A deficit in transport capacity leads to lymphedema. Data on the first clinical experience with a new microsurgical technique of autogenous lymphatic vessel transplantation were reviewed. The technique involves harvesting lymphatic grafts from the patient's thigh, which are then anastomosed in different ways, depending on the site of lymphatic blockade (Figs 18–2 and 18–3).

During a 6.5-year period, 55 patients with lymphedema of the upper or lower extremities underwent autologous lymphatic vessel transplantation; 37 patients had edema of the upper extremity, in 36 of whom it

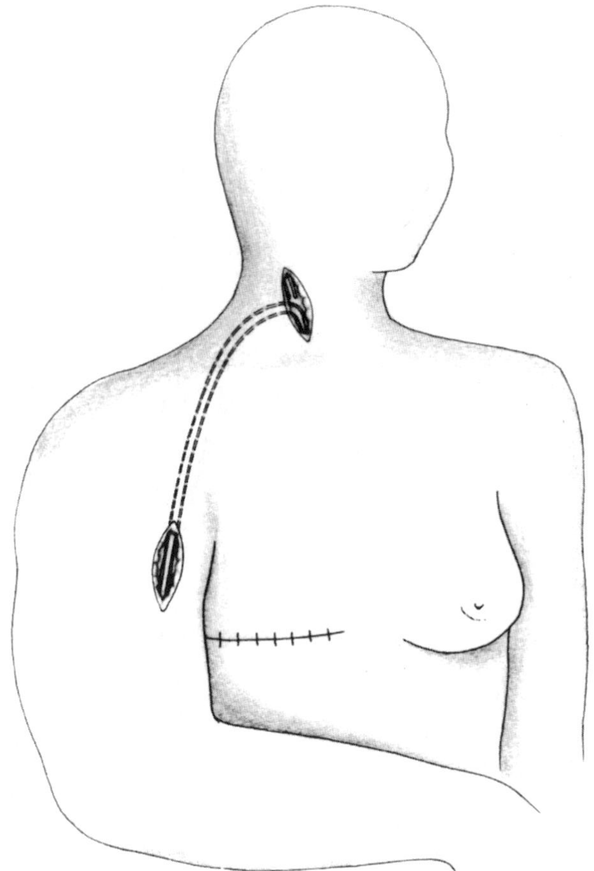

Fig 18–2.—Postmastectomy edema. Lymphatic grafts are interposed between ascending lymphatics at the upper arm and descending deep lymphatics at the neck. (Courtesy of Baumeister RG, Siuda S: *Plast Reconstr Surg* 85:64–74, 1990.)

occurred after mastectomy. Of the 18 patients with lymphedema of a lower extremity, 4 had primary edema, 13 had iatrogenic edema, and 1 had posttraumatic edema; 6 were children or adolescents. The mean interval between onset of edema and lymphatic grafting was 8 years. The functional efficiency and patency of the lymphatic vessel grafts were evaluated by comparing pre- and postoperative volumetric measurements and lymphatic scintiscans.

The mean arm volume in the 36 women with postmastectomy edema decreased from 3,268 cm^3 before operation to 2,509 cm^3 at 2 weeks after operation to 2,436 cm^3 at 2 years. A follow-up of longer than 3 years in 16 women showed a mean decrease to 2,195 cm^3, which was almost similar to the mean volume in normal arms. The mean leg volume in the 12 adults with lower-extremity edema decreased from 11,413 cm^3 before operation to 8,920 cm^3 at 2 weeks after operation to 9,432 cm^3 at 1

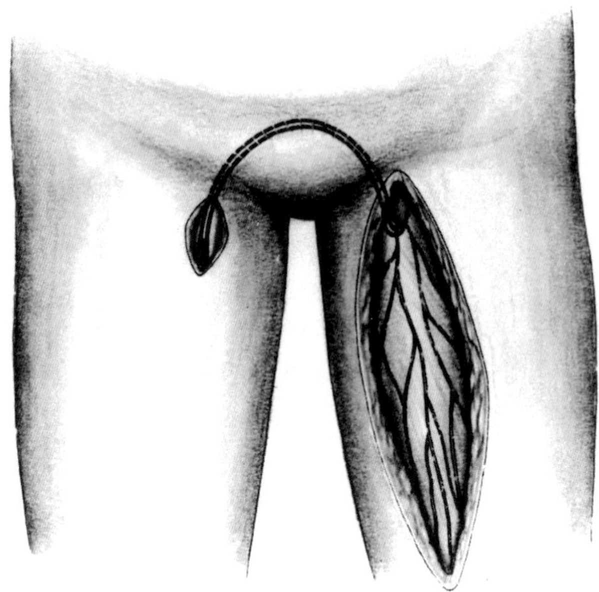

Fig 18.3.—Unilateral lymphedema of lower limb. Lymphatic grafts are transposed by means of the symphysis and are anastomosed with ascending collectors of the affected limb. (Courtesy of Baumeister RG, Siuda S: *Plast Reconstr Surg* 85:64–74, 1990.)

year. Children were followed individually as normal leg volumes vary greatly during growth. These results indicate that nearly 100% patency of the grafted lymphatics can be expected.

▶ The first author, an outstanding microsurgeon, is able to perform lymphatic grafting with patency rates close to 100%, at least in his experiments. In this clinical study of 55 patients, however, only 30 patients had postoperative lymphoscintigraphy to evaluate graft patency and changes in lymph transport capacity. Although the clinical appearance of the extremity and lymphatic transport significantly improved postoperatively, the patency rate of the studied graft was not given by the authors. This group from Munich, however, has provided us with clinical evidence to show that lymphatic grafts stay patent and function for several years after implantation. Patent grafts have been imaged by lymphoscintigraphy in many cases. Because lymph coagulates less than blood, lymphatic grafting probably has a better chance of patency than lymphovenous anastomosis. Also, high venous pressure could not affect the patency of lympholymphatic anastomoses. The paper gives a strong support to the use of lymphatic grafting in the treatment of certain forms of chronic obstructive lymphedema. Technical difficulties in lymphatic microsurgery are considerable, however, thus this operation is still far from routine use. These favorable results need confirmation by other surgical teams and then a correct comparison with conservative compression treatment can be made. This paper brings us a step closer to treating lymphedema. What seems at present impossible, however, is the final goal: to cure this disease.—P. Gloviczki, M.D., Section of Vascular Surgery, Mayo Clinic, Rochester, Minnesota

Adipose Veno-Lymphatic Transfer for Management of Post-Radiation Lymphedema

Pho RWH, Bayon P, Tan L (Singapore Gen Hosp, Singapore)

J Reconstr Microsurg 5:45–54, 1989 18–3

Many techniques have been advocated in the treatment of lymphedema after radiation. Adipose venolymphatic transfer was used to treat a patient with postradiation lymphedema after excision of liposarcoma.

Woman, 55, had gross lymphedema of the leg after 2 resections for liposarcoma and radiotherapy. Despite conservative treatment, the patient had continuing pain and discomfort from the tightness in her calf and thigh. She had repeated attacks of cellulitis. An adipose venolymphatic transfer was performed 4 months after her last attack of cellulitis. The patient was discharged 5 weeks after surgery.

Technique.—Both legs were prepared from the foot up to the groin and suprapubic region. In the donor leg, 1.5 cm of surrounding adipose tissue along the long saphenous vein containing numerous lymphatic channels was isolated and harvested together with the vein. The dissection included the deep fascia, and soft tissue dissection was placed more anteriorly, as it contained more lymphatic channels. The perforator between the deep and superficial systems was ligated and divided. The venous plexus from the long saphenous pedicle and all the intercommunicating branches and perforators in the thigh were divided. The dissection extended to the groin, where the long saphenous vein drains into the femoral vein. A large subcutaneous tunnel was made suprapubically, and the pedicle was tunnelled to the opposite left groin. On the recipient leg a large subcutaneous tunnel was made under the irradiated skin on the medial side of the thigh. The pedicle was tunnelled subcutaneously along the anteromedial aspect of the leg following the long saphenous vein pathway. An incision was made on the posteromedial aspect of the recipient leg, and the posterior tibial artery identified. An end-to-end anastomosis of the distal end of the saphenous vein to the posterior tibial artery was performed to create an arteriovenous fistula in the pedicle. The skin was closed primarily. After the operation, both legs were elevated in elastic stockings.

The patient was discharged after 5 weeks.

▶ As the surgical treatment of lymphedema is frustrating, one must look to new methods to find solutions to the problem. This one, of course, is entirely experimental.

19 Portal Hypertension

Splenic Vein Thrombosis

Simpson WG, Schwartz RW, Strodel WE (Univ of Kentucky)

South Med J 83:417–421, 1990 19–1

Splenic vein thrombosis (SVT) causes localized portal hypertension that results in gastrointestinal (GI) hemorrhage in a high percentage of patients. Splenic vein thrombosis is most often related to inflammatory or neoplastic pancreatic disease. A diagnosis of SVT must be considered in the differential diagnosis of upper GI bleeding, particularly in patients with gastric or gastroesophageal varices.

During a 10-year study period, SVT was documented in 4 women and 2 men aged 42–68 years. Three patients had upper GI hemorrhage and 3 had abdominal pain. Four patients had pancreatitis, including 2 with pancreatic pseudocysts; 1 other had pancreatic carcinoma, and 1 had no pancreatic disease. Three of the 6 patients had an enlarged spleen. Five patients had normal liver function tests; the sixth patient had abnormal liver function tests consistent with acute alcoholic hepatitis.

Four patients had celiac angiography that showed an occluded splenic vein with collateral flow and a patent portal vein (Fig 19–1). All 6 patients underwent splenectomy, with or without additional procedures, to treat the underlying disease process. During a mean follow-up period of 9½ years, the patient with pancreatic carcinoma died at 9 months of recurrent disease. The other 5 patients were alive, and none had experienced further GI bleeding.

Celiac and superior mesenteric artery angiography remains the gold standard for the diagnosis of SVT because it is diagnostic in 100% of the cases. Angiography is essential in the preoperative assessment of patients with suspected SVT because portal vein thrombosis is a contraindication to splenectomy. However, splenectomy is the procedure of choice in the management of SVT because extrahepatic portal hypertension caused by SVT is highly amenable to surgical treatment. Surgical excision of the spleen decreases venous flow through the established collaterals, thus decompressing the system. The surgical outcome is usually good. In contrast, devascularization procedures in the treatment of bleeding resulting from alcohol-associated portal hypertension is associated with a high recurrence of GI hemorrhage.

Splenic vein thrombosis is a curable form of localized portal hypertension that can cause upper GI bleeding. It occurs most often in patients with pancreatic diseases. Splenectomy is the treatment of choice.

▶ In recent years, care of patients with portal hypertension has become less and less the province of surgeons and more and more the domain of gastroen-

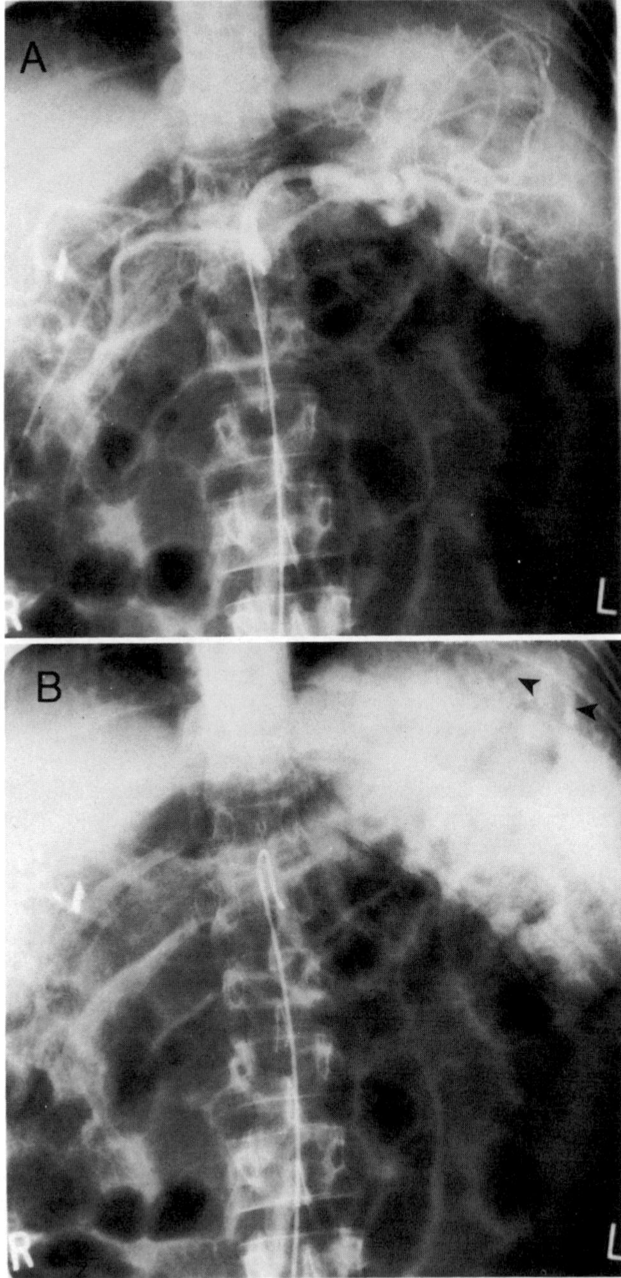

Fig 19–1.—Celiac angiography shows (**A**) splenomegaly and increased pancreatic uptake of contrast material (arterial phase), and (**B**) parenchymal venous pool within the spleen and blood flow through left upper quadrant collaterals *(arrowheads)*. Splenic vein failed to opacify (venous phase). (Courtesy of Simpson WG, Schwartz RW, Strodel WE: *South Med J* 83:417–421, 1990.)

terologists and varicle sclerotherapists. Nevertheless, surgeons remain, as always, ready to treat patients with the complications of less invasive care. Thus the problems of esophageal ulceration, perforation, mediastinitis, esophageal stricture, and failures of sclerotherapy must be addressed surgically and the portal hypertension treated as well. Similarly, splenic vein thrombosis may be best treated by portal decompression with or without splenectomy, and choices of therapy may fall into the hands of the vascular surgeon.

Comfrey Herb Tea-Induced Hepatic Veno-Occlusive Disease
Bach N, Thung SN, Schaffner F (City Univ of New York)
Am J Med 87:97–99, 1989 19–2

The pyrrolizidine alkaloids found in many plants, including comfrey *(Symphytum officinale)*, can act as pulmonary or hepatic intoxicants and cause veno-occlusive disease in the liver. They also have carcinogenic effects in animal models. Comfrey leaves and roots, which are used to brew herbal tea, contain as many as 9 hepatotoxic pyrrolizidine alkaloids, including symphytine and lasiocarpine.

Woman, 47, who complained of abdominal pain and fatigue was told by a homeopathic doctor to drink comfrey tea. After drinking up to 10 cups a day for more than a year and taking comfrey pills by the handful, her serum levels of aminotransferase were raised to twice the normal level. The patient later was hospitalized with massive ascites, hyponatremia, and confusion. A Denver shunt was inserted and she was placed on a low-sodium, fluid-restricted diet. Subsequently, the shunt ceased to function. The initial liver biopsy specimen showed perivenular fibrosis replacing necrotic hepatocytes and mild portal tract fibrosis. Some terminal hepatic venules were narrowed. A biopsy specimen obtained 20 months later showed dense portal tract fibrosis. Most terminal hepatic venules were patent.

Pyrrolizidine alkaloids probably are metabolized in the liver to a toxic substance that causes veno-occlusive disease. Patients should be questioned about all medications, including home remedies, herbal teas, and vitamins. Products sold in health food stores are unregulated and pose a potential health hazard. Consumption of comfrey and its teas should be avoided.

▶ This abstract reports a curiosity. Nevertheless, the case report comes from New York not Bangkok and, as indicated, health food stores are unregulated. Surgeons must be aware of this problem.

Paraprosthetic-Duodenal Fistula Involving a Mesocaval Shunt
Foster WL Jr, Garrett JB, Roberts L Jr, Halvorsen RA Jr (Duke Univ; Durham VA Med Ctrs)
AJR 153:1201–1202, 1989 19–3

Computed tomography is useful in the early diagnosis of aortic graft infections. It is also efficacious in the diagnosis of paraprosthetic-duodenal fistula involving an infected thrombosed mesocaval shunt.

Man, 58, with a history of an H-shaped mesocaval shunt, was admitted for evaluation of fever of unknown origin, abdominal pain, and weight loss. The guaiac test was positive. Abdominal CT showed the mesocaval shunt, complete anterior effacement of the transverse duodenum, and air in the superior mesenteric vein. The biplane inferior venacavogram showed thrombosis of the shunt with a paraprosthetic-duodenal fistula. At surgery, a small purulent cavity at the suture line joining the graft and the duodenal wall, graft erosion into the duodenal wall, and graft thrombosis were noted. The shunt was removed and the duodenum closed. The postoperative course was complicated by septic shock with hypotension bradycardia, and metabolic acidosis. The patient died.

Mesocaval shunt construction involves either direct surgical anastomosis or interposition of an H-graft between the superior mesenteric vein and the inferior vena cava and can be related closely to the transverse third and fourth duodenum. The paraprosthetic-enteric fistula may result from operative ischemia or mechanical factors, with erosion of adjacent bowel wall by the noncompliant, pulsatile graft and subsequent infection. Computed tomography is the procedure of choice in evaluation of a patient with previous vascular surgery and occult sepsis or gastrointestinal blood loss.

▶ To the axiom, "Every prosthesis will fail," we must add, "some will erode adjacent structures."

20 Vena Cava Surgery

Pacemaker-Induced Superior Vena Cava Syndrome: Report of Four Cases and Review of the Literature
Goudevenos JA, Reid PG, Adams PC, Holden MP, Williams DO (Freeman Hosp, Newcastle-Upon-Tyne, England)
PACE 12:1890–1895, 1989 20–1

Superior vena cava (SVC) syndrome is a rare but potentially serious complication of transvenous pacing leads. Data on 4 patients with pacemaker-induced SVC syndrome were reviewed as was the existing literature. One patient was among 3,100 who underwent primary pacemaker insertions performed at the institution and the other 3 were referrals. All patients had evidence of infection preceding the SVC syndrome; 3 had severed retained leads. Venous angiography was useful in showing the site of obstruction.

Data on more than 30 patients with SVC occlusion have been reported. The pathogenesis of SVC occlusion remains unknown, but pathology at the site of obstruction showed thrombosis in most of the patients and fibrotic narrowing in some. Factors that predispose to SVC occlusion include local infection and presence of severed retained leads. The presence of multiple leads does not significantly increase the risk. Symptoms of SVC obstruction occur between 1 month and 15 years after the initial implantation and 15 weeks to 7 years after the last intervention. Venous angiography defines the site of obstruction and extent of collateral circulation, and assesses treatment response. Treatment includes removal of any infected pacemaker apparatus, anticoagulation, and thrombolytic therapy when symptoms are of recent onset. Most patients improve, but angioplasty or surgery may be warranted in some patients to relieve the obstruction.

▶ Subclavian venous thrombosis is common after subclavian vein catheterization by whatever technique. Extension to superior vena cava obstruction is less common but is regularly seen. The consequences of this condition are further explored in subsequent abstracts.

Superior Vena Cava Syndrome: The Myth–The Facts
Yellin A, Rosen A, Reichert N, Lieberman Y (Chaim Sheba Med Ctr, Tel Hashomer, Israel)
Am Rev Respir Dis 141:1114–1118, 1990 20–2

It often is not recognized that many mediastinal disorders other than bronchogenic carcinoma may cause superior caval obstruction. Data were reviewed on 63 patients seen from 1972 to 1987 with superior vena cava (SVC) syndrome. The annual incidence rose steadily during the review period. Seven children younger than 10 years of age were included.

Twenty patients had known disease that produced caval obstruction; half of them had bronchogenic carcinoma. Symptoms were present for a relatively long time before admission but for a shorter time in patients with malignant disease. Ultimately, 52 patients had a diagnosis of malignancy. Surgery was reserved for patients who had treatable vascular problems or a benign mediastinal tumor. Lymphomas were treated with curative intent. Eighty percent of nonterminal patients improved to some degree. Survival was best in patients with benign disorders, followed by those with lymphoma. Patients presenting with SVC syndrome require prompt and comprehensive assessment. Every attempt should be made to achieve a precise tissue or anatomical diagnosis.

▶ As expected, the SVC syndrome is being encountered more frequently. Nonmalignant causes are increasing. The condition was first described by William Hunter in 1757 and aortic aneurysms dominated the cause of the problem until this century. Now, the severity of the SVC syndrome depends on the rapidity of occlusion and the degree of collateral development. Clearly, the more chronic the occlusive process, the less severe the symptomatology. Spontaneous relief of even acute symptoms may occur as collateralization develops further. Severe complications include laryngeal and cerebral edema, and these may require emergency treatment. Respiratory embarrassment is not regularly seen.

Bypass of Superior Vena Cava: Fifteen Years' Experience With Spiral Vein Graft for Obstruction of Superior Vena Cava Caused by Benign Disease

Doty DB, Doty JR, Jones KW (LDS Hosp, Salt Lake City)

J Thorac Cardiovasc Surg 99:889–896, 1990 20–3

Data on 9 patients who underwent surgery for superior caval obstruction were reviewed. Superior vena cava (SVC) syndrome was caused by benign disease in these patients, most often fibrosing mediastinitis with or without caseating granulomas.

Composite spiral vein grafts were made from the patients' saphenous vein, split longitudinally, and wrapped about a stent. The vein edges were joined together to form a conduit 9.5–15 mm in diameter (Fig 20–1). Of the grafts, 6 were from the left innominate vein and 3 from the internal jugular vein; 8 grafts were placed in the right atrial appendage and 1 in the distal superior cava. The patients were followed for up to 15 years after surgery.

Reoperation was necessary in 1 patient because of thrombosis of an innominate vein-graft anastomosis; 2 grafts closed within a year of placement, and 1 patient had recurrent spontaneous venous thrombosis. All patients but 1 remained free of SVC syndrome during follow-up.

The composite spiral saphenous vein graft procedure to bypass the obstructed SVC consistently relieves symptoms of SVC syndrome in patients

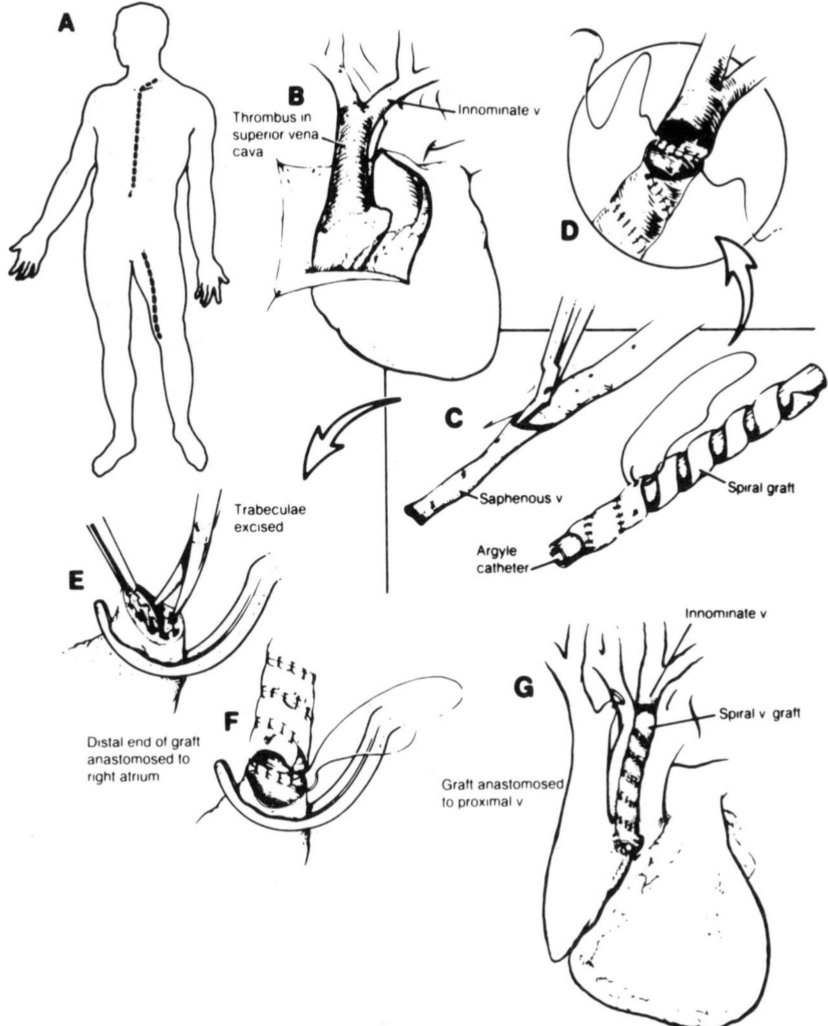

Fig 20–1.—Bypass of SVC with composite spiral vein graft. **A,** midsternal incision with extension to neck if necessary. Simultaneous thigh incision over greater saphenous vein. **B,** pericardium opened to expose right atrial appendage. Innominate vein is mobilized. Biopsy specimen of obstructing process surrounding SVC is obtained. **C,** saphenous vein opened longitudinally, wrapped around stent catheter in spiral fashion, and edges sutured together with 7-0 polypropylene to form composite spiral vein graft. **D,** end-to-end anastomosis of vein graft to innominate vein. **E,** right atrial appendage is excluded, the tip excised, and all trabeculae removed. **F,** anastomosis of vein graft to right atrial appendage. **G,** completed bypass graft. (Courtesy of Lamberth WC, Doty DB: Peripheral Vascular Surgery. Chicago: Year Book Medical Publishers, 1987:317. From Doty DB, Doty JR, Jones KW: *J Thorac Cardiovasc Surg* 99:889–896, 1990.)

with benign disease. Long-term patency is the rule, and the operation is not unduly risky.

▶ In the Mississippi Valley, fibrosing medastinitis would be a cause of the SVC obstructive syndrome, and when prominent CNS symptoms occur, the spiral vein bypass technique described may be a useful adjunct to treatment in selected cases. In a patient with a benign condition who experiences gradual worsening of symptoms, phlebography should be performed bilaterally simultaneously and consideration given to direct SVC reconstruction. At this time, externally supported polytetrafluoroethylene grafts present a reasonable alternative and could be used in patients with slowly growing malignancies.

Reconstruction of the Vena Cava and of Its Primary Tributaries: A Preliminary Report

Gloviczki P, Pairolero PC, Cherry KJ, Hallett JW Jr (Mayo Clinic and Found, Rochester, Minn)

J Vasc Surg 11:373–381, 1990 20–4

The vena cava or its major tributaries, or both were reconstructed in 16 patients aged 8–81 years in 1981–1989. Eight patients had superior

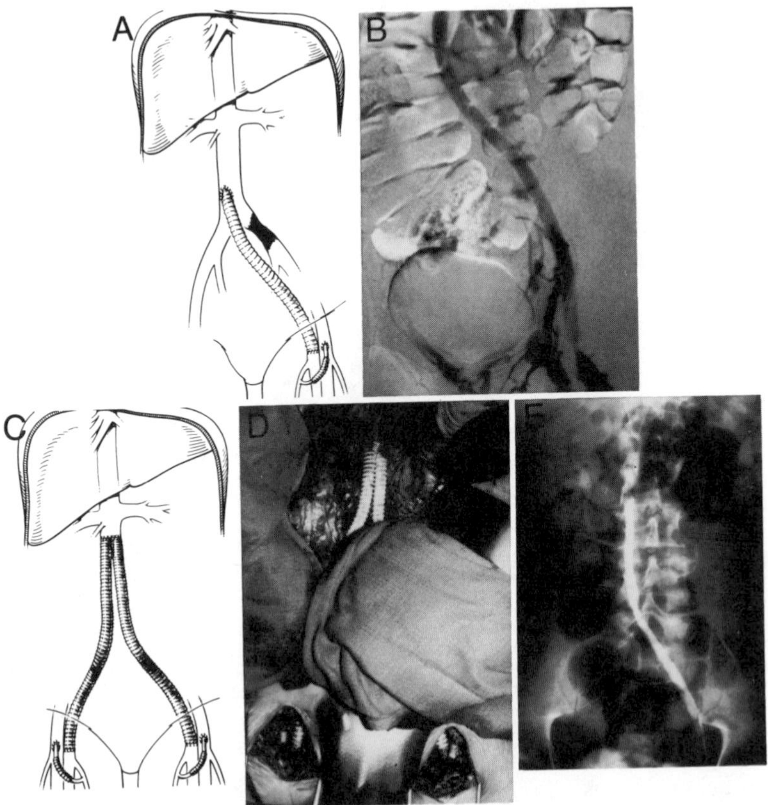

Fig 20–2.—**A**, left femorocaval expanded PTFE graft with a femoral arteriovenous fistula. **B**, postoperative venogram shows patency of the graft. **C** and **D**, artist's conception and intraoperative photograph of a bifemorocaval expanded PTFE graft with bilateral femoral arteriovenous fistula. **E**, left femoral venogram performed at 6 months confirms patency of the graft. (Courtesy of Gloviczki P, Pairolero PC, Cherry KJ, et al: *J Vasc Surg* 11:373–381, 1990.)

vena cava (SVC) syndrome, caused in 2 of them by malignant neoplasms. Two others had membranous occlusion of the inferior vena cava, and 4 had iliocaval venous thrombosis. One patient had undergone iliac vein excision for pelvic neurilemoma, and 1 sustained inferior caval injury during liver transplantation.

The SVC was reconstructed with a spiral saphenous vein graft in 5 patients and with expanded polytetrafluoroethylene (PTFE) in 3. One graft of each type had to be revised, but 7 of the 8 SVC grafts were patent at follow-up. A bifurcated spiral saphenous vein graft was occluded at 3 months. The inferior cava and its tributaries were reconstructed with expanded PTFE in 5 patients, a spiral saphenous vein graft in 2, and Dacron in 1. Four PTFE grafts were patent at follow-up. Two of 3 grafts with a concomitant temporary arteriovenous fistula at the groin were patent (Fig 20–2). One spiral saphenous vein graft was occluded and the other was not evaluable. The Dacron graft occluded, but the patient had only minimal symptoms.

The spiral saphenous vein graft is preferred for reconstructing the SVC. Expanded PTFE grafts give better results in the abdomen. Caval grafting is appropriate for patients who have significant symptoms of venous stasis that cannot be improved with other forms of treatment.

▶ This is destined to be a landmark report simply because the Mayo group is extremely experienced and wisely utilized the spiral vein graft when possible. Their experience indicates that PTFE is a good alternative and may be the graft material of choice wherever extrinsic pressure is to be expected, such as in the abdomen.

Vena Caval Involvement by Renal Cell Carcinoma: Surgical Resection Provides Meaningful Long-Term Survival

Skinner DG, Pritchett TR, Lieskovsky G, Boyd SD, Stiles QR (Univ of Southern California, Los Angeles)

Ann Surg 210:387–394, 1989 20–5

Results of a previous study demonstrated that vena caval extension by tumor thrombus is a potentially curable lesion, provided that complete removal is achieved. A new technique was developed for the safe removal of extensive vena caval thrombi extending up to the right atrium without the need for cardiopulmonary bypass or hypothermic cardioplegia (Fig 20–3). Cardiovascular bypass is advocated for some type III thrombi, but the addition of the pump and heparinization compounds the magnitude of the procedure. A right thoracoabdominal approach is used for tumors arising from either kidney with vascular isolation of the vena cava from its insertion into the right atrium to the iliac bifurcation.

From 1972 to 1988, 56 patients aged 31–76 years with venal caval tumor thrombus secondary to renal cell carcinoma were evaluated. Of these, 53 underwent radical nephrectomy with en bloc vena caval tumor thrombectomy. Subhepatic caval thrombus extension (level 1) occurred

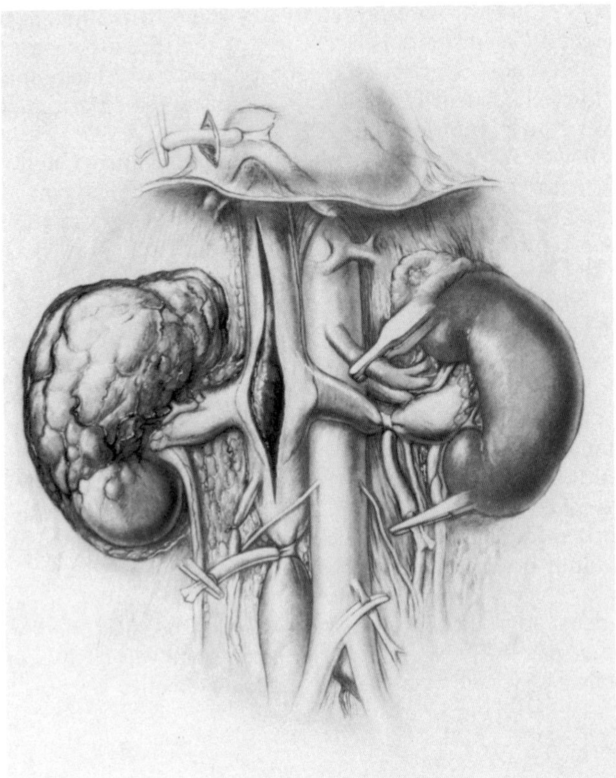

Fig 20–3.—Surgical maneuvers necessary for a safe and effective method of removing all tumor thrombus. For tumors with levels 2 and 3 extension, a vertical pericardiotomy is performed; the phrenic nerve is avoided and a Rumel tourniquet is applied loosely around the intrathoracic inferior vena cava at this level. The superior mesenteric artery is isolated and occluded with a soft Fogarty vascular clamp. The inferior mesenteric artery is similarly occluded. Two Crafoord vascular clamps are placed on the porta hepatis, after which the Rumel tourniquets on the distal vena cava, the contralateral renal vein, and finally the intrathoracic cava are tightened, isolating the vena cava from all venous inflow except for pooled blood within the hepatic system. For left-sided tumors, a soft Fogarty vascular clamp is placed on the right renal artery, thus obviating the need to occlude the right renal vein. (Reproduced by permission from Skinner D, Lieskovsky G, eds: *Diagnosis and Management of Genitourinary Cancer*. Philadelphia, WB Saunders, 1988, p. 699. From Skinner DG, Pritchett TR, Lieskovsky G, et al: *Ann Surg* 210:387–394, 1989.)

in 21 patients, extension into the intrahepatic vena cava (level 2) occurred in 24, and thrombi extending into the heart (level 3) occurred in 8. The 5-year actuarial survival rates for level 1 tumors was 35%; level 2, 18; and level 3, 0%. Complete excision of all grossly recognized tumor was achieved in 75% of patients. The 5-year actuarial survival rates of these patients with successful extirpation was 34% compared with only 8% at 1 year in patients in whom complete resection was impossible. The 5-year actuarial survival rate for patients without metastatic disease recognized before operation was 32%, whereas none of the 27 patients who had metastatic disease at the time of surgery lived for 5 years.

Complete surgical excision of vena caval tumor extension by renal cell carcinoma provides meaningful long-term survival in these patients. Factors affecting survival include level of the vena caval tumor extension, extent of local tissue involvement, whether a complete excision of all tumor was possible, and the presence of metastatic disease. An aggressive, optimistic approach is advocated for patients if there is no preoperative evidence of metastatic disease.

▶ The level of extension of the intracaval thrombus seems to be an important factor in estimating prognosis in patients with malignant tumors extending into the vena cava. Those with tumor thrombus extending only to the level of the hepatic veins have a very favorable prognosis, whereas those with extension proximally do not. There seems to be little evidence that metastatic disease regresses after debulking of the major tumor.

Fiberoptic Examination of the Inferior Vena Cava During Circulatory Arrest for Complete Removal of Renal Cell Carcinoma Thrombus
Hartman AR, Zelen J, Mason RA, Bumpers HL, Washeka R (Univ Hosp, Stony Brook, NY)
Surgery 107:695–697, 1990 20–6

Renal cell carcinoma can invade the inferior vena cava and may extend over its entire length. Profound hypothermic circulatory arrest is an effective means of facilitating the removal of tumor thrombus from the vessel while limiting the amount of blood loss. In 1 man complete removal of

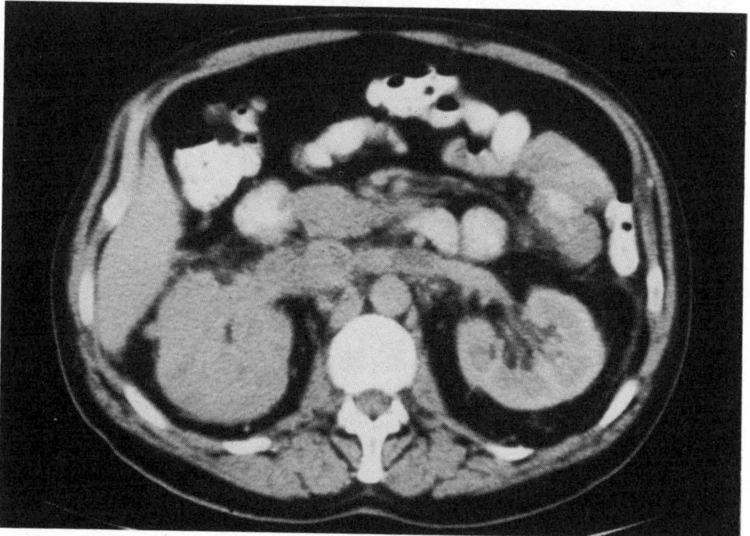

Fig 20–4.—Computed tomography scan demonstrating right renal tumor with extension into right renal vein and inferior vena cava and tumor-thrombus in left renal vein. (Courtesy of Hartman AR, Zelen J, Mason RA, et al: *Surgery* 107:695–697, 1990.)

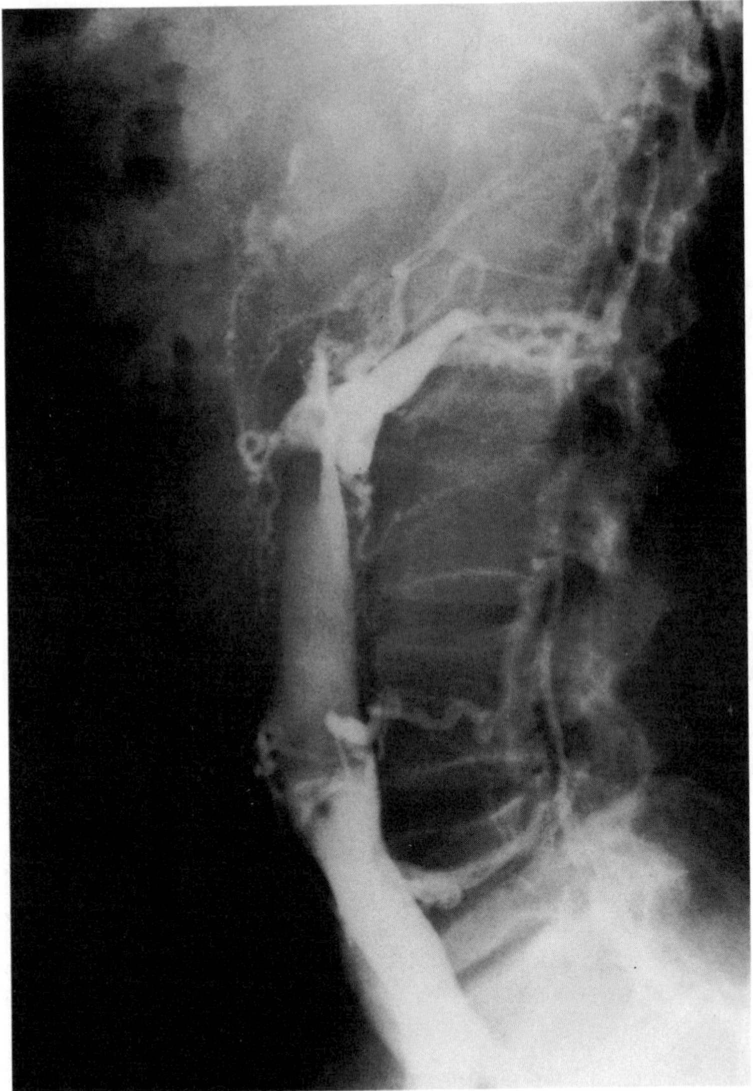

Fig 20–5.—Inferior venacavogram demonstrating lower extent of tumor. There is large venous collateral flow. (Courtesy of Hartman AR, Zelen J, Mason RA, et al: *Surgery* 107:695–697, 1990.)

thrombus was insured by introducing a fiberoptic bronchoscope through the right atrium.

Man, 54, with hematuria, was found to have a large mass that almost completely replaced the right kidney and extended into the inferior vena cava and right renal vein (Fig 20–4). In a venocavogram via the right femoral vein, obstruction was seen at the level of the renal vein, with extensive collateral formation (Fig 20–5). Thrombotic material was present in the vena cava at the level of the hepatic veins. After right radical nephrectomy, cardiopulmonary bypass was instituted via a median sternotomy, avoiding the inferior caval orifice. Profound hypothermia was obtained with venous exsanguination. Thrombotic material was removed from the left renal vein and a balloon catheter was advanced from the vena cava to the right atrium, inflated, and pulled back to deliver tumor thrombus. A fiberoptic bronchoscope, placed in the vena cava via the right atrium, disclosed a large amount of tumor thrombus on the anterior surface of the retrohepatic vena cava. This thrombus was removed. Thrombus also was removed from the right iliofemoral vein. A Greenfield filter was advanced to just below the left renal vein. Circulatory arrest lasted for 73 minutes. The patient was neurologically intact after surgery and end-organ ischemia did not occur. He was discharged on day 9 with warfarin therapy prescribed.

Venacavoscopy is a logical addition to hypothermic circulatory arrest when extensive inferior vena caval tumor thrombus has to be removed. Complete removal of tumor is thereby assured.

▶ Angioscopy is now a common practice in the operating room, supplementing intraoperative arteriographic findings. This technique represents yet another use of the endoscopic technique.

21 Thromboembolism

Trends in Pulmonary Embolism Death Rates for Canada and the United States, 1962–87

Soskolne CL, Wong AW, Lilienfeld DE (Univ of Alberta, Edmonton; Mount Sinai School of Medicine, New York)

Can Med Assoc J 142:321–324, 1990 21–1

The rates of death from pulmonary embolism in Canada for the years 1965–1987 were compared with those of the United States for 1962–1984. Age- and sex-specific death rates were calculated for each year using the 1960 United States population as standard.

In both countries, the age-standardized and sex-specific rates of death caused by pulmonary embolism increased and then decreased, but the Canadian trends in death rates tended to be less pronounced and peaked or plateaued later than the United States rates. The average annual age-standardized death rates for Canada peaked 5 years after those of the United States, whereas the Canadian age-specific death rates peaked 5–10 years after those of the United States. In both countries, men and elderly persons were at higher risk of death from pulmonary embolism.

The decrease in death rates from pulmonary embolism in both countries may be attributed to advances in the prevention and treatment of this lesion. Prevention strategies, such as encouraging a more active lifestyle and targeting high-risk groups, may further reduce mortality from pulmonary embolism in both countries.

▶ Although the epidemiology of pulmonary thromboembolic disease is emphasized in this report, the facts of occurrence are of greater interest to vascular surgeons. Many times, pulmonary thromboembolic death occurs in a young person and follows minor surgical or vascular trauma or even arthroscopy. Care of patients with thromboembolic disease is partly the province of the vascular surgeon, who must be aware of the various modalities of diagnosis and care.

A Prospective Study of Hand-Held Doppler Ultrasonography by Emergency Physicians in the Evaluation of Suspected Deep-Vein Thrombosis

Turnbull TL, Dymowski JJ, Zalut TE (Mercy Hosp and Med Ctr, Chicago; Good Samaritan Hosp, Downers Grove, Ill)

Ann Emerg Med 19:691–695, 1990 21–2

Use of a hand-held Doppler stethoscope is a potentially simple bedside test for deep vein thrombosis (DVT). A prospective study of this device was carried out in 2 community hospitals. Emergency department physicians evaluated 78 extremities in 76 patients by both Doppler ultrasonography and contrast venography. A Medasonics 5.3-MHz Doppler stethoscope was used.

Venography confirmed DVT in 22 extremities. Three falsely negative Doppler studies were obtained, along with 9 false positive studies. The Doppler examination was 85% sensitive and 79% specific, and had positive and negative predictive values of 65% and 92%, respectively. Only 2 of 16 patients with equivocal findings had DVT. Ultrasonography identified all but 1 of 15 proximal thrombi.

The Doppler stethoscope is a highly accurate means of diagnosing DVT at the bedside. It may be useful for confirming thrombosis in high-risk patients whose clinical findings are consistent with DVT.

▶ Although this report focuses on the use of a hand-held, continuous-wave device by emergency physicians, in fact, the vascular surgeon often becomes the evaluating physician in the emergency room, on the hospital ward, and in the office. Fortunately, very few false negative studies are found and the false positive studies only lead to early therapy. The dangerous thrombi are proximal, and the simple technique of Doppler ultrasonography aided in the diagnosis of 14 of 15 such thrombi in this series.

Diagnosis of Deep Vein Thrombosis With Colour-Coded Duplex Sonography

Fobbe F, Koennecke H-C, El Bedewi M, Heidt P, Boese-Landgraf J, Wolf K-J
(Freie Universität Berlin, Germany)

Fortschr Röntgenstr 151:569–573, 1989 21–3

Patients suspected of deep vein thrombosis (DVT) in the lower limbs or pelvic area in whom clinical signs are inconclusive require further investigation. Because of the high risk of pulmonary embolism in these patients, a noninvasive, simple, rapid, and reliable method is needed to confirm the diagnosis. Color-coded duplex sonography has been available for 2 years. As a refinement of conventional duplex sonography, this technique enables simultaneous real-time visualization of soft tissue and blood flow. Whether color-coded duplex sonography provides more accurate diagnostic information than other noninvasive methods, and whether the technique is reliable enough to replace phlebography, were assessed in 49 men and 54 women aged 18–87 years with suspected DVT in 129 legs.

Phlebography was completed within 4 hours of the sonographic examination. The pelvic veins, popliteal veins, and femoral veins were examined. There was 100% agreement between sonographic and phlebographic diagnoses in the pelvic vein and popliteal vein examinations, but sonographic examination gave 2 false positive and 2 false negative results in the femoral vein examinations. The sensitivity of color-coded duplex sonography for detecting fresh venous thromboses in the lower limbs was 96% and the specificity was 97%. It would appear that color-coded duplex sonography can safely replace phlebography.

▶ The diagnosis of DVT must be corroborated by objective techniques, and the duplex scan has emerged as the most attractive of these.

Clinical Significance of Free-Floating Venous Thrombi

Baldridge ED, Martin MA, Welling RE (Good Samaritan Hosp, Cincinnati; Univ of Cincinnati)

J Vasc Surg 11:62–69, 1990 21–4

The incidence, natural history, and clinical significance of free-floating thrombi were studied in a retrospective review of venous duplex scans of 5,238 lower extremities seen during a 2½-year period. Acute deep venous thrombosis (DVT) was diagnosed in 732 patients. Of these, 73 had 82 free-floating thrombi (Fig 21–1); pulmonary embolism was confirmed by ventilation perfusion scanning in 9 of these patients.

Pulmonary emboli were diagnosed before the free-floating emboli were recognized in 7 of these patients, and 2 had pulmonary emboli after the diagnosis of free-floating thrombi. Follow-up duplex scanning was performed on 33 patients during the acute period of 30 days (mean, 7 days); in 18 of these attachment of the free-floating thrombus was observed. In 8 others the free-floating thrombus decreased in size or resolved totally; progression in size of the free-floating thrombus was noted in 3; and persistent thrombus without resolution, propagation, embolism, or attachment was observed in 4.

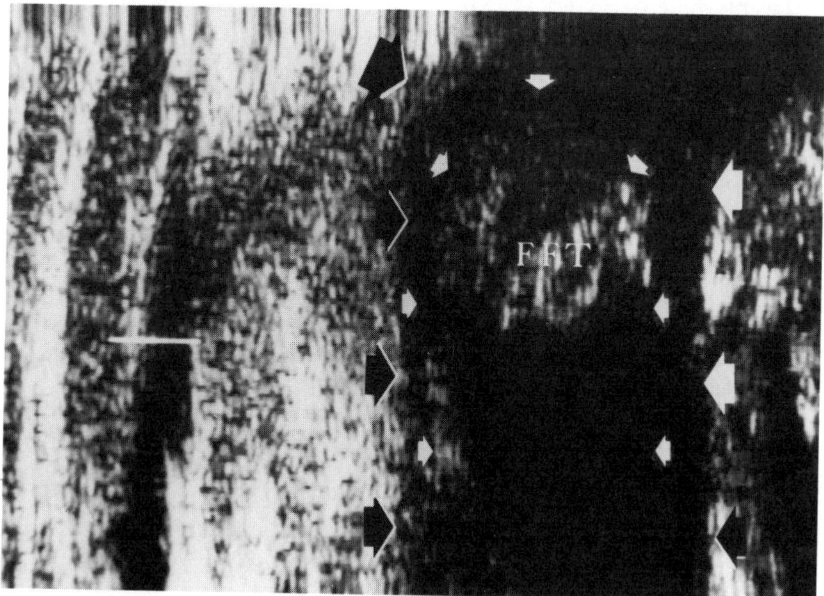

Fig 21–1.—Longitudinal view of free-floating thrombus *(FFT)* in common femoral vein. Note ball-shaped tip indicated by *small arrows; large arrows* indicate vein wall. (Courtesy of Baldrige ED, Martin MA, Welling RE: *J Vasc Surg* 11:62–69, 1990.)

Free-floating venous thrombosis occurs in 10% of acute DVT. Free-floating thrombi are not associated with an increased incidence of pulmonary embolization, and most pulmonary emboli would have occurred by the time free-floating thrombi are recognized. Most free-floating emboli become attached to the wall or resolve. Hence, routine operative treatment of infrainguinal free-floating thrombi is not recommended.

▶ When free-floating thrombi were first seen by duplex technique, they were thought to be very dangerous. This report puts those findings into a pleasant perspective.

Detection of Previous Proximal Venous Thrombosis With Doppler Ultrasonography and Photoplethysmography

Ginsberg JS, Shin A, Turpie AGG, Hirsh J (McMaster Univ, Hamilton, Ont)

Arch Intern Med 149:2255–2257, 1989 21–5

The reliability of venous Doppler ultrasound and photoplethysmography (PPG), 2 noninvasive techniques that can detect venous valvular incompetence, in determining the presence or absence of previous proximal deep vein thrombosis (DVT) was assessed in a blind, retrospective study. Thirty-three patients with objectively confirmed (DVT^+) and 49 with refuted (DVT^-) previous episodes of suspected DVT were included.

Twenty-nine of 33 DVT^+ patients had abnormal findings on PPGs or reflux by venous Doppler ultrasound, or both, whereas 39 of 49 DVT^- patients had normal findings on PPGs and no Doppler reflux. The combined PPG and Doppler ultrasound studies had a sensitivity of 88%, a specificity of 80%, and positive and negative predictive values of 74% and 91%, respectively. Twenty of the 33 DVT^+ patients had abnormal results on Doppler studies (sensitivity, 61%) as compared to 46 of 49 DVT^- patients with normal results (specificity, 94%). The positive and negative predictive values of an abnormal Doppler result were 87% and 78%, respectively.

Moreover, 23 of 33 DVT^+ patients had abnormal results on PPG (sensitivity, 70%), whereas 40 of 49 DVT^- patients had normal findings at PPG (specificity, 82%). The positive and negative predictive values of PPG were 72% and 80%, respectively.

The combination of PPG and venous Doppler ultrasound can reliably predict the presence or absence of previous proximal DVT in most patients. The presence of Doppler reflux is specific for previous proximal DVT, but the absence of a reflux does not exclude it. The combination of abnormal findings at PPG and normal findings on Doppler ultrasound does not reliably predict the presence or absence of previous DVT.

▶ The addition of the PPG to Doppler ultrasonography needlessly complicates the diagnosis of DVT.

Diagnostic Value of the Combination of Ultrasonography–Plethysmography in Deep Vein Thromboses of the Lower Limbs

de Laveaucoupet J, Morel MP, Philippoteau C, Simoneau G, Musset D (Hôp Antoine-Béclère, Paris)

Sem Hôp Paris 66:1399–1406, 1990 21–6

Phlebography is the reference examination for diagnosing deep vein thrombosis (DVT) in the lower limbs; however, the use of contrast medium is not free of potential complications. Noninvasive impedance plethysmography done with the occlusive cuff technique has a sensitivity of 90% to 100% for diagnosing DVT in the proximal part of the leg, but its sensitivity for identifying DVT in the distal part of the leg is insufficient. Several experiences with high-resolution, real-time ultrasonography in the diagnosis of DVT have been reported. A prospective study was

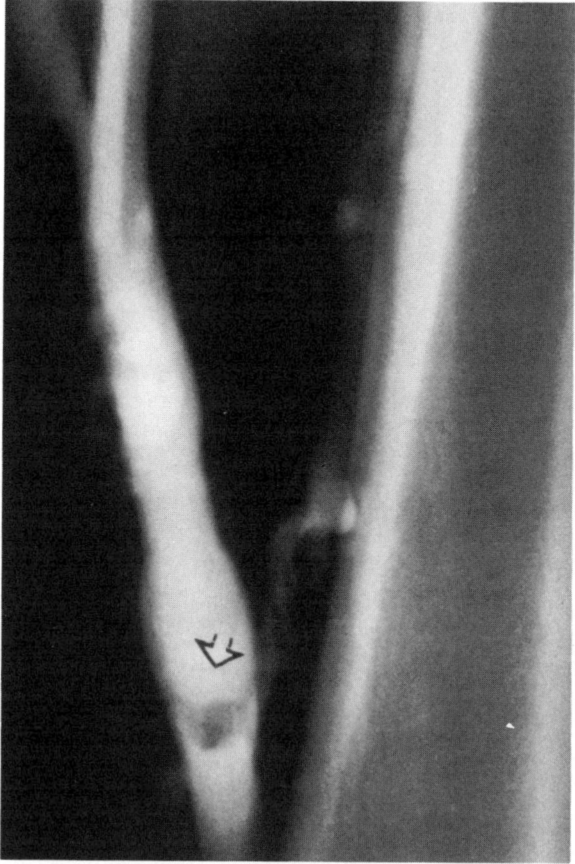

Fig 21–2.—False negative ultrasound: phlebography reveals a floating clot in the left superficial femoral vein. (Courtesy of de Laveaucoupet J, Morel MP, Philippoteau C, et al: *Sem Hôp Paris* 66:1399–1406, 1990.)

done to determine whether the combination of impedance plethysmography and real-time ultrasound would have sensitivity and specificity great enough for diagnosing DVT of the lower extremities so that the venographic examination may be omitted.

Of 39 females and 31 males aged 15–90 years (mean, 62 years), 75% were hospitalized and 25% were examined as outpatients. Indications for examination included either clinical suspicion of DVT or a recent history of pulmonary embolism. Phlebography, real-time ultrasound, and plethysmography of 140 legs were carried out within a 24-hour period, each procedure being performed by different operators. The results were interpreted independently.

Phlebography identified 1 or more DVT in the lower extremities of 33 patients. Ultrasonography could not be performed in 7 legs because of fat or edema in the lower leg, leaving 133 evaluable legs. Ultrasonography missed 12 phlebographically confirmed DVTs, of which 1 was in the internal saphenous vein, 1 in the iliac vein, and 1 in the superficial femoral vein (Fig 21–2). Real-time ultrasound had a sensitivity of 69% and a specificity of 98% for identifying DVT when compared with the reference venographic examination. Impedance plethysmography could not be performed in 15 legs because of ascites, retroperitoneal hematoma, recent abdominal surgery, obesity, or edema, leaving 125 evaluable legs. Plethysmography missed 16 DVTs, for a sensitivity of 57% and a specificity of 90%. When the results of real-time ultrasound and plethysmography were combined, the overall sensitivity for detecting DVT in the lower extremities was 69%, and the sensitivity for detecting DVT in the proximal part of the leg was 90%. The overall sensitivity of the 2 methods combined was 91%.

The addition of plethysmography to ultrasound in the diagnosis of DVT of the lower limbs produced results no better than ultrasound alone. Thus adding plethysmography provides no more information than real-time ultrasound alone, and the venographic examination cannot be safely omitted.

▶ Duplex scanning does not require the addition of plethysmography in diagnosis of DVT.

Deep Venous Thrombosis of Extremities: Role of MR Imaging in the Diagnosis

Erdman WA, Jayson HT, Redman HC, Miller GL, Parkey RW, Peshock RW (Univ of Texas, Dallas)

Radiology 174:425–431, 1990 21–7

Failure to demonstrate central vein involvement and to distinguish acute from chronic changes significantly limits the applicability of current noninvasive imaging techniques in the diagnosis of deep venous thrombosis (DVT) of extremities. The role of spin-echo MRI in the diagnosis of

DVT was determined in 100 patients suspected of having either upper or lower extremity DVT.

In a subset of 36 patients studied prospectively with both MRI and contrast venography, the sensitivity of MRI for DVT was 90%, specificity was 100%, and the kappa level of agreement was .752. Compared with venography, MRI clearly demonstrated a more central extent of the thrombus in all 5 patients with upper extremity DVT and in 13 of 25 patients with lower extremity thrombus.

All 19 patients with upper extremity thrombus had acute disease as evidenced by perivascular edema and nonretracted thrombus on MRI. Among the 40 patients with lower extremity DVT, MRI showed signs of chronic disease such as large collateral vessels, absence of edema, a partially thrombosed lumen, and recanalization in 13 (33%) (Fig 21–3), and acute changes in 27 (67%). Furthermore, MRI showed extravascular

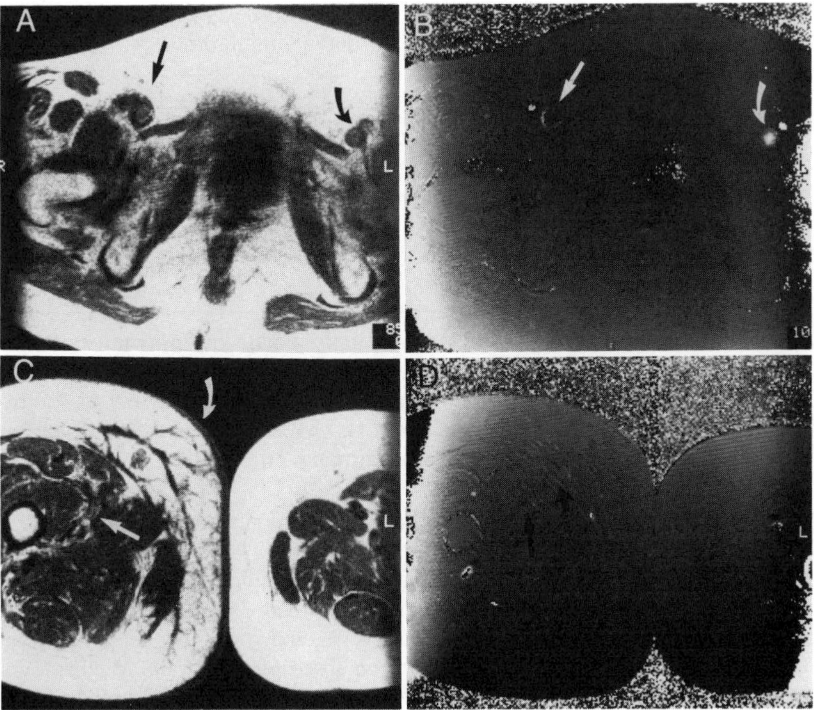

Fig 21–3.—Images of 67-year-old woman with chronic right leg swelling. **A,** axial MRI through right common femoral vein *(straight arrow)* shows distal portion of chronic thrombus. Note absence of perivascular edema and flowing-blood signal void around retracted thrombus. Note how flow artifact in normal left common femoral vein *(curved arrow)* mimics true thrombus. **B,** phase-reconstructed image from **A** confirms flow artifact in left common femoral vein *(curved arrow)*. Note absence of phase shift in retracted thrombus on right side *(straight arrow)*. **C,** axial MRI shows that chronic thrombus involves paired superficial femoral veins *(thin arrow)* and saphenous vein *(thick arrow)*. Note vessels are minimally enlarged and have clear margins and normal perivascular fat signal intensity. Patient's acute symptoms are more related to stasis edema *(curved arrow)* than to thrombophlebitis. **D,** phase-reconstructed image shows no shift in thrombosed superficial femoral vein *(thin arrow)* and saphenous vein *(thick arrow.)* (Courtesy of Erdman WA, Jayson HT, Redman HC, et al: *Radiology* 174:425–431, 1990.)

soft tissue disease to be the cause of the symptoms in 18 of 41 patients without DVT (41%).

The accuracy of MRI in the diagnosis of DVT of the lower extremity is comparable to that of the gold standard, contrast venography. In addition, MRI provides important information about the central extent of the thrombus, differentiation between acute inflammatory and chronic changes, and extravascular soft tissue disease that may explain the symptoms. It can serve as a screening procedure or first-line examination when there is suspicion of upper extremity or pelvic vein thrombosis, a history of previous DVT that necessitates distinction of acute from chronic changes, and when other tests are unavailable.

▶ Experience has taught that CT imaging of venous thrombosis is reliable, and the occasional finding of venous thrombosis in unsuspected areas such as the mesenteric circulation has greatly aided the diagnosis of obscure venous occlusive disease. Now that MRI is becoming increasingly used, it is refreshing to note that the MRI can also detect such occult venous thrombi.

Popliteal Venous Aneurysm Revealed by Pulmonary Embolism: CT Scan, Phlebographic, Tomodensitometric, and Magnetic Resonance Imaging Aspects

De Gennes C, Verny C, Ankri I, Du LTH, de Lassalle EM, Bousquet D, Kieffer E, Godeau P (Hôp Pitié-Salpêtrière, Paris)

J Mal Vasc 14:343–346, 1989 21–8

Venous aneurysms are rare; they usually occur in the major trunks such as the portal vein, the femoral vein, or the renal vein. The first popliteal venous aneurysm was reported in 1976, and a review of the literature yielded only 19 other such reports. Most of the popliteal venous aneurysms developed secondary to pulmonary embolism.

Woman, 45, previously healthy, was admitted with pulmonary embolism. Heparin therapy administered via a pump was initiated. Twenty-four hours later, pain developed in the region of the popliteal vein. Examination disclosed a swelling without pulsation. Doppler ultrasonography revealed a mass with a heterogeneous echostructure in the popliteal venous fossa, and with CT a dense mass was visualized in contact with a dilated and thrombosed popliteal vein. Magnetic resonance imaging showed a mass with a heterogeneous hypersignal in T2 in contact with the popliteal vein, suggestive of a venous aneurysm. Venography confirmed the presence of a partially thrombosed saccular aneurysm. The ileofemoral and caval veins were patent. The patient underwent operation and the aneurysm was opened. The aneurysmal sac contained numerous small fresh blood clots. The aneurysm was not resected but bypassed with an anastomosis. Postoperative treatment included coumarin administration and a compression stocking. Recovery was uneventful, and the patient has had no recurrences of popliteal venous aneurysm or thrombosis.

Because of the risk of embolism, a popliteal venous aneurysm should always be treated surgically, even if the aneurysm is asymptomatic.

▶ Although venous aneurysms are rare, they do occur. When they occur, they may be the source of pulmonary emboli.

Long-Term Heparin Therapy in the Treatment of Acute Venous Thrombosis

Langeron P (Lille, France)
J Mal Vasc (Paris) 14:69–73, 1989 21–9

Although intravenous heparin administration is accepted as standard treatment for deep venous thrombosis (DVT), there is no agreement on the optimal duration of heparin administration. A heparin treatment protocol was developed and the results obtained were evaluated.

Procedure.—After phlebography has confirmed the diagnosis of DVT and its precise extension in a patient, an intravenous heparin infusion of 5,000 international units is administered routinely. Patients with phlebitis not extending beyond the tibial or femorotibial region and with signs of moderate venous obstruction are treated with continuous intravenous heparin for 4–6 days, followed by subcutaneous calcium heparin administration for an additional 1–2 months. Patients with phlebitis extending into the inguinal region and with signs of significant venous obstruction are given intravenous heparin for 10 days, followed by subcutaneous calcium heparin therapy for another 1–2 months. Patients are routinely treated with the very-low-molecular-weight heparin, CY 222.

Follow-up phlebography data were available for 33 patients. Patients who had pulmonary embolism or acute venous stasis were excluded. Of the 33 patients, 11 had major venous obstruction, 14 had moderate venous obstruction, and 8 had minor venous obstruction. Eleven patients improved rapidly with a return to normal or near-normal phlebographic findings within 1 month of heparin therapy. Heparin apparently dissolved the blood clot rapidly and completely in these patients. Improvement in another 6 patients was much slower, with a return to normal or near-normal signs after 2–3 months of therapy. These patients were assumed to have partial lysis of the blood clot in addition to collateral vessels developing. The remaining 16 patients had persistent signs of venous stasis after long-term heparin therapy. A late start of heparin therapy, advanced age, concomitant stroke, the presence of an intracaval (Greenfield) filter, associated arteritis, and advanced cancer were identified as unfavorably affecting the outcome of long-term heparin administration.

▶ Long-term heparin therapy may be necessary in patients with intractable DVT, those with associated malignancy, or those with a florid, inflammatory component.

Heparin for 5 Days as Compared With 10 Days in the Initial Treatment of Proximal Venous Thrombosis

Hull RD, Raskob GE, Rosenbloom D, Panju AA, Brill-Edwards P, Ginsberg JS, Hirsh J, Martin GJ, Green D (McMaster Univ, Hamilton, Ont; Northwestern Univ; Univ of Calgary, Alta)

N Engl J Med 322:1260–1264, 1990 21–10

Commonly, anticoagulant therapy for deep venous thrombosis (DVT) begins with 10 days of the intravenous administration of heparin. Warfarin is added on days 5 to 10 and continued for several months. The relative efficacy of 5 days of heparin treatment was examined in a study of 199 patients with documented acute proximal venous thrombosis. The initial dose of heparin was 40,000 units per 24 hours if the risk of bleeding was low or 30,000 units per 24 hours for high-risk patients.

New symptomatic venous thrombolism was documented in 7% of patients given 10 days of heparin therapy and in 7% of those treated for 5 days. Major bleeding was infrequent and comparably frequent, respectively, in the 2 treatment groups. Two patients treated for 10 days and 3 treated for 5 days had thrombocytopenia.

Heparin therapy for 5 days is as effective as a 10-day course in patients with DVT. A shorter course would allow earlier hospital discharge, and thereby considerable cost savings, without detracting from patient care.

▶ This study goes far toward answering certain questions, but an equally relevant study must be done starting heparin and warfarin simultaneously and discontinuing the heparin when the prothrombin time reaches the therapeutic range. This tactic is in common practice, appears to be useful, and markedly decreases the cost of treatment of thromboembolic disease.

Treatment of Acute Venous Thromboembolism With Low Molecular Weight Heparin (Fragmin): Results of a Double-Blind Randomized Study

Albada J, Nieuwenhuis HK, Sixma JJ (Univ Hosp, Utrecht, The Netherlands)

Circulation 80:935–940, 1989 21–11

Heparin is commonly used in the treatment of acute venous thromboembolism. Although the drug is an effective anticoagulant, it is also associated with a risk of hemorrhage. Low-molecular-weight heparins are effective in preventing postoperative venous thromboembolism in humans and, in animal models, cause less bleeding. In a clinical trial the safety and value of a low-molecular-weight heparin preparation, Fragmin, were compared with those of standard heparin.

The 194 patients were randomly assigned to receive either continuous intravenous heparin (98) or Fragmin (96) for 5–10 days. Patients were classified as having a high or low risk for bleeding on the basis of age, recent surgery, and coexisting medical problems. Doses were adjusted to maintain anti-Xa levels between .3 and .6 unit per mL for those with high risk and between .4 and .9 unit per mL for patients with a low risk.

Major bleeding complications occurred in 13 patients in the heparin group and 10 in the Fragmin group. The total number of bleeding episodes was 118 with heparin and 103 with Fragmin. Thus the difference in bleeding complications between the 2 drugs was not significant. With either drug high-risk patients were more likely to have bleeding. The antithrombotic efficacy of the 2 drugs was similar.

Both standard heparin and Fragmin are effective antithrombotic drugs. The risk of bleeding, however, was not significantly reduced with Fragmin. Results suggest that anti-Xa levels of about .5 unit of Fragmin per mL are optimal to balance the risk of bleeding against the risk of recurrent or progressive thromboembolism.

▶ Low-molecular-weight heparin seems to have few advantages over heparin in the treatment of thromboembolism.

Thrombectomy for Acute Deep Vein Thrombosis: Prevention of Postthrombotic Syndrome

Shionoya S, Yamada I, Sakurai T, Ohta T, Matsubara J (Nagoya Univ; Aichi Med Univ, Nagoya; Kanazawa Med Univ, Japan)

J Cardiovasc Surg 30:484–489, 1989 21–12

The best way to prevent late postthrombotic sequelae after deep venous thrombosis (DVT) of the lower limb remains uncertain. Eighty-nine patients were followed for 1–18 years after acute DVT in 96 lower extremities. Thrombectomy was performed in 43 extremities; 53 others were managed conservatively with urokinase and heparin, followed by warfarin therapy for at least 6–12 months. Most thrombotic sites were in the iliofemoropopliteal or femoropopliteal venous system.

Pigmentation was present in 15% of limbs treated by thrombectomy (Fig 21–4). The revascularized iliac segment consistently reoccluded, but most patients had normal venous valves in the femoropopliteal region

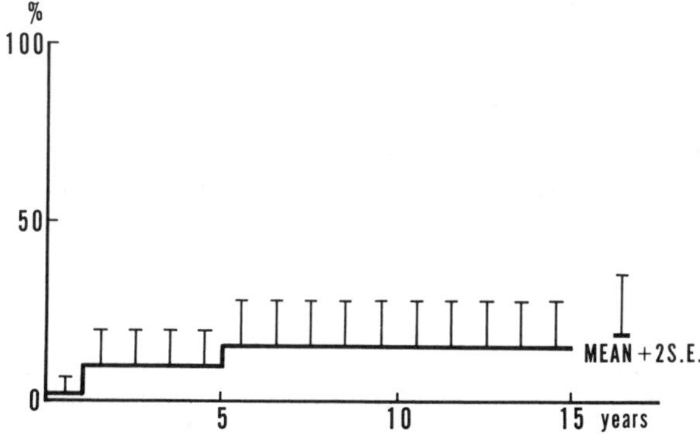

Fig 21–4.—Cumulative incidence of pigmentation at 15 years. (Courtesy of Shionoya S, Yamada I, Sakurai T, et al: *J Cardiovasc Surg* 30:484–489, 1989.)

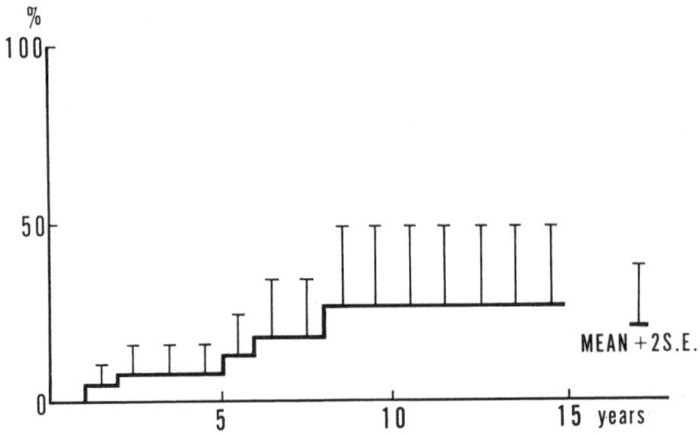

Fig 21–5.—Cumulative incidence of stasis ulcer at 15 years is 27%. (Courtesy of Shionoya S, Yamada I, Sakurai T, et al: *J Cardiovasc Surg* 30:484–489, 1989.)

and remained asymptomatic. After conservative management the cumulative rate of pigmentation was 41%, and 27% of the patients had stasis ulceration by year 15 (Fig 21–5).

Thrombectomy can prevent stasis ulceration. The presence of competent femoropopliteal venous valves appears to prevent ulceration in the lower leg. Fogarty thrombectomy with milking of the extremity can relieve early morbidity and preserve functional venous valves.

▶ Venous thrombectomy continues to be of interest but not in North America.

Surgical Thrombectomy vs Conservative Treatment for Deep Venous Thrombosis: Functional Comparison of Long-Term Results

Gåanger KH, Nachbur BH, Ris HB, Zurbrügg H (Univ of Berne, Bern, Switzerland)

Eur J Vasc Surg 3:529–538, 1989 21–13

The role of surgical thrombectomy in the management of deep venous thrombosis (DVT) remains controversial. Because DVT of the iliofemoral axis treated conservatively is often associated with irreversible damage to valvular competence and consequently chronic venous insufficiency, venous thrombectomy may prove more advantageous given the complete anatomical restoration of the occluded veins. The long-term functional outcome in surgically and medically treated patients with DVT were compared retrospectively to assess the impact of duration and extent of DVT as predictive factors of late outcome in 24 patients who were treated surgically for restoration of venous patency and valvular function and 25 patients who were treated with heparin, orally administered anticoagulants, and compression stockings.

The mean follow-up time was 7.6 years for the surgical group and 7.9 years for the medical group. The frequency of nonfatal pulmonary embolism was roughly equal in both groups (13%). Except for patients operated on for extensive (iliofemoropopliteocrural) DVT, the positive effect of thrombectomy was evident when compared with the medical group. The surgical group led a normal life, without compression stockings and restrictions of any forms of physical activity. In addition, the surgical group had significantly fewer signs of venous hypertension and little or no valvular incompetency, and measurement of the expelled volume and refilling time with dynamic plethysmography after standardized leg work favored the surgical group significantly. These satisfactory late results for the surgical group were significantly superior to conservative management in a subgroup of patients with iliofemoral thrombosis treated within 3 days. In contrast, the advantage of surgery was totally lost among patients operated on for extensive DVT of long duration.

The clinical and hemodynamic long-term effects of surgical thrombectomy are superior to conservative management for iliofemoral thrombosis, particularly when the duration of DVT is 3 or fewer days. The key to successful thrombectomy is early detection and treatment of iliofemoral thrombosis within the first 3 days.

▶ As venous thrombectomy has fallen into disuse in North America, it is important to recognize that well-documented series of cases point out the advantages of performance of iliofemoral thrombectomy when the diagnosis can be made within 3 days of the onset.

Thrombectomy or Thrombolysis in the Treatment of Deep Vein Thrombosis? Long-Term Functional Results

Frisch N, Fieve G, Schmidt Cl, Laprevotte MC, Larcan A, Frisch R (Centre Hospitalier Régional et Universitaire Hôp Central, Nancy, France)

J Mal Vasc 14:294–298, 1989 21–14

Early aggressive treatment in patients with acute iliofemoral venous thrombosis using either thrombectomy or thrombolysis decreases the risk of postthrombosis functional impairment. However, the mortality rate associated with surgical thrombectomy is approximately 3.5%, and with thrombolysis, approximately 2%. Furthermore, thrombolysis results in a reported 13% incidence of severe hemorrhagic complications.

A retrospective study compared the long-term functional results after thrombectomy and thrombolysis in the treatment of acute iliofemoral venous thrombosis in 78 patients; 52 underwent thrombectomy and 26 were treated with urokinase and plasminogen infusion for 48 hours. Functional outcome was assessed on a 9-point clinical scoring system that rated the presence of functional impairment, edema, and circulation in the legs. Patency and valvular status were assessed with Doppler ultrasonography and plethysmography.

There were 3 early deaths in the thrombectomy-treated group, 1 of which was attributed to pulmonary embolism. Thirteen patients with early recurrence of thrombosis required long-term heparin therapy, but none underwent reoperation. Within 6 weeks nearly 50% of the patients had a recurrence of thrombosis, but none required operation. After a median follow-up of 4½ years, 40 of the 50 survivors had satisfactory functional results. Only 5 patients had symptoms of phlebitis; 8 patients had claudication or venous ulcers. In 46% of the patients valve damage occurred that significantly lowered their functional scores.

Three thrombolysis-treated patients had major hemorrhagic complications, resulting in the death of 1. In 60% of the patients improvement was noted radiographically immediately after urokinase therapy, but radiographic improvement was not always synonymous with clinical improvement. After 4 years of follow-up, 85% of the patients had good functional results. None had leg ulcers, but 37% had valvular damage. The difference in late functional results between the 2 groups was statistically not significant.

▶ Other studies have failed to show that thrombolysis is clearly better than anticoagulant treatment. Comparing thrombolytic therapy with surgical therapy now seems to indicate that the lytic therapy is again not noticeably better. The fundamental question, of course, is whether or not surgical intervention is clearly superior to anticoagulant therapy.

Percutaneous Balloon Occlusion of Surgical Arteriovenous Fistulae Following Venous Thrombectomy

Endrys J, Eklöf B, Neglén P, Zýka I, Peregrin J (Kuwait Univ, Kuwait)

Cardiovasc Intervent Radiol 12:226–229, 1989 21–15

Percutaneous balloon occlusion of surgically created femoral arteriovenous fistulas (AVFs) after thrombectomy was carried out in management of acute iliofemoral venous thrombosis.

Technique.—The ipsilateral femoral artery is punctured for catheter entry. After selective femoral arteriography, the balloon-tipped catheter is inserted through the sheath into the superficial femoral artery. The balloon is positioned just above the AVF and partially inflated with dilute contrast material. When the balloon is within the AVF, it is inflated to its occlusive volume. After repeat arteriography confirms complete occlusion of the AVF, the balloon is detached.

The technique was successful in closing the AVF permanently in 25 of 28 patients. In 1 of the failures there was significant stenosis of the proximal AVF. Implanted balloons were reduced to 50% of their original diameter after an average of 7 weeks. No signs of recanalization were noted. Complications included displacement of the embolized balloon in 3 patients and a hematoma in 1, but all complications occurred during the early developmental period of the procedure. No patients required surgical intervention.

Percutaneous balloon occlusion is a successful and simple method of AVF closure. Using the contralateral femoral artery for catheter entry simplifies the procedure and may prove more advantageous.

▶ Eklof has made a significant contribution in devising the nonsurgical closure of the AVF performed for venous thrombectomy. This tactic is equally important in performing direct venous reconstruction for chronic venous stasis.

Total Hip Replacement and Deep Vein Thrombosis: A Venographic and Necropsy Study

Planès A, Vochelle N, Fagola M (Clinique Radio Chirurgicale du Mail, La Rochelle, France)

J Bone Joint Surg 72-B:9–13, 1990 21–16

The natural venographic pattern of deep venous thrombosis (DVT) after total hip replacement was evaluated in 745 consecutive patients, all of whom received heparin prophylaxis. Bilateral venography was performed

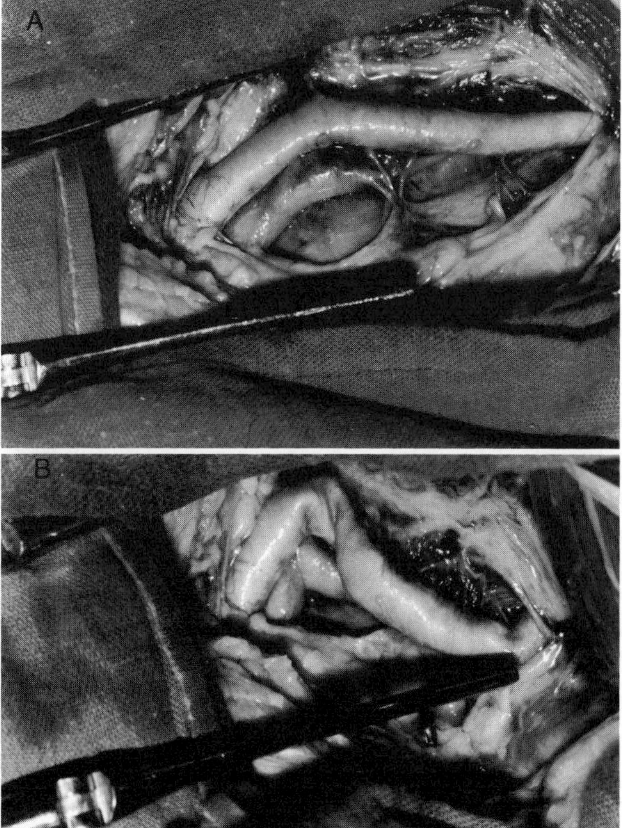

Fig 21–6.—Two examples of folding and kinking of the vessels in necropsy specimens. **A,** the original exposure; **B,** with flexion and adduction of the thigh. The femoral artery (above the vein) would normally be protected by internal blood pressure and pulsation, but the femoral vein is unprotected. (Courtesy of Planès A, Vochelle N, Fagola M: *J Bone Joint Surg* 72-B:9–13, 1990.)

12–15 days after hip replacement. Also, necropsy studies were performed on 5 fresh cadavers to ascertain the manner in which femoral veins may be damaged during hip arthroplasty.

Recent DVT was diagnosed in 81 patients, 23 of whom had distal DVT; 44 others had isolated proximal thrombosis, 5 had both proximal and distal DVT, and 9 had extensive thrombosis from calf to thigh. The unoperated-on leg was involved in 9 patients. During simulated total hip replacement in cadavers, all femoral veins became kinked or folded when the hip was adducted and flexed at the time of preparation of the femoral canal (Fig 21–6); this occurred regardless of whether the anterior or posterior approach was used.

Compared with previous reports, heparin effectively reduced the incidence of distal and contralateral thromboses, but not proximal femoral thrombosis. It appears that distal and proximal DVT occur as separate entities after total hip replacement. The latter may be related to the local damage resulting from specific hip positions during hip replacement. This could be reduced by minimizing trauma to the femoral veins with careful management of the hip during replacement surgery.

▶ As vascular surgeons are not usually involved in suggesting prophylaxis of DVT in patients with hip replacements, this abstract may be of marginal interest. However, it was selected for inclusion here because it is beautifully illustrated, proposes a new mechanism of venous thrombosis, and could be called to the attention of our orthopedic colleagues.

Graduated Compression Stockings in the Prevention of Postoperative Deep Vein Thrombosis

Jeffrey PC, Nicolaides AN (Groote Schuur Hosp, Univ of Cape Town, South Africa; St Mary's Hosp Med School, London)

Br J Surg 77:380–383, 1990 21–17

About 40 years ago, increased venous flow was shown to follow local compression applied to the lower limbs. However, compression of the leg with elastic bandages may also result in the garter effect and delayed venous emptying. Doppler flow velocity measurements have demonstrated that stockings designed with relatively low pressure (18 mm Hg at the ankle decreasing to 6.5 mm Hg at the upper thigh) increase blood velocity in the femoral vein. The role of graduated elastic compression stockings in the prevention of postoperative deep vein thrombosis (DVT) was assessed.

Early studies of below-knee elastic stockings and cylindrical tubular stockings showed little value in preventing postoperative DVT. Graduated compression stockings, however, reduced the condition by approximately 60% when compared with controls. Because multiple factors are involved, compression stockings have been used in conjunction with low doses of heparin and intermittent calf compression. With such combination therapy, the incidence of postoperative DVT has been reduced by up to 85%.

Currently, there are numerous contraindications in the claims for various prophylactic regimens. Management must be tailored to fit individual requirements, with the risks of thromboembolism weighed against potential bleeding complications. Graduated compression stockings, however, are suitable for all levels of risk, relatively inexpensive, and easy to use. Nevertheless, patients with peripheral vascular disease should be monitored to make certain that ischemia is not aggravated by the compression. Low-risk patients may need only the stockings, whereas those at high risk may require 2 additional prophylactic agents.

▶ As old methods of prophylaxis and therapy are associated with complications, it is important to note the admonition of the authors of this article, who point out that patients with occlusive arterial disease should be watched very carefully so that ischemia is not aggravated by prolonged, albeit low, pressure compression.

Effectiveness of Intermittent Pneumatic Leg Compression for Preventing Deep Vein Thrombosis After Total Hip Replacement

Hull RD, Raskob GE, Gent M, McLoughlin D, Julian D, Smith FC, Dale NI, Reed-Davis R, Lofthouse RN, Anderson C (Univ of Calgary, Alta; Chedoke-McMaster Hosps, Hamilton, Ont)

JAMA 263:2313–2317, 1990 21–18

In a randomized trial to evaluate the effectiveness of sequential intermittent calf and thigh compression for preventing venous thrombosis, 310 consecutive patients who were undergoing total hip replacement were assigned to a pneumatic compression or control group. Compression began in the recovery room, with pressures of 50–65 mm Hg being produced for a total of 35 seconds and continued for 2 weeks or until hospital discharge.

Compression cuffs were worn for a mean of 10½ days. Deep venous thrombosis was detected in 49% of the control patients and in 24% of the compression group. The respective rates of proximal venous thrombosis were 27% and 14%. One control patient had documented pulmonary embolism. One patient in the study group had compression withdrawn when traction was necessary after operation and subsequently died of massive pulmonary embolism.

Sequential intermittent leg compression significantly lowered the risk of venous thrombosis after elective total hip replacement in this study. Previous studies have suggested that this measure is potentially cost effective. Case finding is a costly approach to averting pulmonary embolism.

▶ There is no doubt that sequential, intermittent leg compression lowers the risk of venous thrombosis, but it is terribly disappointing to find breakthroughs and even fatal pulmonary thromboembolic complications in patients who are carefully monitored during such prophylaxis. The final and totally effective method of prophylaxis of deep venous thrombosis continues to be elusive.

Value of the Ventilation/Perfusion Scan in Acute Pulmonary Embolism: Results of the Prospective Investigation of Pulmonary Embolism Diagnosis
PIOPED Investigators
JAMA 263:2753–2759, 1990 21–19

A sample of 933 patients undergoing ventilation-perfusion lung scanning were studied prospectively. Pulmonary angiography was carried out in 755 patients, and 33% of these had pulmonary embolism. The patients were aged 18 or older and were seen at 6 clinical centers in a 20-month period. Lung scans were done using radioxenon and ^{99m}Tc-macroaggregated albumin.

Lung scans were 98% sensitive overall in detecting pulmonary embolism but only 10% specific. All but 14 of 116 patients with high-probability scans and definitive angiograms had pulmonary embolism, but only a minority of those with pulmonary embolism had high-probability scans. Embolism was present in one third of the patients with intermediate-probability scans and definitive angiograms. The angiographic and follow-up findings suggested that pulmonary embolism occurred in 12% of patients with low-probability lung scans.

Although a high-probability lung scan usually indicates pulmonary embolism, only a minority of affected patients have such scans. A low-probability scan makes pulmonary embolism unlikely if supported by the clinical picture. A normal or nearly normal scan makes acute pulmonary embolism very unlikely.

▶ The greatest value of a ventilation/perfusion scan is that a normal scan rules out pulmonary embolism. Even so, 4% of patients with normal or near-normal perfusion lung scans were found to have pulmonary emboli, a rather surprising finding. As stated in the editorial by R. C. Bone (1) on the V/Q scan, the emperor is incompletely attired. When there is significant doubt, a pulmonary angiogram should be done.

Reference

1. Bone RC: *JAMA* 263:2794, 1990.

Preliminary Clinical Experience With the Titanium Greenfield Vena Caval Filter
Greenfield LJ, Cho KJ, Pais SO, Van Aman M (Univ of Michigan; Univ of Maryland; Ohio State Univ)
Arch Surg 124:657–659, 1989 21–20

Mechanical protection against pulmonary thromboembolism is frequently needed instead of or as an adjunct to anticoagulation. A new titanium model of the Greenfield vena caval filter was evaluated in 40 patients aged 17–94 years at 3 institutions. The titanium filter is slightly larger than the standard stainless steel filter. It can be loaded into a 12-F diameter carrier system instead of the 24-F stainless steel filter.

Twenty-four patients had percutaneous insertions from the right femoral vein, 11 from the left femoral vein, and 2 from the right internal jugular vein. At laparotomy, operative access was attained in 1 patient each from the right femoral, right jugular, and a lumbar vein. Insertion was completed in all but 1 patient. Postoperative femoral vein thrombosis occurred in only 1 patient. Three patients had distal filter migration without sequelae. There were no cases of proximal migration.

The new titanium Greenfield vena caval filter is easier to insert than previously used filters. The sheath technique prevents misplacement. Distal migration can be prevented by techniques to promote hook engagement at the time of insertion.

▶ The percutaneous Greenfield filter is now available and will gradually become the method of choice in interrupting the vena cava. The transvenous device has already proven itself with regard to efficacy and safety, and it is hoped that the percutaneous device will have an equal record of success.

Initial Clinical Experience With an Endoluminal Spiral Prosthesis for Treating Complicated Venous Thrombosis and Preventing Pulmonary Embolism

Jakob H, Oelert H, Schmiedt W, Teusch P, Iversen S, Hake U, Schild H, Maass D (Mainz Univ Hosp, Germany)

Tex Heart Inst J 16:87–94, 1989 21–21

Conventional treatment methods may be unsuccessful in patients with complicated venous thrombosis or recurrent pulmonary embolism. An endoluminal spiral prosthesis was developed to maintain patency after venous reconstruction in patients with complicated venous thrombosis; the modified stent can be used as a filter to prevent pulmonary and carotid artery embolism. The prosthesis is a 1-way system consisting of a double- or triple-helix spiral, measuring 8 mm in diameter and composed of a surgical steel alloy.

The study group included 12 men and 2 women whose mean age was 50 years. The patients divided into 2 groups according to their primary diagnosis and the purpose of the prosthesis. The 8 patients in group I had extensive iliofemoral or caval thrombosis; all had marked swelling in 1 or both legs. After balloon angioplasty and surgical thrombectomy or embolectomy, the endoluminal spiral stent was implanted to prevent elastic recoil of the vessel. Of the 6 patients in group II, 4 had recurrent pulmonary embolism, 1 had massive pulmonary embolism, and 1 paradoxical bilateral carotid artery embolism. Surgical thrombectomy or embolectomy was performed in 4 patients; 2 had no treatment other than the stent. Because of their higher risk for pulmonary or carotid artery embolism, the endoluminal stent was modified to serve also as a caval filter.

At a mean period of 20 months postoperatively, 12 of the 14 patients remain alive. The 2 deaths, 1 in each group, were not related to device failure. There was no operative mortality or postoperative embolism. Patients available for late follow-up had patent stented vessels. Endoluminal stenting with an expandable spiral prosthesis appears to be a promising approach in the management of a difficult surgical problem.

▶ New endocaval devices will have to prove themselves better than the Greenfield filter if they are to achieve general utility.

Analysis of Benefit of Anticoagulation After Placement of Kimray-Greenfield Filter

Jones B, Fink JA, Donovan DL, Sharp WV (Akron City Hosp, Ohio)

Surg Gynecol Obstet 169:400–402, 1989 21–22

The Kimray-Greenfield venal caval filter has gained widespread acceptance as a tool to prevent pulmonary embolism when medical anticoagulation fails or produces complications. When indicated, anticoagulants usually are begun again after the filter has been placed. A retrospective trial was carried out to compare the thromboembolic and postphlebitic complications in 68 patients who continued to take anticoagulants after filter placement with those in patients who did not. After placement of the Kimray-Greenfield filters in the 25 women and 43 men, 26 patients received anticoagulant therapy and 42 did not.

Three patients receiving anticoagulants and 6 who did not had significant swelling of the leg. Two patients receiving anticoagulants and 2 who did not had recurrent deep venous thrombosis. No significant differences in outcomes between the 2 treatment groups were observed.

These findings are consistent with previous observations indicating no correlation between the use of anticoagulant therapy after filter placement and recurrent thromboembolism or stasis sequelae. Because medical anticoagulation is associated with complications, it should be discontinued in all patients after Kimray-Greenfield filter placement.

▶ Many patients require placement of a Greenfield filter because of anticoagulant complications. Therefore, it is refreshing to be reminded that such anticoagulation is not requisite.

Phlegmasia Cerulea Dolens, a Complication After Placement of a Bird's Nest Vena Cava Filter

Aruny JE, Kandarpa K (Brigham and Women's Hosp, Boston; Harvard Med School)

AJR 154:1105–1106, 1990 21–23

Phlegmasia cerulea dolens (PCD) is a combination of venous thrombosis with painful ischemia, loss of distal pulses, and purple ecchymosis. Massive edema and deep cyanosis can involve a large part of the extremity. Thrombosis of the deep and superficial collateral venous channels precludes venous return. The iliofemoral venous system is totally thrombosed and the terminal vena cava usually is involved. One man had PCD after placement of a Greenfield inferior vena caval filter.

Man, 50, with adenocarcinoma of the lung and brain metastases and a new neck mass also had upper gastrointestinal bleeding. He suddenly became short of breath and reported pleuritic chest pain. A lung scan indicated a high likelihood of pulmonary embolism. Hematochezia continued despite full systemic anticoagulation. Heparin was stopped and a bird's nest vena caval filter was implanted uneventfully. After 24 hours both legs were weak and the patient reported lower back pain. The legs were very swollen, blue, and cold, and no pulses were palpated. Autopsy showed thrombosis of the inferior vena cava extending into both popliteal veins. Widespread metastases were present throughout the thorax and abdomen, and there were pulmonary emboli of varying age. Primary follicular thyroid cancer was discovered. There was no evidence of caval perforation.

Caval perforation and filter migration were not factors in the development of PCD in this patient. A tight configuration of the mesh may have allowed a large thrombus fragment to be trapped. At the same time, a hypercoagulable state secondary to malignancy could have promoted caval thrombosis and extension of thrombus into the veins of the lower extremities.

▶ Severe distal venous thrombosis was seen occasionally following vena cava clip placement. Such a devastating complication has been virtually eliminated by the general acceptance of the Greenfield filter. To have this complication reappear as other endovenous devices are being developed is disappointing, to say the least.

Technique of Pulmonary Thromboendarterectomy for Chronic Pulmonary Embolism

Daily PO, Dembitsky WP, Iversen S (Univ of California, San Diego)
J Cardiac Surg 4:10–24, 1989 21–24

Resolution of embolic material often occurs after severe acute pulmonary embolism. However, in a small percentage of patients, incomplete resolution of the emboli may result in severe chronic pulmonary arterial obstruction. The majority of reports of surgical treatment have emphasized unilateral thoracotomy with distal pulmonary arteriotomies, with an average mortality rate of 22%. An alternative surgical technique was developed for treatment of chronic pulmonary embolism using median sternotomy for bilateral pulmonary thromboendarterectomy (PTE) with cardiopulmonary bypass, deep hypothermia, and circulatory arrest. The major indication for PTE was the demonstration of a proximal location of pulmonary arterial obstruction by pulmonary arteriography.

From 1984 to 1988, 103 patients underwent bilateral PTE in which this standardized approach was used. The mean age was 50 years. Associated procedures included coronary artery bypass grafting in 8 patients, tricuspid valve annuloplasty in 2, mitral valve replacement in 3, aortic valve replacement in 1, and closure of a patent foramen ovale or atrial septal defect in 49. The hospital mortality rate was 11.7%, compared with approximately 25% for heart-lung transplantation, the only therapeutic alternative for chronic pulmonary embolism. The survival rates at 3 years and 5 years were 85% and 80%, respectively, with bilateral PTE, compared with 53% and 33%, respectively, for heart-lung transplantation. Bilateral PTE should be the surgical procedure of choice for chronic pulmonary embolism.

▶ The San Diego group under Daily has made momumental contributions to the therapy of chronic venous hypertension caused by repetitive pulmonary embolization. Their technique is profusely illustrated in the original article abstracted here.

22 Primary Varicosities

The Incidence and Sites of Medial Thigh Communicating Veins: A Phlebographic Study

Tung KT, Chan O, Lea Thomas, M (St Thomas' Hosp, London)

Clin Radiol 41:339–340, 1990 22–1

Varicography has shown that incompetent communicating veins in the thigh are a frequent cause of recurrent varicosities after surgery on the long saphenous vein. Sites of potentially incompetent communicating thigh veins were studied in 100 consecutive saphenograms done before arterial bypass surgery on the lower extremity in patients not known to have venous disease. The mean age was 63 years. Studies were done using iopamidol 300.

Communicating veins were present on the medial aspect of the middle third of the thigh in 61% of extremities. In 11% there was more than 1 communicating vein in this region. Communicating veins were found in the lower thigh in about one fourth of the extremities. In only 1 extremity was there such a vein in the upper third of the thigh. Eleven percent of the legs had no communicating veins. In nearly one third of the cases there was partial or complete duplication of the long saphenous vein in the thigh.

Varicography appears to be necessary before surgery for recurrent varicose veins to define sites of incompetent or potentially incompetent communicating veins. Ligation of the saphenofemoral junction will not obliterate communicating veins that may already be, or will become incompetent. Stripping of a duplicated vein will eliminate only those communicating veins that connect with the stripped segment.

▶ Selection of several articles for abstracting in this section of the YEAR BOOK reflects the increasing interest of surgeons in the treatment of the problems of primary venous stasis. Further, it reflects the interest of patients in going to a specialist for care of their vascular problem. This abstract focuses on the Hunterian midthigh perforating vein, which is so important to the greater saphenous reflux syndrome. The implication is that vascular surgeons know that gross greater saphenous reflux necessitates removal of the greater saphenous vein at least to knee level. When this is done, it may be necessary to identify the source of a cluster of varicosities in the midthigh, as simple removal of the saphenous vein may not be sufficient to rid the patient of that important area of localized venous stasis.

Varicose Vein Surgery Using a Pneumatic Tourniquet: Reduced Blood Loss and Improved Cosmesis

Thompson JF, Najmaldin A, Royle GT, Clifford PC, Farrands PA, Webster JHH (Royal South Hants Hosp, Southampton, England)

Ann R Coll Surg Engl 72:119–122, 1990 22–2

The value of using a pneumatic tourniquet was assessed in 100 consecutive patients with clinically evident saphenofemoral incompetence and varicosities. Bilateral varicose veins were present in 21 patients. In some patients, saphenofemoral flush ligation and multiple lower leg avulsions were performed with the leg exsanguinated, using a Rhys-Davies cuff, and ischemia was maintained with a pneumatic tourniquet. In others the same surgery was performed but with a 30-degree head-down tilt only.

Blood loss was significantly less when a tourniquet was used (13 vs. 133 mL). Bruising at 3 weeks was comparable in the 2 groups, but cosmetic results were significantly better in the tourniquet group as judged by an independent observer. More than 90% of the patients in both groups were pleased with the outcome of surgery.

Use of a pneumatic tourniquet is a helpful adjunct to surgery for varicose veins. Blood loss is substantially reduced, and the cosmetic results may be improved.

▶ The suggestion of tourniquet use during varicose veins surgery reappears repeatedly in the surgical literature. Another way of reducing blood loss is 30-degree elevation of the lower extremity during varicose vein surgery. Recognition that hematoma and, specifically, blood adjacent to muscle and fascia, is morbid dictates need for the surgeon to address this problem and prevent the complication.

Hookers and French Strippers: A Technique for Varicose Vein Surgery

Chester JF, Taylor RS (Epsom District Hosp, Epsom, Surrey, England)

Br J Surg 77:560–561, 1990 22–3

A large proportion of varicose vein surgery is performed for cosmetic reasons, although the surgical techniques used often yield far from cosmetic results. Certain modifications of standard surgical methods are both efficient and highly cosmetic.

Technique.—Meticulous preoperative marking of the varicose veins is essential. Once marked, a circular stamp is used to outline the proposed incision points while the patient's leg is in the fetal position. When the limb is restored to the extended position, the circles turn into ellipses. The direction of the long axes of the ellipses vary from patient to patient and in different parts of the leg. The surgeon places small stab incisions along this longitudinal axis so that there is minimal tension on the incision. This results in a virtually invisible scar. When the incisional guideline is drawn with a pen, the position of the line will be maintained in whatever position the limb is placed. The stamping procedure is not appropriate for across joint lines, where better results are attained with transverse incisions. In patients with saphenofemoral incompetence, the above-knee segment of the long saphenous vein is stripped. Further above and/or below-knee varicosities are removed by multiple avulsions. The stripper developed by Hardillier is used. The head of this stripper is no wider than its shaft, and only a small incision is needed to retrieve it. The incision is placed in the direction indicated by one of the elliptical marks. An unravelled swab attached to a hole in the proximal end of the stripper allows the instrument to pass distally, permitting stripping of the long saphenous vein with immediate compression of the tunnel. This decreases bleeding and hematoma formation. Distal division of the long saphenous vein precedes its retrieval from the groin wound. Multiple avulsions are performed using a Beaver knife to make 2-mm incisions in the premarked ellipses. Specially constructed hooked forceps are used to hook out segments of vein from within each wound. Forceps are gently introduced through each incision and then turned in each direction without pulling against the wound edges until the vein is grasped. Each vein segment is seized by mosquito forceps and the avulsions completed without recourse to inserting the forceps into the wound, which can cause stretching.

These modifications have produced very satisfactory cosmetic results. They represent a significant advance in the operative treatment of lower limb varicosities.

▶ The French method of using 5-cm or 10-cm wide gauze strips attached to the stripper decreases hematoma formation in the tunnel as the long saphenous vein is stripped from above downward. Note that retrieval of the gauze strip, the stripper, and the vein is achieved from the proximal incision, thus minimizing the size of the distal incision. The distal incision can, in fact, be made quite small. The special hooked forceps are of interest. They are simply miniature, curved, Ochsner or Kocher forceps.

Surgeons must compete with sclerotherapists for cosmetic benefit to the patient as they treat venous stasis.

Treatment of Varicose and Telangiectatic Leg Veins With Hypertonic Saline: A Comparative Study of Heparin and Saline

Sadick NS (New York Hosp-Cornell Univ)

J Dermatol Surg Oncol 16:24–28, 1990 22–4

Data on 800 patients who underwent treatment for varicose and telangiectatic veins with hypertonic saline were reviewed. Half of the patients were treated with hypertonic saline, 23.4% sodium chloride with heparin, 100 μm/cc, and the other half were treated with hypertonic saline alone. All patients were followed for 1 year.

The groups did not differ significantly in the incidence of thrombophlebitis (.5% vs. .25%), microthrombosis requiring puncture evacuation (6.25% vs. 4.5%), postsclerotic pigmentation (2.5% vs. 3%) or matting (.75% vs. .75%). There were no significant differences in objective clini-

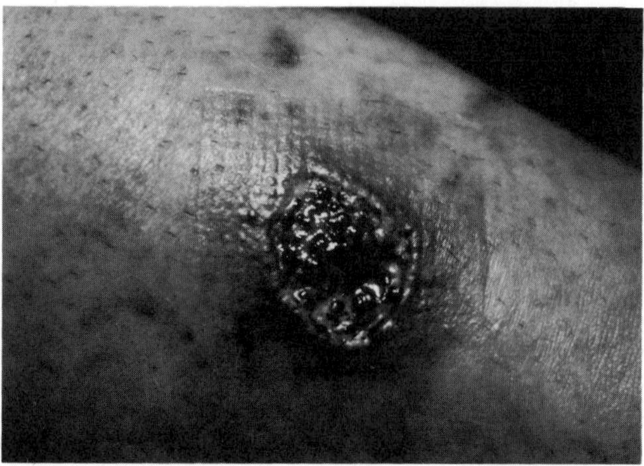

Fig 22–1.—Granulating ulceration secondary to sclerotherapy extravasation necrosis. (Courtesy of Sadick NS: *J Dermatol Surg Oncol* 16:24–28, 1990.)

cal improvement or complication rate between patients treated with postsclerotherapy compression and those treated without occlusion. Extravasation necrosis occurred in only 1 (.125%) patient (Fig 22–1). Other complications included transient cramping (19%), postsclerosis pigmentation (15%), thrombophlebitis (.4%), thrombus formation (5%) particularly in large-caliber veins, and postsclerotic telangiectatic mats. Urticaria/angioedema, arrhythmias, and hypoglycemia did not occur.

Sclerotherapy with hypertonic saline is an effective treatment of varicose and telangiectatic leg veins. Heparin may not be used in treating veins smaller than 1 mm in diameter. In the treatment of medium to large caliber veins, it is important that involvement of the lesser or greater saphenous systems should be treated surgically, and the use of more concentrated sclerosant solutions, heparin, and postsclerotherapy compression are recommended.

▶ It was Foley (1) who suggested heparin adding to the hypertonic saline solution, and this study confirms its value. Note the emphasis by this dermatologist on the fact that saphenous reflux should be treated surgically.

Reference

1. Foley WT: *Cutis* 15:665, 1975.

Resolution of Pain Associated With Varicose and Telangiectatic Leg Veins After Compression Sclerotherapy

Weiss RA, Weiss MA (Johns Hopkins Univ)

J Dermatol Surg Oncol 16:333–336, 1990 22–5

Painful Symptoms and Degree of Improvement After Treatment*

Symptom	No. of Patients	% Relief of Symptoms (No. of Patients)
Burning of area†	(57)	93% (53)
Swelling	(42)	83% (35)
Pain along vein	(66)	86% (57)
Throbbing	(37)	86% (32)
Night cramps	(46)	70% (32)
Tiredness	(67)	85% (57)

*For all categories, $P < .01$.

†Painful symptoms and degree of improvement after treatment. The *burning* symptom is associated with a specific group of visibile varicosities or telangiectasias. This can be exacerbated by prolonged standing as can any of the other symptoms. *Swelling* refers to edema in an area of a leg or protrusion or bulging of a group of varicosities or telangiectasias. *Pain along vein* is any type of painful sensation following a visible pattern of varicosities or telangiectasias. *Throbbing* refers to a pulsating vein along the leg regardless of the presence of a visible varicosity or telangiectasia. With *night cramps,* a patient awakens at night with a cramping sensation or muscle spasm. *Tiredness* refers to a sensation of fatigue bordering on a dull ache or a sensation of "heaviness" as described by patients. This fatigue was the most common symptom. Most patients had several symptoms concomitantly.

(Courtesy of Weiss RA, Weiss MA: *J Dermatol Surg Oncol* 16:333–336, 1990.)

The prevalence of pain in patients with telangiectasis and varicosities prompted a trial of sclerotherapy for reducing leg pain and discomfort. More than half of 215 patients undergoing sclerotherapy reported various painful symptoms involving areas of telangiectasia or varicosities. A questionnaire was returned by 215 patients who previously had received 1 or more treatments with hypertonic saline. An average of 3–5 treatments per region were administered.

Good to excellent cosmetic improvement was achieved in 85% of patients. Temporary burning or cramping pain was frequent, but very few patients stopped treatment for this reason. Many women reported less discomfort after sclerotherapy (table); this was especially true when large clusters of telangiectasis and small varicosities had caused significant pain on prolonged standing or during the menses. The overall reported rate of pain relief was 85%.

Pain from varicosities is significantly relieved in most patients with sclerotherapy. Patients with pain limited to a single varicosity or a group of varicosities or telangiectasias are especially likely to respond.

▶ This interesting study reports a result that most physicians who do sclerotherapy have found to be true—that patients with painful "spider" veins have amelioration of symptoms after sclerotherapy. Even though their results were obtained through a retrospective patient survey and the patients had a mixed bag of telangiectasias and varicose veins, the authors' overall success in pain relief was impressive at 85%. Perhaps this information will be helpful in convincing third-party payers of the noncosmetic benefit of sclerotherapy performed even if the vein is small.—Julie Freischlag, M.D., UCLA School of Medicine, Los Angeles

Compression in the Treatment of Leg Telangiectasia: A Preliminary Report

Goldman MP, Beaudoing D, Marley W, Lopez L, Butie A (Univ of California, San Diego; North American Society of Phlebology Multictr Cooperative Group)

J Dermatol Surg Oncol 16:322–325, 1990 22–6

Postsclerosing compression is common practice in treating varicose veins, but it is not routine when treating smaller leg veins or spider veins. The value of immediate postinjection compression was studied in 37 women undergoing bilaterally symmetrical superficial leg telangiectasias less than 1 mm in diameter, not associated with larger vessels. Several different sclerosing solutions were used. A compression stocking was applied to 1 extremity for 72 hours, starting 2 hours after injection.

Compression promoted the clinical resolution of vessels located distally on the leg; in the thigh, it provided little advantage over noncompression management. Telangiectatic matting was noted only 3 times. Postsclerotherapy hyperpigmentation occurred in 28.5% of legs when graduated compression stockings were used and in 40.5% of control extremities. In addition, calf and ankle edema was reduced by the use of compression stocking.

Use of a medium-strength compression stocking enhanced the resolution of distal telangiectasias in these women and lessened postsclerotherapy hyperpigmentation and edema. Different compression techniques might empty treated veins more completely.

▶ Goldman's work is increasingly informative. He has produced a volume of literature, abstracted in previous YEAR BOOKS, that has proven to be practical. This essay on compression contains much wisdom and introduces to surgeons unfamiliar with the complication the phenomenon of telangiectatic matting.

Surgeons are accustomed to treating patients with elastic bandaging and may find this technique easier than the application of stockings. The need for compression is emphasized by this study, however.

Varicose Veins: Optimum Compression After Surgery and Sclerotherapy

Shouler PJ, Runchman PC (Royal Naval Hosp, Haslar, Gosport, Hants, England)

Ann R Coll Surg Eng 71:402–404, 1989 22–7

Graduated compression stockings are used after varicose vein surgery, but the optimum compression pressure remains to be defined. Of 99 patients who underwent varicose vein surgery, 48 were randomly assigned to use low compression (15 mm Hg compression at the ankle) and 51 to use high compression (40 mm Hg compression) stockings after surgery. In another study, 62 patients treated by sclerotherapy were randomly assigned to either an Elastocrepe bandage with a high compression stocking or high compression stocking alone. The stockings were worn for 6 weeks.

Both low and high compression stockings were equally effective in reducing bruising and thrombophlebitis after varicose vein surgery. However, low compression stockings were more comfortable. Similarly, high compression stockings alone and Elastocrepe bandages with stockings were equally effective in reducing thrombophlebitis after sclerotherapy, although a stocking alone was more comfortable. In a subgroup of patients in whom compression was left in place continuously or removed, there were more good results among those with uninterrupted compression, but the incidence of thrombophlebitis was similar in both groups.

▶ Although this study is not absolutely definitive, it does provide confirmation that low-level compression is acceptable and that continuous compression is advisable after surgery and sclerotherapy.

Pulsed-Dye Laser Treatment of Leg Telangiectasia: With and Without Simultaneous Sclerotherapy

Goldman MP, Fitzpatrick RE (Univ of California, San Diego)

J Dermatol Surg Oncol 16:338–344, 1990 22–8

Laser treatment of leg telangiectasis is an alternative to sclerotherapy and a possible means of avoiding telangiectatic matting. Specific laser-induced endothelial damage may also limit hyperpigmentation, another result of excessive endothelial damage with red blood cell extravasation and perivascular inflammation.

Thirty consecutive women with red leg telangiectasis less than .2 mm in diameter were treated with a pulsed dye laser at 585 nm. Energies from 6 J/cm^2 to 8.5 J/cm^2 were delivered through a 5-mm spot size to the entire telangiectasia. The pulse duration was 450 microseconds. In addition, 7 patients with telangiectatic matting after sclerotherapy were treated with the laser. Twenty-seven patients having large telangiectatic flares or symmetric patches were treated with combined laser therapy and sclerotherapy using Polidocanol in concentrations of .25% to .75% or with the laser alone.

No telangiectatic matting followed laser treatment alone in 101 treated sites. Hyperpigmentation consistently resolved within 4 months of treatment. The most effective laser energies were in the range 7–8 J/cm^2. Telangiectatic matting failed to respond to laser treatment in only 1 instance. When the 2 treatments were compared, complications, including superficial ulceration, were more frequent with combined laser therapy/sclerotherapy than with laser treatment alone.

The pulsed dye laser is an effective approach to telangiectasia and to telangiectatic matting. Combining laser treatment with sclerotherapy has no apparent advantage over sclerotherapy alone, but it causes significant complications.

▶ In essence, this study suggests that the complication of telangiectatic matting is best treated by laser, but that the laser itself has no great advantage over sclerotherapy in treating the primary telangiectatic webs.

Determination of Incidence and Risk Factors for Postsclerotherapy Telangiectatic Matting of the Lower Extremity: A Retrospective Analysis

Davis LT, Duffy DM (King/Drew Med Ctr, Los Angeles; Univ of California, Los Angeles)

J Dermatol Surg Oncol 16:327–330, 1990 22–9

Telangiectatic matting refers to the appearance of vessels less than .2 mm in diameter peripheral to sclerotherapy sites, most often in the thigh. This change may sometimes be permanent and may be resistant to repeat sclerotherapy. Risk factors were examined in 2,120 patients undergoing sclerotherapy for leg telangiectases.

Telangiectatic matting occurred in 16% of the patients. More of those with matting were overweight, were receiving hormones, and had a family history of spider veins. They had a longer duration of spider veins compared to findings in patients without matting. Leg swelling was less frequent in patients with matting, and there was no significant difference with regard to excessive standing.

Vessel formation may be a normal repair phenomenon after sclerotherapy. Persisting matting may reflect an exaggerated healing response, analogous to hypertrophic scarring or postinflammatory hyperpigmentation. Genetic and metabolic factors may significantly influence the expression of telangiectatic matting.

▶ Although neoangiogenesis or telangiectatic matting may be a normal repair phenomenon after sclerotherapy, it is highly undesirable. The common thread running through the abstracts in this section is that the complications of treatment of primary venous stasis must be minimized if good results are to be obtained.

Aneurysmal Transformation of the Venous System in Venous Angiodysplasia of the Limbs

Vollmar JF, Paes E, Irion B, Friedrich JM, Heymer B (Univ of Ulm, Germany)

VASA 18:96–111, 1989 22–10

Klippel-Trenaunay (KT) syndrome and Servelle-Martorell (SM) syndrome are rare congenital disorders characterized by venous angiodysplasia of the upper and lower extremities. In approximately 80% of patients with these syndromes, venous valves are partially or totally lacking. The availability of new radiographic techniques has helped to clarify the venous pathology and hemodynamic consequences of these disorders. Chronic deep venous insufficiency and venous reflux are the most important signs. Fusiform and cylindric aneurysms of the venous system were long considered a rare occurrence in these syndromes. The incidence and presentation of venous abnormalities, including aneurysm transformation in patients with 1 of the congenital angiodysplasias, were reviewed.

During a 35-year period, KT-type angiodysplasia was diagnosed in 76

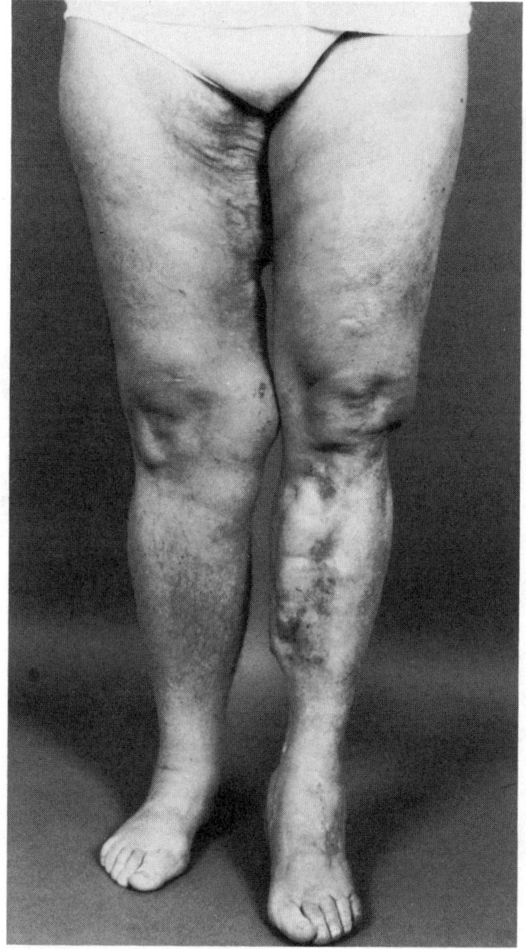

Fig 22–2.—Angiodysplasia of the Servelle-Martorell type with shortening of the left lower leg and foot with fixed pes equinus can be seen. There are cavernous hemangiomas in the area of the malleolus and on the planter side of the foot. Scar tissue formation is shown after several operations on the left lower leg, left knee, and inner right thigh. (Courtesy of Vollmar JF, Paes E, Irion B, et al: *VASA* 18:96–111, 1989.)

patients and SM-type angiodysplasia in 31 (Figs 22–2 and 22–3). In 57 patients (75%) with KT and 19 (61%) with SM the diagnosis had been made before age 1 year. The lower limbs were significantly more often involved than the upper extremities. Deep venous abnormalities of the lower limbs were present in 96% of the KT patients and in all SM patients. Forty-two patients had asymptomatic aneurysms of subcutaneous veins, deep veins, and communicating veins in the lower extremities. The average age when venous aneurysm formation was first seen was 30 years. Cylindric aneurysms were more common than fusiform aneurysms.

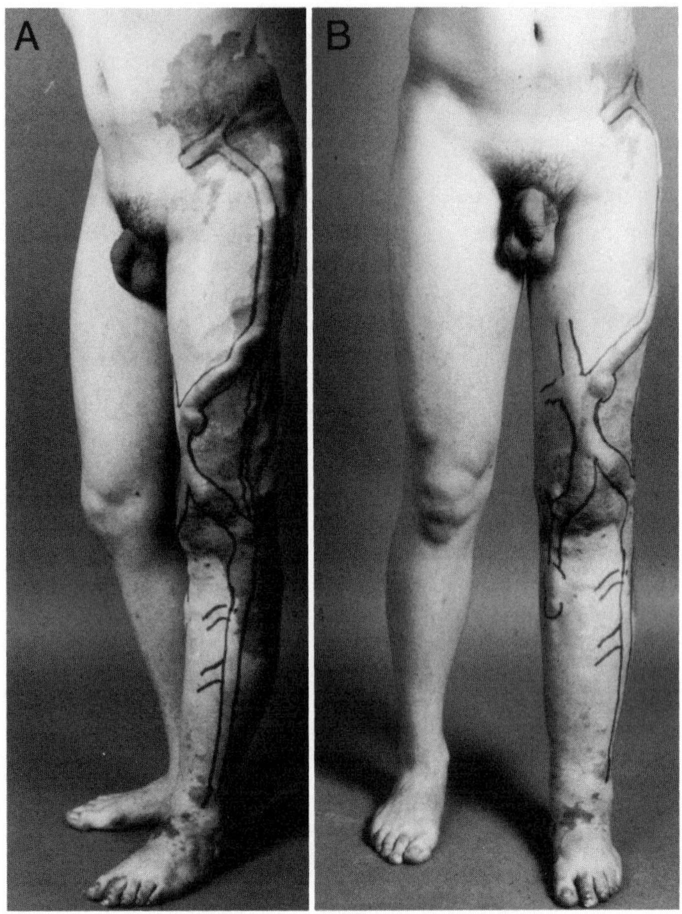

Fig 22–3.—Map-shaped nevus flammeus extends from the left hip region to the middle of the lower leg. There is evidence of prominent atypical major sinuses surrounding persistent lateral marginal veins (high-grade hypoplasia of the popliteal vein). Shortening of the lower leg and of the longitudinal axis of the left foot is shown. There is extensive cavernous hemangioma on the lateral circumference of the knee and lower leg (Servelle-Martorell type). (Courtesy of Vollmar JF, Paes E, Irion B, et al: *VASA* 18:96–111, 1989.)

The popliteal vein, external iliac vein, and communicating veins between them were most often involved.

None of the patients experienced local thrombosis, pulmonary embolism, or rupture of a venous aneurysm during follow-up, and most aneurysms remained asymptomatic. Conservative treatment, which is preferred, may include the use of external compression bandages or compression stockings. Surgical intervention should be limited to the treatment of aneurysmal complications or pathologic short-circuit flow in some drainage veins. Antireflux procedures (e.g., venous valve transfer from the brachial vein) are still under clinical investigation.

▶ Varicose veins may be part of the clinical manifestation of congenital venous malformation. Surgeons must be aware of this condition. Only the tip of the iceberg is seen in this abstract. Vollmar's massive experience is displayed in full in the original article. Fortunately, Vollmar stresses conservative therapy for these conditions and reserves surgical intervention only for complications.

23 Chronic Venous Insufficiency

Quantification of Venous Reflux by Means of Duplex Scanning
Vasdekis SN, Clarke GH, Nicolaides AN (St Mary's Hosp, London)
J Vasc Surg 10:670–677, 1989 23–1

Measuring the refilling time of veins has shown a correlation between skin changes in the legs and reflux; however, this measurement provides only an indication of severity rather than a true quantitative measurement of reflux. Duplex scanning was used to quantify reflux and determine its relationship to symptoms in 47 legs in 46 patients with symptomatic varicose veins.

In 45 limbs reflux was present in only 1 vein; in 28 limbs there was reflux in the long saphenous vein; in 9, the short saphenous vein; and in 8, the femoropopliteal vein. In 1 limb, reflux was found in the long saphenous, short saphenous, and femoropopliteal veins, and in another it was found on the long and short saphenous veins. There were skin changes in 19 limbs. The median reflux in these limbs was 30 mL/sec, whereas in limbs without changes, it was 10 mL/sec. In limbs with reflux of more than 10 mL/sec, skin changes were common whether reflux was in the superficial or deep system but were infrequent when reflux was less than 10 mL/sec.

The use of duplex scanning to quantify venous reflux will help in studying the history of chronic venous insufficiency and in evaluating the outcome of surgery. However, other factors need to be studied to explain why skin changes do not occur in about one third of patients with high reflux values.

▶ There has been a need for precision in assessing venous stasis, and this technique contributes to a solution of that problem. The method is not difficult to perform, provides definitive information regarding precise reflux, and, in general terms, correlates with the patient's clinical status. Other laboratories have also explored this method and have verified its utility.

Age-Related Rather Than Ulcer-Related Impairment of Venous Function Tests in Patients With Venous Ulceration
Höhn L, Chiarenza S, Schmied E, Bounameaux H (Univ Hosp of Geneva, Switzerland)
Dermatologica 180:73–75, 1990 23–2

The assessment of patients with venous leg ulcers is not well standardized. During the past 20 years numerous noninvasive methods for evaluating chronic venous insufficiency (CVI) have been proposed, but their role in the diagnosis of CVI has not been established. Various noninvasive tests of venous function and skin oxygenation were evaluated systematically in 6 men and 6 women aged 51–93 years with unilateral venous leg ulcers, 12 age- and sex-matched hospitalized patients who had no evidence of venous insufficiency of the legs, and 12 young healthy volunteers aged 24–45 years.

The duration of ulceration ranged from 2 weeks to 25 years. Ulcer sizes ranged from 1 cm^2 to 18 cm^2. There were signs or symptoms of chronic venous insufficiency of the contralateral leg in 10 patients. None of the patients had a history of deep vein thrombosis. Each study participant underwent venous occlusion plethysmography to measure maximal venous outflow and venous capacitance, Doppler ultrasound, photoplethysmography to measure venous filling time, transcutaneous oxygen tension determinations, and measurement of arterial pressure at the great toe.

There was no difference between the leg with a venous ulcer and the leg without a venous ulcer in any of the tests studied. Patients with leg ulcers had significantly higher maximal venous outflow values in both legs than their matched controls had (Fig 23–1). Venous capacitance values were also higher in patients with leg ulcers than in controls, but the difference did not reach statistical significance because of large interindividual variations among controls. There was no difference between patients and controls for any of the other tests. However, there were striking differences between the older and the younger controls. Older con-

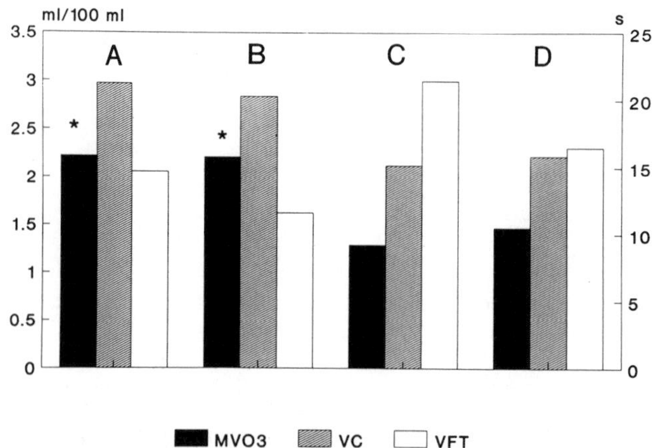

Fig 23–1.—Comparison of ulcer patients with their matched controls. Mean values (n = 12 legs) of maximal outflow in the first 3 outflow seconds *(MVO3)*, venous capacitance *(VC)* (both expressed in mL/100 mL), and venous filling time *(VFT)* assessed by photoplethysmography *(PPG)* (expressed in seconds. *A* and *B* concern the ulcer patients (*A* leg with ulcer) and *C* and *D* concern the age- and sex-matched controls *(C* corresponding to *A)*. Asterisk indicates *P* <.05. (Courtesy of Höhn L, Chiarenza S, Schmied E, et al: *Dermatologica* 180:73–75, 1990.)

trols had significantly reduced maximum venous outflow, shorter venous filling times, lower transcutaneous partial oxygen pressures at calf level, and higher venous pressure in the posterior tibial vein, compared with younger controls. These findings suggest that the changes in various noninvasive venous function tests observed in patients with CVI are mostly age related.

▶ The severe venous stasis syndrome, referred to as CVI in this abstract, has increasingly been disassociated with previous venous thrombosis. Clearly, it is important to recognize the postphlebitic venous stasis limb and distinguish it from the limb without previous venous thrombosis, as one is amenable to valve repair and the other is not. It is apparent that advancing age correlates with increasing venous stasis, and this helps to explain the onset of venous insufficiency stigmata in older patients.

CT of Swollen Legs

Vaughan BF (St Andrews Hosp, Adelaide, South Australia)

Clin Radiol 41:24–30, 1990 — 23–3

Previous studies have suggested that a single CT scan of a swollen leg shows characteristic details that enable a differential diagnosis not possible by venography. The diagnostic value of using a single axial slice through the mid calf of a swollen leg was investigated in a CT study.

Since 1985, 64 patients with a swollen leg or legs underwent CT examination according to an established protocol; 10 patients who did not have swollen legs served as controls. After a scout film was taken, a single 10-mm thick axial slice was taken through the upper third of the calf of both legs. No contrast medium was used. The cross-sectional area of the subfascial muscle compartment was calculated by standard method-

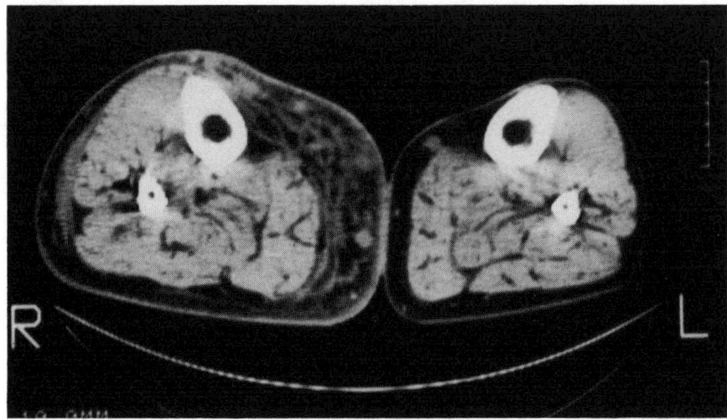

Fig 23–2.—Chronic venous insufficiency *(R)*. Man, aged 55 years. Long-standing femoral vein thrombosis. There is chronic subcutaneous lymphedema, marked skin thickening caused by recurrent erypsipelas, enlarged superficial veins, and an increased cross-sectional muscle area; *right,* 76 cm^2; *left,* 61.7 cm^2. (Courtesy of Vaughan BF: *Clin Radiol* 41:24–30, 1990.)

ology. Indications for CT examination included acute or chronic deep venous thrombosis, venous incompetence, lymphatic obstruction caused by malignant disease, elephantiasis caused by filariasis, hematoma, popliteal cyst extension, and chronic bilateral swelling of unknown origin.

The CT scans from all 8 patients with acute deep venous thrombosis showed increases in the subcutaneous layer and signs of lymphedema, varying from patient to patient, depending on the interval from onset and the degree of ambulation and treatment. The CT scans from 3 patients with chronic deep venous thrombosis showed large increases in the cross-sectional muscle area caused by previous deep venous thromboses, enlarged veins, and advanced changes of lymphedema in the subcutaneous layer (Fig 23–2). Scans from 4 patients with venous insufficiency caused by an incompetent superficial venous system but patent deep veins showed lymphedema in an increased superficial layer and enlarged superficial veins. Of 20 patients with chronic bilateral lower limb swelling of unknown origin, 9 had signs of lymphedema with increases in the subcutaneous layer and interstitial fibrosis and skin thickening (Fig 23–3). In the other 11 patients enlarged homogeneous fat-density subcutaneous layers were seen on scans; 2 of these had lymphatic hypoplasia confirmed by lymphography. The 6 patients with lymphatic obstruction secondary to malignant disease had fluid in the interstitial tissues and areas of water density in enlarged subcutaneous layers (Fig 23–4). The 1 patient with elephantiasis caused by filariasis had a honeycomb pattern in the calf. The scans from 4 patients with popliteal cyst extensions showed fluid collections between muscle planes.

A 10% increase in the cross-sectional muscle area of a swollen leg appears to be diagnostic of deep venous thrombosis. In this study, a single CT scan was capable of differentiating complicated popliteal cysts, hematomas, and lymphedema.

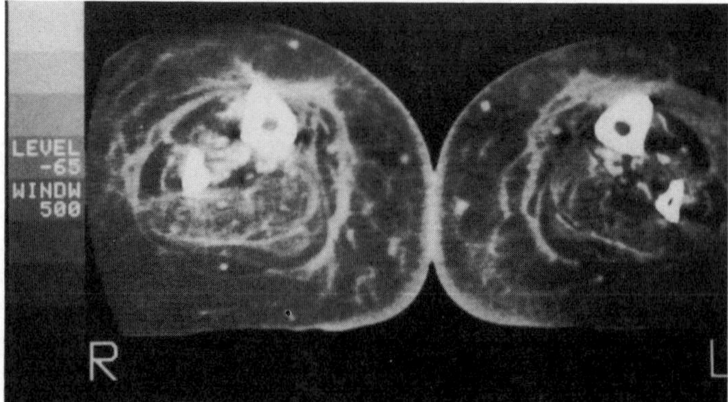

Fig 23–3.—Lymphedema praecox. Very marked increase in the subcutaneous layer, with interstitital fibrosis and skin thickening. Attenuation between fibrous strands, −120 HU. (Courtesy of Vaughan BF: *Clin Radiol* 41:24–30, January 1990.)

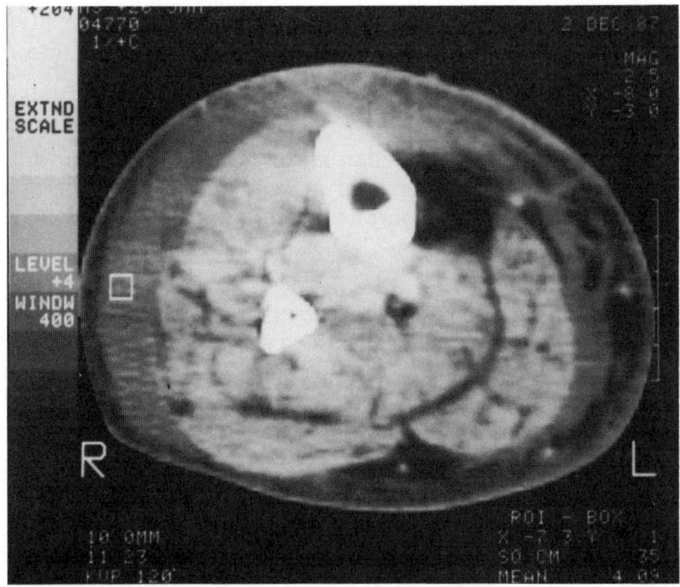

Fig 23–4.—Acute lymphedema. Man, aged 55 years, with lymph node involvement with carcinoma of the prostate. Increased subcutaneous layer, fluid in the interstitial tissue, and a water density collection laterally. Attenuation in box, +4.09 HU. (Courtesy of Vaughan BF: *Clin Radiol* 41:24–30, January 1990.)

▶ Assessment of the swollen limb must be complete before therapy is chosen. Computed tomography adds to other testing modalities in providing additional useful information.

On the Edema-Preventing Effect of the Calf Muscle Pump
Stick C, Grau H, Witzleb E (Univ of Kiel, Germany)
Eur J Appl Physiol 59:39–47, 1989 23–4

Edema is rarely observed in healthy persons. To determine what mechanisms counteract the development of edema in the lower extremities when in the upright position, extravascular volume changes in the calf were measured during lying, standing, sitting, and cycle ergometer exercise using the mercury-in-Silastic strain gauge method. Low-pass filtering was used to remove movement artifacts during muscular exercise.

When changing body position from lying to standing, a 2-stage change in calf volume was noted, consisting of rapid initial filling of the capacitance vessel followed by a slow but nearly linear increase in calf volume during motionless standing. This slow increase continued during sitting with the legs dependent. In contrast, slow continuous decreases in calf volume were observed during cycle ergometer exercise. The rates of increase in calf volume were .17% per minute during standing and .12% per minute during sitting. In contrast, mean decreases in calf volume during 18 minutes of cycling were −1.6% at 50 W workload and −1.9% at 100 W; the difference was significant.

These findings demonstrate the edema-protective effect of the calf muscle pump. During exercise, 3 factors account for the reduced calf volume: a reduction in venous pressure resulting in reduced effective filtration pressure; increased lymph flow that removes fluid and osmotically active colloid proteins from the interstitial space; and an increase in muscle tissue pressure during muscle contraction, resulting in reduced capillary filtration.

▶ A strong calf muscle pump may compensate for some degree of venous reflux, but when valves in the communicating veins become incompetent, there is failure of the calf pump and all of the late stigmata of chronic venous stasis will be present. External compression aids markedly in the treatment of calf pump failure, as does closure of the relevant perforating veins. Primary muscle dysfunction may also contribute to calf pump failure.

Pathogenesis of Venous Ulceration in Relation to the Calf Muscle Pump Function

Christopoulos D, Nicolaides AN, Cook A, Irvine A, Galloway JMD, Wilkinson A (St Mary's Hosp, London; Hull Royal Infirmary, Hull, England)

Surgery 106:829–835, 1989 23–5

Air plethysmography allows the quantitative measurement of venous reflux as reflected by the average filling rate of the veins on standing from the supine position, the ejection fraction of the calf muscle pump as a result of 1 tiptoe movement, and the residual volume fraction after 10 tiptoe movements. To investigate the pathogenesis of venous ulceration in terms of calf muscle pump action, 30 normal lower extremities, 110 with primary varicose veins, 34 with deep venous incompetence, and 31 with deep venous occlusions, with or without reflux, were studied.

The incidence of ulceration increased significantly with increasing severity of reflux and decreasing values of the ejection fraction of the calf muscle pump. A poor ejection fraction (less than 40%) was associated with a high incidence of ulceration, even in extremities with minimal reflux. In contrast, a good ejection fraction (more than 40%) significantly reduced the incidence of ulceration in extremities with moderate to severe reflux. The residual volume fraction, which expressed the combined effect of venous reflux and ejection fraction with rhythmic exercise, showed a good correlation with the incidence of ulceration and measurements of ambulatory venous pressure.

Air plethysmography allows complete assessment of the action of the calf muscle pump and provides an accurate method of identifying the hemodynamic factors responsible for ulceration. Ulceration results from both increased reflux and reduced ejection fraction in extremities with primary varicose veins, from reduced ejection fraction in extremities with deep venous incompetence, and from marked reflux in extremities with deep venous occlusion.

▶ The air plethysmography referred to in this article and abstract quantitates calf muscle pump failure and, once again, emphasizes the importance of reflux through incompetent valves. It is duplex scanning, however, that is precise in identifying and quantifying individual venous conduit reflux.

Intravenous Prostaglandin E_1 in the Treatment of Venous Ulcers: A Double-Blind, Placebo-Controlled Trial

Rudofsky G (Univ of Essen, Germany)

Vasa Suppl 28:39–43, 1989 23–6

An effective drug regimen for the treatment of chronic venous leg ulcers refractory to conventional therapy is not yet available. Numerous studies have reported the efficacy of prostaglandin E_1 (PGE_1) in the treatment of leg ulcers caused by arterial incompetence. There is some evidence to suggest that PGE_1 may also be effective in the treatment of chronic venous leg ulcers.

The efficacy of intravenously administered PGE_1 in the treatment of resistant venous leg ulcers was assessed in 19 men and 25 women aged 39 to 79 years who had not responded to conventional therapy for at least 4 months and whose ulcer state had remained unchanged for at least 3 weeks. The ulcer diameter was at least .5 cm. All patients had postthrom-

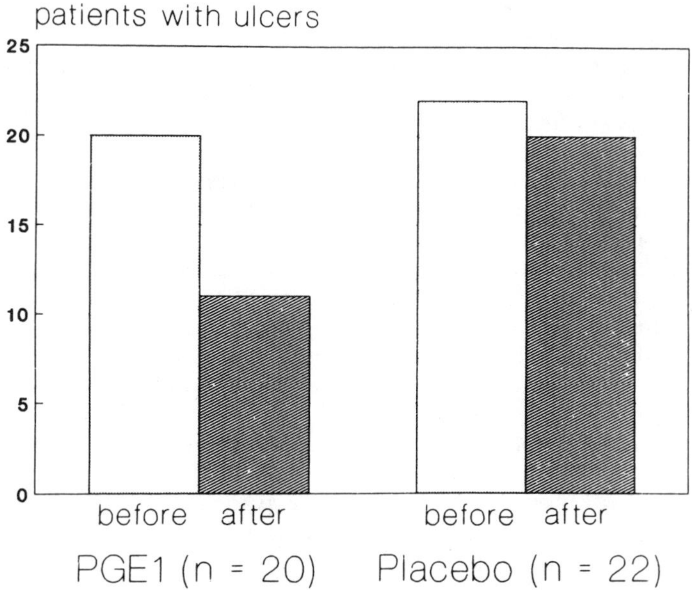

Fig 23–5.—Comparison of complete healing of venous ulcers in PGE_1-treated patients and placebo-treated patients. (Courtesy of Rudofsky G: *Vasa Suppl* 28:39–43, 1989.)

botic syndrome with insufficiency of the perforant veins. Patients with mixed arterial and venous ulcers were excluded. After a 14-day wash-out phase, 20 patients were randomly assigned to daily intravenous infusions of 3 ampules of 60 μg PGE_1, and 22 patients received daily intravenous infusions of 3 ampules of placebo. The treatment period was 6 weeks.

Mean ulcer scores improved by 70.4% in the PGE_1-treated patients as compared with a 23.8% improvement in the placebo-treated patients. Clinical symptoms improved proportionately. Eight (40%) of 20 PGE_1-treated patients had complete healing of their leg ulcers, compared with only 2 (9%) of 22 placebo-treated patients (Fig 23–5). Edema resolved completely in 17 (85%) of the PGE_1-treated patients, but in only 7 (35%) of the placebo-treated patients. Calf cramps resolved with PGE_1 treatment in 12 of 15 patients, compared with 6 of 12 placebo-treated patients. Statistical analysis of all parameters indicated a significant difference in therapeutic success in favor of PGE_1. No side effects were observed. Prostaglandin E_1 appears to be an effective therapy for the treatment of refractory venous leg ulcers.

▶ It appears that prostaglandins are therapy in search of a condition.

Treatment of Skin Ulcers With Cultured Epidermal Allografts

Phillips TJ, Kehinde O, Green H, Gilchrest BA (Boston Univ; Harvard Med School)

J Am Acad Dermatol 21:191–199, 1989 23–7

Treating skin ulcers in elderly, diabetic, paraplegic, or other debilitated patients can be difficult. Keratinocytes from neonates have been found to be more responsive to mitogens than those from older donors. Thirty-six nonhealing skin ulcers in 23 patients were treated with cultured allogeneic epidermal sheets derived from neonatal foreskin.

Complete healing occurred in 26 (73%) ulcers within 8 weeks, with a mean healing time of 3.3 weeks. In the remaining 27% there was a decrease in size of 35% to 93% within 8 weeks. Pain was markedly relieved within 24 hours of grafting in 30 painful ulcers. The cultured epidermal sheets apparently acted by stimulation of host keratinocytes to divide and migrate instead of by permanent acceptance of the allograft. Twenty-three of the 26 ulcers that healed within 8 weeks (88.5%) remained healed for 10–18 months, with an overall mean duration of healing of 13 months.

Cultured allografts derived from neonatal foreskin can be helpful in the treatment of difficult skin ulcers. Such allografts offer the advantages of rapid growth in culture and immediate availability. They obviate skin biopsies, are simple to apply, and can be stored for future use. The grafting procedure is painless.

▶ Allografts in general provide a fine biologic dressing.

Leg Ulcers: Ambulatory Treatment and Results
Hördegen KM (Basel, Switzerland)
Schweiz Med Wochenschr 119:1264–1269, 1989 23–8

The incidence of venous leg ulcers in developed nations is approximately 1% to 2%. Some studies have reported a 60% deep vein etiology and a 40% varicose vein etiology, whereas others found a deep vein etiology in only 30% to 40% of their patients. However, the pathogenesis of leg ulcers has important prognostic ramifications. Varicose veins can be treated by injection of sclerosing agents, resulting in rapid subsequent healing of most leg ulcers. On the other hand, the treatment of leg ulcers secondary to deep vein thrombosis is usually much less successful. The records of 85 patients who received ambulatory treatment for leg ulcers were studied retrospectively.

The study population consisted of 59 women (mean age, 66 years) and 26 men (mean age, 58 years) who were treated for leg ulcers. Nine patients had no history of vascular disorders, 16% had a history of deep vein thrombosis, and 84% had a history of varicose veins. Most patients (72%) had jobs that required long periods of continuous standing or sitting. Approximately 42% of the women and 50% of the men were being treated for a recurrence of leg ulcers. All patients underwent noninvasive Doppler ultrasound examinations of the lower limbs. The 3-pronged approach to ambulatory treatment involved the use of compression bandages and elastic stockings, sclerotherapy when indicated, and local treatment of the ulcer and the eczematous skin around it. Zinc ointment was applied directly on the ulcer, and cortisone ointment was applied to any local eczema.

After 2–3 months of aggressive ambulatory treatment, 66 of the ulcers had healed, 12 were improved, 2 were unchanged, and 5 had become worse. Most ulcers in younger patients healed within 2 months from the start of treatment. Four of the 7 patients whose ulcers were not improved had concomitant arterial occlusive diseases. The other 3 patients were very elderly, nonambulatory individuals with extensive postphlebitic involvement. Only 3 of the 75 leg ulcers (4%) for which the underlying venous pathogenesis was identified and incorporated into the treatment approach did not heal spontaneously with ambulatory treatment. Thus the overall success rate for treating venous ulcer on an ambulatory basis in this group of patients was 96%.

When treating venous leg ulcers it is most important to identify the underlying pathogenesis and take it into consideration when planning treatment for the patient.

▶ This article clearly shows that the majority of patients (96% of this series) with venous leg ulcers can be treated successfully on an ambulatory basis by combining sclerotherapy, local ulcer treatment, and the use of compressive bandages. The authors also validly highlight the need to study the arterial blood supply of patients whose venous ulcers do not respond to an ambulatory treatment program (4.7% of series). However, the study is retrospective and as such does not depict which of the treating modalities, or combinations thereof, is most effective in achieving healing. The study also fails to indicate how the rate of healing can be enhanced by combining treatment methods. A follow-up study done prospectively to answer the posed questions would be welcome indeed.—Luis A. Queral, M.D., Director, Maryland Vascular Institute, Baltimore

---

Oxpentifylline Treatment of Venous Ulcers of the Leg

Colgan M-P, Dormandy JA, Jones PW, Schraibman IG, Shanik DG, Young RAL (St James Hosp, Dublin; St George's Hosp, London; Univ of Keele, Staffordshire; Birch Hill Hosp, Rochdale, Lancashire, England; Trinity College, Dublin; et al)

Br Med J 300:972–975, 1990 23–9

The pathophysiology of venous ulcers of the leg is poorly understood. No proven pharmacologic treatment is yet available. White blood cell accumulation in dependent legs of patients with venous hypertension has been proposed as a possible mechanism responsible for the typical trophic skin changes. Oxpentifylline has fibrinolytic effects and influences the behavior of white blood cells. A 4-center, prospective, double-blind, randomized, placebo-controlled clinical trial was conducted to determine the effect of oxpentifylline on the healing of venous leg ulcers in 80 patients, none of whom had evidence of arterial disease.

Patients were randomly assigned to oxpentifylline, 400 mg 3 times a day by mouth, or to a matching placebo. Treatment was continued until the ulcer headed, up to a maximum of 6 months. A standardized 2-layer method of bandaging that produced adequate graduated compression was used in all patients. A computerized system was used to measure the ulcer area from tracings.

Nine placebo-treated patients (21%) and 3 oxpentifylline-treated patients (8%) dropped out of the study. After 6 months of follow-up, 23 oxpentifylline-treated patients and 12 placebo-treated patients had complete healing of the reference ulcer. Life-table analysis showed that the proportion of ulcers healed at 6 months was 64% in oxpentifylline-treated patients and 34% in placebo-treated patients. The difference was statistically significant. Minor side effects were reported by 45% of the oxpentifylline-treated patients and 33% of the placebo-treated patients. Oxpentifylline appears effective for healing venous ulcers of the leg when added to a standard regimen of compression bandaging.

▶ Adjuncts to compression therapy in treating leg ulcers come and go.

Reconstructive Surgery for Deep Vein Valve Incompetence in the Lower Limb

Eriksson I (Univ Hosp, Uppsala, Sweden)

Eur J Vasc Surg 4:211–218, 1990 23–10

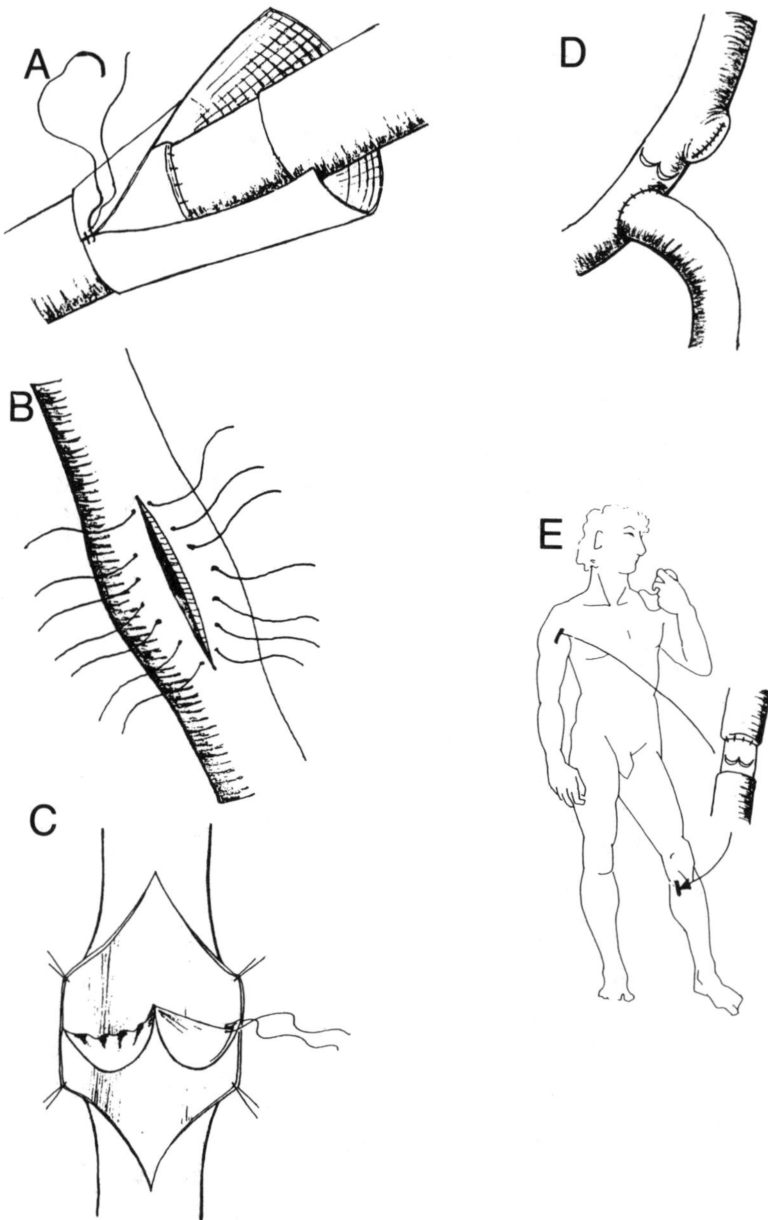

Fig 23–6.—Schematic drawings of various methods of valve reconstruction. **A,** external cuff encircling a valve or a transplanted vein segment; **B,** vein wall plication; **C,** valvuloplasty according to Kistner's method; **D,** transposition of incompetent superficial femoral vein into competent profunda femoris vein; and **E,** principle of valve transplantation. (Courtesy of Eriksson I: *Eur J Vasc Surg* 4:211–218, 1990.)

Indications for deep venous valve surgery have varied, but a lack of response to conventional treatment of deep venous incompetence (DVI) is the usual reason. A variety of methods have been described for the surgical management of DVI (Fig 23–6).

Initially successful results using the gracilis muscle tendon as an "external valve" could not be replicated. Use of a Dacron cuff about the vein has its advocates. Valvuloplasty has been proposed for repairing leaking valves in nonthrombotic DVI. In cases of secondary DVI this approach is not feasible, however, because the valves are scarred and retracted. Valve transposition has been used to correct both primary and secondary DVI of the superficial femoral vein when a neighboring vein has a competent proximal valve. Valve transplantation may be especially useful in the management of severe secondary DVI. Postoperative venous thrombosis has been less frequent than expected. Heparin generally is given, and graded compression stockings also are indicated.

Presently, valve surgery is limited to patients with intractable venous symptoms. In the future, the indications for valve reconstruction might shift toward earlier intervention before the muscle pump is permanently damaged.

▶ This reference is given to interested vascular surgeons so that the original article can be obtained. It provides a thoroughly complete summary of the current status of deep venous reconstruction.

Visual Vignettes

▶ The 1989 YEAR BOOK OF VASCULAR SURGERY contained an abstract of an article by Grigg and Wolfe and reproduced their figure (pp 170–171). The editorial comment at that time was that this ingenious technique looked to be very useful. The utility of the idea had been recognized by LoGerfo and his colleagues and the editors of the *Journal of Vascular Surgery* when they published the description of the procedure some 8 months earlier. These figures (Figs 1, 2, and 3) are being reproduced again in this edition of the YEAR BOOK OF VASCULAR SURGERY because the apparent simultaneous generation of the idea on both sides of the Atlantic Ocean suggests its value and utility.

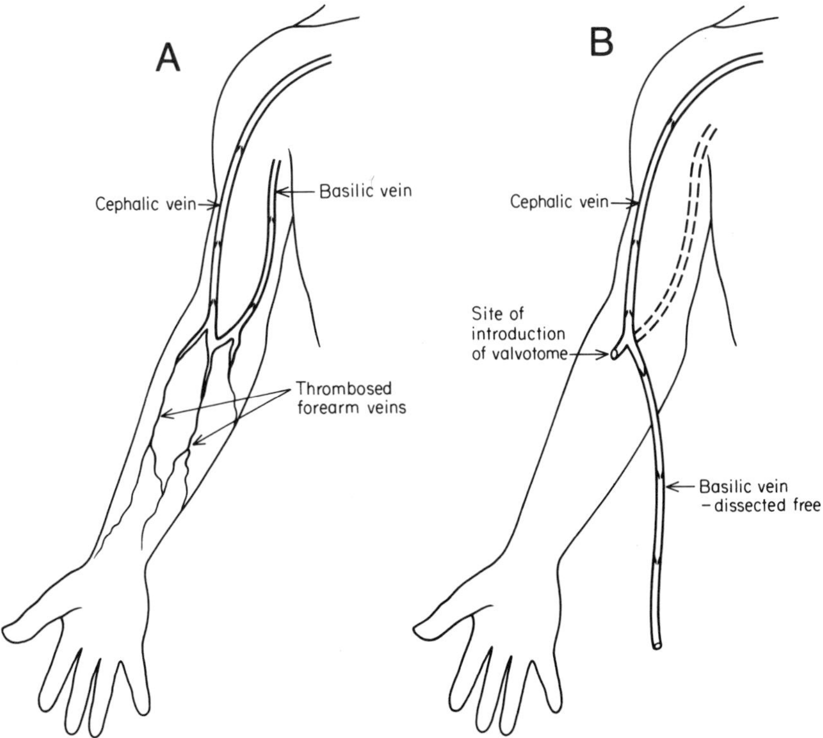

Fig 1.—Diagramatic representation of **A,** the upper arm vein anatomy and **B,** after mobilization of the basilic vein showing the eventual orientation of the graft. (Courtesy of Grigg MJ, Wolfe JHN: *Eur J Vasc Surg* 2:49–52, 1988.)

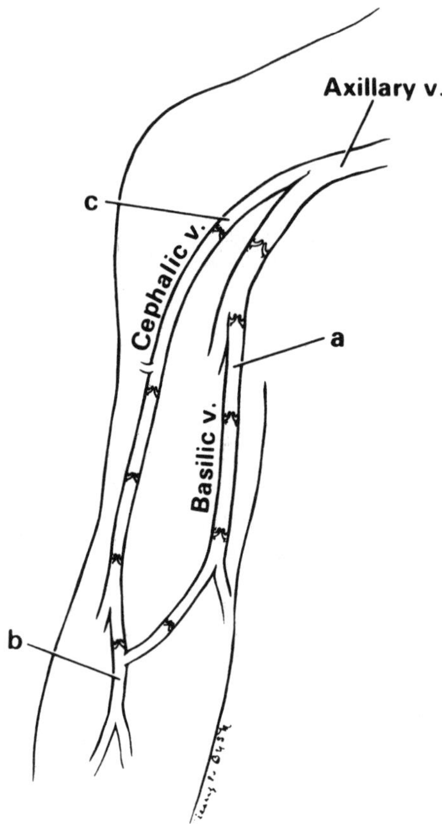

Fig 2.—Anatomy of upper arm veins. Three points (*a, b,* and *c*) have been labeled for orientation in subsequent figures. Point *(b)* is the location at which the cephalic vein is divided in the forearm. The divided stump will later be used for insertion of the valvulotome. (Courtesy of LoGerfo FW, Paniszyn CW, Menzoian J: *J Vasc Surg* 5:889–891, 1987.)

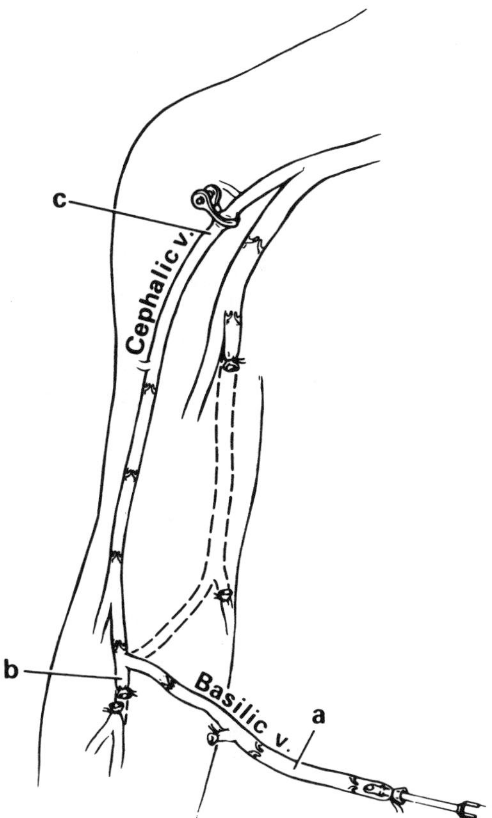

Fig 3.—Harvesting of arm veins with mobilization of basilic vein to become the inflow segment. The end of the vein is cannulated to facilitate subsequent valvulotomy. Before cannulation the end of the basilic vein may be everted so that the first valve can be excised with a scissors. (Courtesy of LoGerfo FW, Paniszyn CW, Menzoian J: *J Vasc Surg* 5:889–891, 1987.)

Subject Index

A

B

C

D

E

F

G

H

I

K

L

O

P

R

S

T

U

V

W

X

Y

Author Index

A

B

F

G

H

I

J

K

L

O

P

Q

R

S

T